Health Financing Revisited
A Practioner's Guide

Health Financing Revisited

A Practioner's Guide

Pablo Gottret

George Schieber

The World Bank

ISBN-10: 0-8213-6585-1
ISBN-13: 978-0-8213-6585-4
eISBN-10: 0-8213-6586-X
eISBN-13: 978-0-8213-6293-8
DOI: 10.1596/978-0-8213-6585-4

Library of Congress Cataloging-in-Publication data has been applied for.

Contents

v

Boxes

Figures

Tables

Foreword

Global health policy is at the forefront of the international policy agenda. Globalization, the international community's commitment to reduce poverty and achieve the Millennium Development Goals (MDGs), the intervention of new foundations with significant resources, as well as health threats such as severe acute respiratory syndrome and avian flu, have sparked significant increases in funding for global health from both traditional and new sources. Recipient countries have also made commitments to increasing resources for public financing of essential health services to reach the MDGs. This represents both a great opportunity and a major challenge to all donors and recipient countries alike.

There is a tremendous gap between rich and poor countries with respect to health spending and health needs. Developing countries account for 84 percent of the global population and 90 percent of the global disease burden, but only 20 percent of global gross domestic product (GDP) and 12 percent of all health spending. High-income countries spend about a hundred times more on health on a per capita basis than low-income countries: even after adjusting for cost of living differences, high-income countries are spending about 30 times more on health. Worse still, more than half of the spending in poor countries comes from out-of-pocket payments by consumers of care—a highly inequitable form of financing because it hits the poor hardest and denies all individuals the type of financial protection from the costs of catastrophic illness provided by public and private insurance mechanisms. In addition, most poor countries are unable to provide their citizens with a basic package of essential health services.

This inequity has tremendous consequences for the health status of the world's poor. Low-income countries are still facing major disease burdens from preventable and treatable communicable diseases, in addition to the financing problems associated with sustained increases in population growth, life expectancies, and disease burdens related to noncommunicable diseases. These factors not only disproportionately affect the poor, but also increase health care costs and impede productivity and economic growth.

Middle-income countries are struggling to achieve universal coverage of essential services and provide their populations with financial protection against catastrophic spending, while facing increasing health costs caused by demographic and epidemiological transitions and the implementation of new technologies. Most middle-income countries have embarked on reforms to deal with these problems by enhancing revenue collection and risk pooling efforts and improving the efficiency of health care spending.

International recognition of these global health inequities by the Group of Eight, the European Commission, and the United Nations, as well as global public health threats and support for countries to reach the MDGs, have resulted in significant increases in development assistance overall and development assistance for health in particular after almost a decade of decline in the 1990s. Nonetheless, much larger increases in donor assistance—estimated to be on the order of $25 billion to $70 billion a year—are needed to provide the world's poor with essential services and for countries to reach the health MDGs.

But more resources alone will not lead to better results unless the global community squarely faces the challenge of strengthening the implementation capacity of health systems so that resources translate into better health outcomes for the poor. Despite improvements in access to health care services as a result of global programs, recent experiences in scaling up assistance through these programs have also highlighted the presence of significant implementation bottlenecks— macroeconomic, governance, institutional, health systems-specific—that inhibit the effective, efficient, and equitable use of development assistance for health.

To mitigate the effects of implementation bottlenecks, donors as well as recipients must be held mutually accountable for their promises, behaviors, and results. Donor countries will need to meet their aid commitments, harmonize their efforts, increase the predictability and longevity of aid flows, and reconcile national political interests with global needs. Countries need to do their part to ensure that increased public spending "buys" better health and human development outcomes for the poor. Recipient countries need to improve governance and their macroeconomic and budgetary management capacity, reduce corruption, ensure that they have functioning health systems supported by long-term sustainable financing and effective partnerships with nongovernmental providers, and achieve results in terms of improving their human development indicators.

In middle-income countries and even some large low-income countries, donors play only a minor role in the financing of health systems, and major increases in external resources for health in these countries are unlikely. Under these circumstances, certain factors become important public sector priorities, including ensuring equitable, efficient, and sustainable financing; developing effective and equitable risk pooling and prepayment mechanisms; improving regulatory capacity to deal with market failures; ensuring appropriate governance arrangements; getting better value for money through allocative and technical efficiency gains; targeting financing to the poor and vulnerable; and learning from the experiences of the high-income countries.

This report provides an overview of health financing tools, policies, and trends, with a focus on challenges facing developing countries. While all health financing systems should seek to improve health status, provide financial protection against catastrophic illness costs, and satisfy their participants, the evidence reviewed here reveals that there is no single "road" for achieving these goals. Countries operate within highly variable economic, cultural, political, demographic, and epidemiological contexts. The development of their health delivery and financing systems—and the optimal solutions to the challenges they face—will continue to be influenced by these and other historical country-specific factors. Nonetheless, countries can learn from each other's health financing efforts. This report highlights some key lessons in this area and provides policy recommendations based on underlying economic principles, political environments, socioeconomic conditions, and institutional realities, not buzzwords, slogans, and magic bullets. It also highlights the remaining and anticipated challenges for developing countries and their global partners.

Jacques Baudouy
Director, Health, Nutrition, and Population
The World Bank

Acknowledgments

This report was prepared by Pablo Gottret and George Schieber. Other joint authors are Nicole Tapay, Axel Rahola, Marko Vujicic, Lisa Fleisher, Margaret Maier, Eduard Bos, Emi Suzuki, Paolo Belli, Mark Bassett, Abdo Yazbeck, Reinhard Busse, Jonas Schreyögg, and Christian Gericke. The report also contains written contributions from Agnes Soucat, John Langenbrunner, Cristian Baeza, Daniel Kress, Farasat Bokhari, Ginny Hsieh, Jumana Qamruddin, Qiu Fang, Ricardo Bitran, Vijaysakar Kalavakonda, and Yunwei Gai. Charito Hain and Philomena Williams supported the editing and formatting. The work was carried out under the general direction of Jacques Baudouy and Kei Kawabata.

The authors are indebted to the peer reviewers—Peter Berman, Mukesh Chawla, Oscar Picazo, and Anand Rajaram—as well as Alex Preker, Pia Schneider, and Adam Wagstaff who also provided written comments on the report. The econometric work also received comments and suggestions from Mead Over and Santiago Herrera. The team would also like to express its appreciation to Paul Gertler who provided strategic policy direction for the report.

The report was edited by Susan Graham as well as Bruce Ross-Larson, Carol Rosen, and Jodi Baxter, with Communications Development Incorporated. Book production and printing was handled by the World Bank's Office of the Publisher.

The work was supported in part by the government of the Netherlands, through the World Bank–Netherlands Partnership Program.

Acronyms and Abbreviations

CBHO	community-based health organization
CPIA	country policy and institutional assessment (World Bank)
DAC	Development Assistance Committee (OECD)
DfID	U.K. Department for International Development
DRG	diagnostic-related groups
FDI	foreign direct investment
G-8	Group of 8 (countries)
GDP	gross domestic product
GFATM	Global Fund to Fight AIDS, Tuberculosis and Malaria
GP	general practitioner
HIPC	Heavily Indebted Poor Country
HIV/AIDS	human immunodeficiency virus/acquired immune deficiency syndrome
IDA	International Development Association (World Bank)
IFF	international finance facility
ILO	International Labour Organization
IMF	International Monetary Fund
MAMS	maquette for multisectoral analysis
MBB	marginal budgeting for bottlenecks
MP	Millennium Project (Millennium Development Goal needs assessment)
MTEF	medium-term expenditure framework
NGO	nongovernmental organization
NHS	national health survey
OECD	Organisation for Economic Co-operation and Development
PEPFAR	U.S. President's Emergency Plan for AIDS relief
PER	public expenditure review
PETS	public expenditure tracking survey
PHI	private health insurance
PRSC	poverty reduction support credit
PRSP	poverty reduction strategy paper
SDR	special drawing right
STEP	Strategies and Tools against Social Exclusion and Poverty
VAT	value added tax
WHO	World Health Organization

Overview

Health is now widely recognized as a basic human right, and the urgency of some global health issues has pushed global health policy to the top of the international agenda. With globalization comes the flow of ideas, capital, and people across borders, which has profound implications for the spread and treatment of disease. The epidemics of HIV/AIDS and SARS, the potential impact of avian flu, and the international public goods dimensions of public health make global health policy both a national security issue and a foreign policy issue. Furthermore, it has become clear that the Millennium Development Goals cannot be achieved without massive infusions of new overseas development assistance, much of it targeted to health.

These issues have produced new global health policy dynamics among multilateral and bilateral donors, the new financiers (such as the Bill and Melinda Gates Foundation), the new global programs (such as the Global Fund to Fight AIDS, Tuberculosis, and Malaria), and recipient countries. Multilateral and bilateral institutions and foundations, nongovernmental organizations (NGOs), and joint donor initiatives are helping countries to finance, rationalize, and operationalize health reforms.

The international community must live up to its promise to scale up development assistance and make it predictable and sustainable. Nevertheless, it is ultimately the developing countries that must face the challenges of organizing their institutions and health financing systems to provide sufficient financial resources, ensure equitable access to effective health interventions, and protect their people against health and income shocks. These reforms must be based on social and macroeconomic realities and especially on good governance.

This report provides an overview of health financing policy in developing countries. It is a primer on major health financing and fiscal issues, intended to assist policy makers and all other stakeholders in the design, implementation, and evaluation of effective health financing reforms. The health sector is an extremely complex one, and reformers must be prepared to deal with its complexities when designing and implementing health policy reforms.

The report assesses health financing policies from the perspectives of the basic financing functions of collecting revenues, pooling resources, and purchasing services. It evaluates these functions for their capacity to improve health outcomes, provide financial protection, and ensure consumer satisfaction—in an equitable, efficient, and financially sustainable manner.

There are various well-known models for implementing these basic functions—national health service systems, social health insurance funds, private voluntary health insurance, community-based health insurance, and direct purchases by consumers. More important than the models, however, are three basic principles of public finance:

- *Principle 1.* Raise enough revenues to provide individuals with a basic package of essential services and financial protection against catastrophic medical expenses caused by illness and injury in an equitable, efficient, and sustainable manner.
- *Principle 2.* Manage these revenues to pool health risks equitably and efficiently.
- *Principle 3.* Ensure the purchase of health services in ways that are allocatively and technically efficient.

All health financing systems try to follow these principles, but the evidence reviewed here shows that there is no single road. Countries operate within highly different economic, cultural, demographic and epidemiological contexts, and the development of their health provision and financing systems—and the optimal solutions to the challenges they face—will continue to be heavily influenced by these and other historical factors as well as political economy considerations. Even so, countries can learn from both the successes and the failures of each other's health financing efforts.

The numbers

Globally there exists an enormous mismatch between countries' health financing needs and their current health spending. Developing countries account for 84 percent of global population and 90 percent of the global disease burden, but only 12 percent of global health spending. The poorest countries bear an even higher share of the burden of disease and injury, yet they have the fewest resources for financing health services.

These underlying population and epidemiological dynamics will have profound effects on the economies and future health needs of all countries. The world's population will grow to a projected 7.5 billion by 2020 and to 9 billion by 2050. Most of this growth is expected to occur in developing countries. Low-income countries face the highest rates of growth; the populations in 50 of the poorest countries will double by 2050.

The shift in demographics (high but declining rates of population growth and increased life expectancies) as well as the trend toward noncommunicable diseases and injuries will dictate the needs and service delivery systems in low-

and middle-income countries. Over the next 20 years, changes in population size and structure alone will increase total health care spending needs by 14 percent in Europe and Central Asia; 37 percent in East Asia and the Pacific; 45 percent in South Asia; 47 percent in Latin America and the Caribbean; 52 percent in Sub-Saharan Africa; and 62 percent in the Middle East and North Africa. Excluding Europe and Central Asia, developing countries will face 2–3 percent annual increases in health care expenditure needs (or pressures) from demographics alone.

High but declining rates of population growth coupled with longer life expectancy means that developing countries will face significant increases in population in all age ranges, particularly the elderly range. As a result of population momentum, larger numbers of individuals will enter the work force. Whether this will be a "demographic gift" of faster economic growth or a "demographic curse" of greater unemployment and social unrest will depend on government policies that foster economic and labor force growth. Industrial structures need to be in place and employment patterns established for domestic resource mobilization and specific health financing efforts.

Patterns and effectiveness of current health spending

Global health spending in 2002 was $3.2 trillion, about 10 percent of global gross domestic product (GDP). Only some 12 percent of that, $350 billion, was spent in low- and middle-income countries. High-income countries spend about 100 times more on health per capita (population-weighted) than low-income countries—30 times if one adjusts for cost of living differences. Worse still, more than half of the meager spending in low-income countries is from out-of-pocket payments by consumers of care—the most inequitable type of financing because it hits the poor hardest and denies all individuals financial protection from catastrophic illness that public and private insurance mechanisms provide.

The public share of total health expenditures changes with income category: the public share is 29 percent in low-income countries, 42 percent in lower-middle-income countries, 56 percent in upper-middle-income countries, and 65 percent in high-income countries. (In 2003, the World Bank defined countries as low-income when their GNI was less than $766; countries with a GNI per capita between $766 and $9,385 were considered middle-income; and $3,035 was the dividing line between lower-middle-income and upper-middle-income countries.)

Social health insurance institutions are a very limited source of health care spending in low-income countries. They accounted for only some 2 percent of total spending on health in low-income countries, 15 percent in lower-middle-income countries, and 30 percent in upper-middle-income and high-income countries. In Sub-Saharan Africa only 2 percent of all public spending on health (less than 1 percent of total health spending) is through social insurance institutions and in South Asia 8 percent (less than 2 percent of total health spending).

For the private share of spending, the poorer the country the larger the amount that is out of pocket: 93 percent in low-income countries (more than 60 percent of the total); some 85 percent in middle-income countries (40 percent of the total); and only 56 percent in high-income countries (20 percent of the total). Such figures in the low- and middle-income countries are troublesome because they imply that out-of-pocket expenditures, the most inequitable source of health financing, predominates in these countries.

External sources account for 8 percent of health spending in low-income countries and less than 1 percent in middle-income countries (according to population-weighted expenditure information). But on a country-weighted basis, external sources account for 20 percent of total low-income country health spending. In 12 countries in Sub-Saharan Africa, external sources finance more than 30 percent of total health expenditures.

How effective is this spending for health outcomes? Various studies document a range of effects—from no impacts, to limited impacts, to impacts for only specific interventions. Greater improvements in health outcomes are associated with stronger institutions and higher investments in other health-related sectors, such as education and infrastructure.

A new econometric analysis performed for this study finds strong impacts of government health spending on maternal mortality and child mortality; direct health spending effects are larger than those found for public investments in infrastructure, education, and sanitation. The analysis also shows that parallel investments in infrastructure and education further reduce infant and child mortality, supporting the need for a cross-sectoral approach to reach the Millennium Development Goals for health. Economic growth also has a large impact on health outcomes—both by directly improving outcomes and by generating increased resources that can be mobilized by governments for increased public spending.

Another important finding is that external donor assistance has a limited direct impact on health outcomes. Development assistance for health has a direct impact on under-five mortality, after controlling for volatility. But it does not affect maternal mortality directly—it does so only indirectly, through its effect on government health spending. This outcome is not surprising given the fungibility of aid, the off-budget nature of a significant amount of aid, the exclusion of much aid from the balance of payments, and the fact that much aid has gone to debt forgiveness and technical assistance.

Health financing functions and sources of revenues

There are myriad ways for countries to design and implement policies to collect revenues, pool risks, and purchase services. *Risk pooling* is the collection and management of financial resources so that large unpredictable individual financial risks become predictable and are distributed among all members of the pool. *Pur-*

chasing refers to the many arrangements for buyers of health care services to pay health care providers and suppliers.

The success of countries in carrying out these functions has important implications for

- funds available (now and in the future) and the concomitant levels of essential services and financial protection,
- fairness (equity) of the revenue collection mechanisms to finance the system (basing financial access on need rather than ability to pay),
- economic efficiency of revenue-raising, in not creating distortions or economic losses in the economy,
- levels of pooling and prepayment (and the implications for risk and equity subsidization),
- numbers and types of services purchased and consumed and their effects on health outcomes and costs (allocative efficiency),
- technical efficiency of service production (producing each service at its minimum average cost),
- financial and physical access to services (including equity in access).

Collecting revenue

Revenue collection in developing countries is the art of the possible, not the optimal. Although there are numerous public and private sources for raising revenues, the institutional realities of developing countries often preclude the use of the most equitable and efficient revenue-raising mechanisms. Revenue-raising capacities increase as country incomes increase (as a result of greater formalization of the economy, greater ability of individuals and businesses to pay, and better tax administration). Low-income countries collect some 18 percent of their GDP as government revenues, severely limiting their ability to finance essential public services. For example, a country with a per capita GDP of $300 can collect $54 per capita (18 percent of GDP) for all public expenditure needs—defense, roads, airports, electricity, sewage systems, pensions, education, health, and water. Middle-income countries raise some 23 percent of their GDP from government revenues, and high-income countries, 32 percent.

Pooling risk

Risk pooling and prepayment are critical for providing financial protection. Pooling health risks enables the establishment of insurance and improves citizens' welfare by allowing individuals to pay a predetermined amount to protect themselves against large unpredictable medical expenses.

There are various ways for governments to finance public health insurance programs, and each should be assessed on the basis of equity, efficiency, sustainability, administrative feasibility, and administrative cost. Most low- and middle-income countries have multiple public and private pooling arrangements, and governments should strive to reduce fragmentation (and thereby improve equity and efficiency), lower administrative costs, and provide the basis for more effective risk pooling and purchasing.

Resource allocation and purchasing

Resource allocation and purchasing mechanisms determine for whom to buy, what to buy, from whom, how to pay, and at what price. Purchasing includes the many arrangements used by purchasers of health care services to pay medical care providers. A variety of arrangements exists: some national health services and social security organizations provide services in publicly owned facilities where staff members are salaried public employees; sometimes individuals or organizations purchase services through direct payments or through contracting arrangements from public and private providers. Other arrangements combine these approaches.

Resource allocation and purchasing procedures have important implications for cost, access, quality, and consumer satisfaction. Efficiency gains (both technical and allocative) from purchasing arrangements provide better value for money and thus are a means of obtaining additional "financing" for the health system.

Purchasing has taken on increased importance because donors want to be assured that new funding to scale up services is being used efficiently. Moreover, the efficiency of a system has important financial implications for long-term fiscal sustainability and for governments to find the "fiscal space" in highly constrained budget settings for large increases in public spending. Indeed, health financing policies (collection, pooling, and purchasing) must be developed in the context of a government's available fiscal space.

Fiscal space

Large proposed increases in public health spending must be considered in the context of the available *fiscal space*—the budgetary room that allows a government to provide resources for a desired purpose without any prejudice to the sustainability of its financial position. (Fiscal space is at the center of the current debate over the purported negative impacts of International Monetary Fund (IMF) programs that preclude countries from using the increased grant funding for health investments and recurrent health expenditures, such as hiring additional health workers).

In principle, a government can create fiscal space in the following ways:

- through tax measures or by strengthening tax administration;
- cutting lower-priority expenditures to make room for more desirable ones;
- borrowing resources, either from domestic or from external sources;
- getting the central bank to print money to be lent to the government; or
- receiving grants from outside sources.

Creating fiscal space requires a judgment that the higher short-term expenditure, and any associated future expenditures, can be financed from current and future revenues. If financed by debt, the expenditure should be assessed for its impact on the underlying growth rate or its impact on a country's capacity to generate the revenue to service that debt.

Risk pooling mechanisms

Policy makers must assess the most appropriate mechanisms to pool health risks and provide financial protection to their populations. The challenge for low- and middle-income countries is to somehow direct the high levels of out-of-pocket spending into either public or private pooling arrangements, so that individuals will have real financial protection. Four main health insurance mechanisms are used to pool health risks, promote prepayment, raise revenues, and purchase services:

- State-funded systems through ministries of health or national health services
- Social health insurance
- Voluntary or private health insurance
- Community-based health insurance

While the features of each financing mechanism differ significantly, no one method is inherently better than another. So, policy makers must examine the context and determine which method constitutes the best means for developing a strong health financing system in terms of equity, efficiency, and sustainability. It is important to be pragmatic and ensure that the mechanisms chosen are aligned with country-specific economic, institutional, and cultural characteristics.

Ministry of health/national health service systems

Ministry of health or national health service–style systems generally have three main features. First, their primary funding comes from general revenues. Second, they provide medical coverage to the country's entire population. Third, their services are delivered through a network of public providers. (In most low- and middle-income countries, ministries of health function as national health services and generally exist alongside other risk pooling arrangements, so they are not the sole source of coverage for the entire population).

The features of national health services give them the potential to be equitable and efficient. Their broad coverage means that risks are pooled broadly, without the dangers of risk selection inherent in more fragmented systems. And unlike other systems, they rely on a broad revenue base. National health service–style systems also have the potential for efficient operation. Most are integrated and under government control, and they have less potential for the high transaction costs that arise from multiple players. But when power is decentralized or shared with local authorities, and when the decision-making authority is unclear, coordination problems can ensue.

Provision under the pure national health service model is through public facilities and personnel, but in practice there is much variability—many governments contract services from nongovernmental organizations, faith-based organizations, and other private providers. Whether public provision is more efficient, equitable, and sustainable than private provision is a question not of ownership but of the underlying delivery structures and incentives facing providers and consumers.

Although national health service systems have the theoretical benefit of providing health care to the entire population free of charge (except for any applicable user fees), the reality is less encouraging. Reliance on general government budgets is vulnerable to the vicissitudes of annual budget discussions and changes in political priorities. And in most low-income developing countries, public health spending as a share of the budget is low.

Health services in many low- and middle-income countries are primarily used by middle- and high-income households in urban areas because of access problems for the rural poor. In addition, the poor tend to use less expensive local primary care facilities, whereas the rich disproportionately use more expensive hospital services. Public provision of health services may also face problems of corruption and inefficiencies caused by budgets that do not generate the appropriate incentives and accountability—which has led many governments to split financing from provision.

To exploit the potential strengths of national health service–style systems, it is important for developing countries to improve the capacity to raise revenue, the quality of governance and institutions, and the ability to maintain the universal coverage and reach of the system. It is also important to take specific measures to target spending to the poor, such as increasing the budget allocations for primary care. But the system must not neglect the needs of the middle- and high-income populations—that way, they can maintain political support and deter the middle- and high-income populations from opting for privately financed providers at the expense of supporting the public system.

Social health insurance systems

Social health insurance systems are generally characterized by independent or quasi-independent insurance funds, a reliance on mandatory earmarked payroll contributions (usually from individuals and employers), and a clear link between these contributions and the right to a defined package of health benefits. In many countries, coverage has been progressively extended to subpopulations and then to the whole population.

The state generally defines the main attributes of the system, although funds are generally nonprofit and supervised by the government. The number of funds varies by country. Where there are multiple funds, mechanisms are often used to compensate for different risk profiles across funds, and administrative costs are generally higher. Some countries are reducing the number of funds to maximize risk pooling and to benefit from economies of scale.

The payroll base of much of the funding of social health insurance systems insulates them from budgetary negotiations that may subject national health service systems to more variable funding. Yet social health insurance contributions alone may not be adequate to fully fund health care costs, especially if the system is intended to cover a broader population than those who contribute. Social health insurance systems may thus require an infusion of resources from general tax revenues. Additional subsidies may come from external aid or other earmarked taxes.

The equity of social contribution financing depends on the presence or absence of contribution ceilings and other features, but some studies have concluded that such financing is less progressive than general revenue financing, or at best as progressive. Social contributions may also have a deleterious effect on employment and economic growth if they increase labor costs (as might happen if employers are unable to offset the added cost by reducing wages).

Social health insurance systems often cover only a limited population (for example, those in large formal sector enterprises), at least at their inception, and it is difficult to add informal sector workers to the covered population. When successfully implemented, they often have strong support from the population, which perceives them as private and stable in their management and finances.

Social health insurance systems sometimes are more difficult to manage because they involve more complex interactions among players. They can also confront cost escalation and difficulties in paring back benefits. And their less integrated nature does not lend itself to efficient treatment of chronic diseases and preventive care.

What preconditions might lead to the successful development of social health insurance systems in developing countries?

- *Level of income and economic growth.* The systems often begin in lower-middle-income countries, and expansions to universal coverage generally occur during periods of strong economic growth.
- *Dominance of formal sector versus informal sector.* The systems are easier to administer in countries with a high proportion of industrial or formal sector workers, because employers will likely have a formal payroll system for contributions.
- *Population distribution.* The systems are successful in countries with growing urban populations and increased population density but face slower implementation in countries with a large rural population.
- *Room to increase labor costs.* Countries where the economies can tolerate increased payroll contributions without negative effects on employment and growth are better candidates for such systems.

- *Strong administrative capacity.* The ability to implement a social health insurance system without excess administrative costs—and in a transparent, well-governed fashion—is critical for population support and for financial and political sustainability.
- *Quality health care infrastructure.* The systems can be successful only if the services they fund are available and of good quality, which will support membership in the scheme and avoid a system where the wealthier populations opt for a separate, privately financed system and do not provide needed political support.
- *Stakeholder consensus in favor of social health insurance, together with political stability and rights.* Societies that place a high value on equity and solidarity are likely to support the redistributive aspects of such systems. But significant differentials in contributions may not be tolerated in systems where solidarity plays a less prominent role.
- *Ability to extend the system.* Governments seeking to expand their social health insurance systems must design realistic and progressive goals that reflect the operating context. These goals include the ability to encourage the affiliation of informal sector workers and the means to collect regular contributions from them. Transparent and participatory schemes are more likely to garner population support. And governments may need to subsidize the extension of social health insurance to the poor.

Countries aiming to implement social health insurance systems face formidable challenges but also have the potential to reap significant rewards. It is important to examine the specific socioeconomic, cultural, and political contexts and determine whether the setting and the timing are right for implementing such a system.

Community-based health insurance

Community-based health insurance schemes have existed for centuries. They were the precursors to many of the current social health insurance systems, such as those in Germany, Japan, and the Republic of Korea, and they are currently prevalent in Sub-Saharan Africa. The schemes can be broadly defined as not-for-profit prepayment plans for health care that are controlled by a community that has voluntary membership. Most community-based health insurance schemes operate according to core social values and cover beneficiaries excluded from other health coverage.

There is evidence that such schemes reduce out-of-pocket spending, and one study found that they contributed to greater use of health resources. They may also fill gaps in existing schemes (as for informal workers in Tanzania) and form part of a transition to a more universal health care coverage system.

But the protection and sustainability of most community-based health insurance schemes are questionable. They are often unable to raise significant resources because of the limited income of the community, and the pool is often small, making it difficult to serve a broad risk-spreading and financial protection function. The schemes' size and resource levels make them vulnerable to failure. They are also placed at risk by the limited management skills available in the community, and they have limited impact on the delivery of health care, because few negotiate with providers on quality or price. They also cannot cover the poorer parts of the population—even small premiums may be out of reach for the poor.

Government intervention could improve the efficiency and sustainability of such schemes through subsidies, technical assistance, and links to more formal financing arrangements. But community-based health insurance is not likely to be the "magic bullet" for solving the bulk of health financing problems in low-income countries. It should be regarded more as a complement to, rather than a substitute for, other forms of strong government involvement in health care financing.

Private or voluntary health insurance

Private or voluntary health insurance often supplements publicly funded coverage, especially in high-income countries. Private health insurance is paid for by non-income–based premiums (not tax or social security contributions). Voluntary health insurance is defined as any health insurance paid for by voluntary contributions. Although the two types of coverage are distinct, most private health insurance markets are also voluntary—except in a few countries, such as Switzerland and Uruguay, where the purchase of private coverage is mandatory for all or a part of the population.

There are several roles that private/voluntary health insurance can play in a country's public or social coverage:

- Primary—as the main source of coverage for a population or subpopulation
- Duplicate—covering the same services or benefits as public coverage, but differing in the providers, time of access, quality, and amenities
- Complementary—covering cost-sharing under the public program
- Supplementary—for services not covered by the public program

Private/voluntary health insurance markets have been somewhat controversial, partly because they often reach wealthier populations and have been the subject of market failures, such as adverse selection by covered individuals and "cream skimming" of better health risks by insurers. Nonetheless, at least in countries of the Organisation for Economic Co-operation and Development (OECD), such markets have been found to promote risk pooling of resources that are often otherwise paid out of pocket, to enhance access to services when public or mandatory financing is incomplete, and in some cases to increase service capacity and promote innovation.

Yet private/voluntary health insurance has limits. A study of OECD countries found financial barriers to access because of affordability and premium volatility. Such insurance can contribute to differential access to health care services in some countries. It has done little to reduce cost pressures on public systems. Nor has it made significant contributions to quality improvements, except in a few countries.

The complexity of private/voluntary health insurance markets raises questions about their relevance and feasibility in low-income countries. They may be more plausible options in middle-income countries with large literate and mobile urban populations. Some of the challenges and market failures associated with these markets can be addressed through regulations that mandate certain insurer actions (on acceptance of applicants and premium calculations) and minimize or rectify market failures. Yet these regulations can be difficult to implement and enforce. And they presuppose regulatory resources, political backing, and well-functioning financial and insurance markets. It can also be challenging to strike the most appropriate balance between access and equity concerns and desires to promote an efficient and competitive marketplace.

In sum, each of the pooling mechanisms discussed here raises challenges and must be considered in the country context. While national health services and social health insurance have different institutional eligibility and financing criteria, they both face the same issues of ensuring adequate and sustainable financing in an equitable and efficient manner. Future contingent liabilities are a concern for both systems even if national health services in theory have a wider revenue base than payroll contributions. Policy makers need to focus on underlying principles—maximizing risk pooling and assuring equitable, efficient, and sustainable financing—not on labels or generic models.

Development assistance for health

Large increases in official development assistance and development assistance for health will be needed to assist poor countries in providing essential services to their populations and scaling up to meet the Millennium Development Goals. After almost a 25 percent decline in the 1990s, official development assistance has once again started to increase. In 2003 it was 0.25 percent of gross national income (some $70 billion), still well short of the Monterrey target of 0.7 percent and the Millennium Project's estimated need of 0.54 percent. Much of the increase has been devoted to debt relief and technical assistance.

Development assistance for health has increased significantly over the past few years, to more than $10 billion in 2003. Most of the recent increases have been focused on Africa and on specific diseases and interventions. Given the renewed efforts of countries to meet their Monterrey commitments from the European Union and Group of Eight as well as the large amounts of assistance pledged to meet the Millennium Development Goals, issues concerning the impact, absorption, use, and sustainability of this external assistance have been receiving attention.

Increased assistance on the order of $25–70 billion a year will be needed to achieve the Millennium Development Goals for health. Although official development assistance is of critical importance, accounting for 55 percent of all external flows to Africa, it accounts for only 9 percent of such flows to other developing regions. In those regions foreign direct investment, workers' remittances, and other private flows account for 91 percent of external flows. It is essential for policy makers to focus on these critically important external sources of funding as well as official development assistance.

Global programs, generally focused on specific diseases or interventions, have been responsible for the bulk of the recent increases in external health assistance, representing 15–20 percent of development assistance for health. Global partnerships and private funding are becoming a more important part of the picture, whereas the United Nations' organizations and development bank roles are relatively constant.

Aid effectiveness and absorption

Large increases in donor funding for health, much of it for recurrent spending, raise important questions about the ability of countries to absorb these funds, the predictability and maturity of these funds, and the ability of countries to sustain services once donor funding stops.

With most of the recent increases in development assistance for health directed to specific diseases and interventions, there is growing concern about the disease- and intervention-specific focus of aid. Such a focus can be very effective in resource-scarce environments. But as health systems develop, waste and efficiency can result from separate delivery silos for different diseases. And given the severe human resources constraints in many African countries, aid programs compete with each other to hire away the few skilled professionals needed to run the public health system. It is important for the ongoing work on health systems to address this issue; evidence-based policy recommendations as opposed to the conventional wisdom and conceptual arguments should drive much of this debate.

A recent study of 14 poverty reduction strategy papers (PRSPs) found that 30 percent of external aid did not enter into the balance of payments, and another 20 percent was entered into the balance of payments but not the government budget. Of the remaining 50 percent, only 20 percent was for general budget support. For governments to effectively implement their "country-owned" programs, they need the flexibility to manage these funds. Donors and countries need to seek ways to funnel this increased external funding through general budget support and to finance gaps in the recipient countries' programs as much as possible.

Aid's fungibility implies that governments may divert domestic resources to other uses given the presence of donor funding in priority areas (such as primary care). Once donor funding stops, governments may face difficulties in reallocating resources to these priority areas, which could lead to their underfunding. Donors must exercise care in analyzing the impact of their own resources, which may not actually attain the intended outcomes. They must also give serious consideration to supporting government budgets directly, through budget support for an agreed program, rather than to directly financing projects that may crowd out the government's own resources. Budget support for existing government programs must be predictable, committed over longer maturities to ensure continuity, and facilitate planning.

Large increases in development assistance for health to low-income countries (promised and actual) raise questions about whether countries can make effective use of new aid flows. Absorptive capacity has macroeconomic, budgetary, management, and service delivery dimensions. It also rests on critical macro conditions: good governance, lack of corruption, and sound financial institutions. Also critical are human resources for public sector management and for service delivery. Both donors and recipient countries need to develop a better understanding of these constraints and provide an evidence-based system for dealing with them.

Realities of government spending and policy levers

One of the most significant challenges to improving health system performance in developing countries is weak public sector management, particularly at the district or municipal level. Empirical analyses support direct correlations among the quality of policies and institutions, absorptive capacity, and the country's ability to improve certain health outcomes through increased government health spending. Several tools have been developed to improve public sector management.

Poverty reduction strategy papers, poverty reduction support credits, and medium-term expenditure frameworks

To receive concessionary funding assistance from the World Bank and IMF, all low-income countries are required to base their macroeconomic and sectoral reforms on a poverty reduction strategy, embodied in a poverty reduction strategy paper (PRSP). In theory PRSPs are designed to strengthen country ownership, provide a poverty focus for country programs; establish a coordinated framework for the World Bank and IMF and other development partners; and improve governance, accountability, and priority-setting.

Evidence to date has been mixed. PRSPs have encouraged a results-oriented approach but have fallen short as a roadmap for integrating sectoral strategies into the macroeconomic framework, understanding micro-macro linkages, and linking medium- and long-term operational targets. The process could be more inclusive, and the focus could be sharper for capacity building and for monitoring and evaluation. PRSPs become meaningful only if priorities feed into the annual budget process. Ownership by countries and their external partners is still problematic. And external partners have not adapted their procedures to the PRSP process in a coordinated manner.

Poverty reduction support credits (PRSCs), one of the World Bank's major general budget support vehicles for implementing PRSPs, are intended to provide medium-term support, encourage donor harmonization, improve resource predictability, and reinforce country ownership. They have been found to facilitate coordination between central and line ministries, as well as among donors. In addition, they have limited conditionalities. Further progress could be made in streamlining policy matrices and improving monitoring and evaluation.

Medium-term expenditure frameworks (MTEFs) combine macroeconomic models projecting revenues and expenditures in the medium term with "bottom-up" reviews of sector policies—a tool to optimize intrasectoral allocations in the context of annual budget processes. To date, these frameworks have not improved macroeconomic balances or increased budgetary predictability for line ministries. But there is some limited evidence that they have led to reallocations to priority sectors.

An analysis of countries implementing PRSPs, PRSCs, and MTEFs produced several examples of good practices. These practices include (1) establishing clear priorities and criteria within the PRSP through an iterative process that involves line ministries and the central government; (2) conducting annual reviews of progress by sector; and (3) having a credible process for budget preparation by the ministry of finance and the cabinet, along with medium-term assurances of budget levels for each sector. Even so, PRSPs remain a work in progress.

Public expenditure reviews and public expenditure tracking surveys

Public expenditure reviews (PERs) and public expenditure tracking surveys (PETS) assist countries in developing public expenditure strategies and tracking expenditures.

PERs seek to provide objective analysis of public spending issues. They analyze and project tax revenues, the level and composition of public spending, and intersectoral and intrasectoral allocations, as well as review financial and nonfinancial public enterprises and the governance structure and functioning of public institutions. In the health sector, PERs have revealed important information about budget execution and have shown disparities between disbursements and amounts budgeted through the MTEF.

PETS track the flow of government resources to determine the amount that actually reaches the service delivery level. They have uncovered significant leakages (as high as 90 percent) in the education and health sectors, leading governments to improve public sector management. A review of PETS in African countries found nonwage funds to be more susceptible to leakage than salaries, and it showed leakage occurring at specific levels of governments. This information can help in creating and targeting more efficient interventions.

Health financing challenges in low-income countries

Most low-income countries are being severely challenged to provide essential services to their populations and to provide financial protection. Without substantial increases in external assistance, meeting the Millennium Development Goals is highly unlikely.

Most regions will not reach the Millennium Development Goals for health because of slow progress in the 1990s. In Africa the declines in child mortality of some 0.5 percent a year since 1990 will have to accelerate to declines of 8 percent a year to reach the target of halving childhood mortality by 2015. Similarly, East Asia and the Pacific will need to improve previous annual reductions of 2.7 percent to 5 percent. Neither increased health spending nor growth alone will do the job. Reaching the goals requires growth and a multisectoral effort. For example, India would need a 15 percent annual economic growth rate from 2000 to 2015 to reach the goals on the basis of growth alone. Rwanda would need a twentyfold increase in public spending on health to achieve the Millennium Development Goals on the basis of public health spending alone.

Mobilizing domestic resources and deciding on user fees

Some countries can improve their domestic resource mobilization efforts, particularly as there appear to be such wide ranges for countries at the same income levels. Various estimates suggest that countries can possibly generate an additional 1–4 percent of their GDPs in government revenues. This is an important area of focus, given the poor revenue performance of many low-income countries in the past decade.

User fees have been a contentious source of financing in low-income country settings. In most cases they have occurred spontaneously as a result of the scarcity of public financing, the prominence of the public system in the supply of essential health care, the government's inability to allocate adequate financing to its health system, the readiness of the poor and nonpoor to pay fees as a way of reducing the travel and time costs of alternative sources of care, the low salaries of health workers, the limited public control over pricing practices by public providers, and the lack of key medical supplies such as drugs. User fees are likely to remain in place until governments are ready and more able to mobilize greater funding for health care.

A blanket policy to remove user fees could do more harm than good by removing a small but important source of revenue at the health care facility level. Until low-income country governments can mobilize alternative (and more equitable) financing mechanisms, the global community should focus on helping countries design policies that can foster access by the poor to health-enhancing services and protect the poor and near-poor from catastrophic health spending. User fees can be harmonized to achieve these objectives if they reduce financial barriers to the poor by improving the quality of public services, reducing waiting time, reducing the need for costly self-medication, or substituting lower-priced quality public services for more expensive private care.

Conditional cash transfers provide direct cash payments to poor households, contingent on behaviors such as completing a full set of prenatal visits or attending health education classes. They thus represent a negative user fee. The evidence, largely from middle-income countries, suggests that well-designed conditional cash transfers have the potential to improve health outcomes and reduce poverty with relatively modest administrative costs. But additional research is needed to determine whether such programs can be effective in low-income settings.

Securing more external funding

Donor funding will be critical for most countries to meet the Millennium Development Goals. Donors need to reduce the volatility, improve the predictability, and improve the longevity of aid. They also need to ensure that a larger proportion of aid goes to countries as general budget support and to resolve the health systems, fragmentation, coordination, and sustainability issues raised by disease- and intervention-specific aid. And they need to deal with capacity constraints. Increased debt relief will provide countries with additional fiscal space and resources to fund programs. There are, however, important questions about how this debt relief will be financed by donors and used by countries.

Improving risk pooling

To improve financial protection, low-income countries must improve risk pooling. Because private out-of-pocket payments are such a large share of total spending, governments should improve risk pooling though the most viable and effective methods. These methods can include more effective risk pooling through the ministries of health financed by the general budget—and the use of social health insurance, voluntary health insurance, or community-based health insurance—with caveats and enabling conditions kept in mind.

The most globally prominent and straightforward way to increase risk pooling in most low-income countries is through ministries of health acting as national health services. General government revenue–based systems represent the main source of health care funding in 106 of 191 members of the World Health Organization. However, the problems with national health service systems overall, and particularly in low-income countries, have been well documented. Issues of management, accountability, corruption, incentives, underfunding, and misallocation of expenditures are common. The results are limited access to and poor quality of health services as well as limited financial protection against catastrophic health expenditures, particularly for the poor in rural areas. Thus whether a country can take advantage of the substantial strengths of this approach depends heavily on the country's general revenue base, the public sector's management capacities, the public's views about the availability and quality of government services, and the public's willingness to use general government revenues for this purpose.

Social health insurance has the potential not only to improve risk pooling but also to bring additional funding into the health sector. It exists in some 60 countries, mostly high- and middle-income countries. The question is whether social health insurance is the best mechanism in a low-income country setting. Payroll taxes are not the most efficient source for funding a health system, particularly when formal sector employment may be only 10–15 percent of the total. And ministries of health may offer more financial protection than social health insurance.

Proponents of social health insurance argue that giving contributors a clear stake in the system, earmarking funds to protect health expenditures, and improving efficiency through competition on the purchasing side are sufficient justifications to pursue it. At issue are the preconditions for social health insurance: a growing economy and level of income capable of absorbing new contributions, a large payroll contribution base and thus a small informal sector, a concentrated beneficiary population, and good administrative and supervisory capacity.

Voluntary health insurance can also increase risk pooling using private funding. But it accounts for less than 5 percent of private health spending in low-income countries, and it clearly fares poorly on equity grounds. In most middle- and high-income countries, it generally supplements other types of public insurance. Its scope for promoting significant amounts of financial protection in low-income country settings is likely to be quite limited for several reasons: individuals lack purchasing power, financial markets are generally not well developed, and the ability of low-income countries to set up the complex regulatory structures needed for an effective voluntary health insurance market is questionable.

Community-based health insurance may provide some marginal benefits in increased risk pooling and resources, but alone is unlikely to significantly improve financial protection in low-income settings.

Increasing the efficiency and equity of public spending

Low-income countries need to increase the efficiency and equity of all public spending, including health spending. Given budget constraints and difficulties in generating additional fiscal space, low-income countries are likely to have a larger and more equitable impact on health outcomes if they select a very basic universal package of public and merit goods, including some treatment services that have been proven effective in advancing toward the Millennium Development Goals. The financing of other interventions should be targeted. Studies of equity show large imbalances in the benefit incidence of public spending on health. So low-income countries must improve their targeting of expenditures to those interventions that have the greatest marginal impact on the poor. Low-income country governments also need to do a better job in purchasing. Whether this job involves decentralization, contracting out, or developing efficiency-based provider payment incentives and systems, countries need to get better value for money spent.

Health financing challenges in middle-income countries

The focus of middle-income countries is now on universal coverage, financial protection, and health system efficiency. But these countries still have poverty and income inequality, as well as challenges in literacy, education, employment, and social security. Their health spending, while not insignificant (6 percent of GDP), is substantially below the average for high-income countries (10 percent). They also rely heavily on out-of-pocket expenditures, which account for some 40 percent of all health spending. High out-of-pocket payments, higher but still limited revenue-raising capacities, generally fragmented financing systems, and inefficient purchasing arrangements pose significant constraints to universal coverage and better risk pooling.

Middle-income countries are attempting to increase risk pooling and reduce fragmentation in their multiple pooling arrangements by

- subsidizing the premiums of the poor and sometimes informal sector workers through general revenues,
- expanding pools though mandatory inclusion of other groups and integration of private health insurance funds,
- creating single actual or virtual pools.

Purchasing reforms are a critical part of most middle-income country reform efforts. Most reforms follow the general principles of separating finance from provision, having money following patients, and using incentive-based provider payment systems. Although there is a wealth of experimentation with purchasing reforms, few have been rigorously evaluated, and in many cases results have not lived up to expectations because of the lack of reforms in public sector management and civil service laws.

The main policy recommendations for middle-income countries are to

- View efficient and equitable revenue mobilization as a top priority for health, because it is critical that funding be sustainable and commensurate with long-term needs resulting from the health transition. Count on domestic revenues for the bulk of financing because most development assistance for health is focused on low-income countries.
- Promote increased risk pooling on grounds of equity, financial protection, and allocative and technical efficiency. Start by pooling the almost 40 percent of total health spending that is out of pocket. As the first step, integrate informal workers by providing the right incentives.
- Provide maximum financial protection and universal coverage by consolidating multiple risk pools. The associated benefits are greater purchasing power and greater efficiency through reduced transaction costs.
- Focus on designing appropriate benefit packages for covered populations because these packages affect the efficiency of risk pooling, the level of financial protection, and allocative efficiency. Standard benefit packages should have the right mix between the breadth and depth of coverage, so that trade-offs among universal coverage, financial protection, costs, and health outcomes are well balanced.

- Be parsimonious with health spending to expand coverage to more people. Consider increasing overall system efficiency by reforming service purchasing functions and by instituting incentive-based payment mechanisms. Furthermore, payment policies should be in line with overall cost containment and cost-effectiveness objectives.

The specific form of insurance schemes is of less importance than a focus on improving the specific financing functions of revenue collection, risk pooling, and service purchasing. Depending on the context, a combination of insurance schemes may be necessary to accomplish the dual goals of universal coverage and financial protection.

Although there is no "best" strategy to achieve universal coverage, improve financial protection for all, and increase efficiency and quality through more effective purchasing arrangements, policy makers in middle-income countries should focus their immediate attention on improving health services and health coverage for the very poor and vulnerable. Learning what mechanisms have worked well in other countries is necessary for informing reform efforts. Success can occur only when proven financing strategies are adapted to a country's socioeconomic and political context.

Learning from high-income countries

High-income countries have a rich history of health financing reforms as their systems have evolved from community-based voluntary insurance arrangements to formal public insurance funds to social or national health insurance–based financing systems. Nearly all high-income countries, with the exception of the United States, have achieved universal or near universal health coverage. The tax-financed systems have been in place for some time, the social insurance systems more recently. Political will was critical to achieving universal coverage, along with economic growth. As most high-income countries have achieved universal coverage, recent reform activities have tended to focus on efficiency gains through purchasing arrangements, rather than on revenue collection and pooling.

Although high-income countries operate in very different contexts from low-income countries, their experiences furnish some lessons for lower-income countries:

- Economic growth is the most important factor in the move toward universal coverage.
- Improved management and administrative capacity is critical in expanding coverage, as is strong political commitment.
- For low- and middle-income countries transitioning to universal coverage, general revenues and social health insurance contributions are the two principal sources of public funding. Both accumulate public revenues into one or several

pools. Because the critical issue is pooling, whether a social health insurance or national health service system is ultimately chosen is of secondary importance.

- Voluntary and community-based financing schemes can serve as tests for countries as they seek to expand the role of prepaid health coverage schemes.
- Broader risk pooling mechanisms, instead of fragmented, smaller risk pools, can contribute significantly to effective and equitable financing of health coverage.

Products and services must be evaluated for their effectiveness and cost-effectiveness within the context of particular countries' coverage systems. To facilitate the affordability of such efforts, cooperation among similar countries should be encouraged, possibly led by one or more international organizations.

1

Health transitions, disease burdens, and health expenditure patterns

In rich and poor countries alike, health needs are changing in response to lower fertility rates, longer life expectancies, and the shifting burden of illness toward chronic diseases and injuries. These demographic and epidemiological transitions will pose health challenges for countries at every income level. In high-income countries, aging populations, rapidly increasing health costs, and shrinking numbers in the workforce will put increasing pressure on publicly financed health care systems. In some middle-income countries and in most low-income countries, which already are hard pressed to provide even the most basic health services, meeting projected health needs is likely to require additional funds from external financing sources.

Developing countries account for 84 percent of global population, 90 percent of the global disease burden, and 20 percent of global GDP, but only 12 percent of global health spending (Mathers, Lopez, and Murray, forthcoming). Health financing policies designed to ameliorate these disparities are subject to numerous and ever-changing conditions, as populations change, disease burdens shift, new infectious diseases emerge, and societies cope with civil and economic unrest. This unstable policy baseline means that health financing decisions must be firmly based on evidence but also flexible enough to contend effectively with uncertainty. These decisions will affect the demand and supply of health services, the health needs of individuals and populations, and the availability of financial and technical resources to meet those needs. Despite wide variation among countries, key lessons can be learned from analyzing the evidence:

- The ongoing health transition in many developing countries—which encompasses demographic changes, such as lower fertility and longer life expectancy, as well as epidemiological changes, such as the shifting burden of illness toward noncommunicable diseases and injuries[1]—will have profound effects on the quantity and type of health services needed. These trends will increase cost pressures on health care systems in most developing countries.
- High but declining rates of population growth, coupled with increases in life expectancy, mean that developing countries will face significant increases in

population in the medium term, particularly among the working-age population and the elderly.

- Low-income countries are struggling under a large burden of communicable disease, while also confronting increases in the prevalence of noncommunicable diseases and injuries, a trend that will likely continue for some time. The availability of resources to meet these numerous health needs is limited. The international community will have to make a considerable effort to raise levels of donor assistance for health and to ensure that adequate resources are available for low-income countries to increase spending for essential health services and to meet the Millennium Development Goals.

- Middle-income countries, some with growing working-age populations, will be challenged to provide adequate employment. Whether this burgeoning population will be a demographic gift bearing economic growth or a curse bringing more unemployment and social unrest will depend on whether government policies foster economic and labor force growth. Communicable diseases among younger populations will still lead to high demands on the health system, while increased life expectancy will heighten demand on the other end of the age spectrum.

- High-income countries will also have to contend with growing proportions of the elderly and rapidly rising health expenditures. These countries face serious concerns about how a declining working-age population can support the health and social services demanded by increasing numbers of elderly, as well as the large and growing contingent liabilities of publicly financed health and pension systems.

- Though cross-country comparisons of health expenditure data are complicated by wide variations across countries, a paucity of reliable national data, and multiple data sources, it is clear that as per capita income levels rise, the public share of total health spending increases, while private and out-of-pocket shares decrease. This trend translates into greater pooling of resources and financial protection. At the lower end of the income spectrum, out-of-pocket spending accounts for the bulk of total health spending.

This chapter assesses the impacts of the demographic and epidemiological transitions, explores the complex relationships between these transitions and disease burdens, and provides estimates of the impact of these transitions on health expenditures. Current patterns of health spending by region and income class are analyzed, and the global discrepancy between health financing needs and current expenditures is discussed.

Demographic dynamics

The size and composition of the world's population have changed dramatically in the past century and will continue to change in the coming decades. The number of people who will be demanding health services is expected to increase as a result of these changes. The size of the productive population that could support health financing schemes will also change, and this has important implications for health financing decisions.

Global population

Population projections can indicate the future development of a population when certain assumptions are made about the future course of fertility, mortality, and migration. They can be helpful in estimating the impact of population change on health systems.

The world's population, which was about 2.5 billion in 1950, reached 6 billion by the end of 1999 and is projected to reach 7.5 billion by 2020 and 9 billion by 2050 (figure 1.1).[2] The world is now adding about 75 million people each year; nearly all world population growth until 2050 is projected to occur in developing countries. In contrast, the population of the developed countries is expected to remain close to its current size. Although projected population growth patterns have different implications for developed and developing countries, most countries will have difficulty generating sufficient revenues to adequately address the health needs of their increasing and aging populations.

Demographic change and health spending

All countries are experiencing varying degrees of demographic change. In general, high-income countries have low fertility and low mortality, and most of the

FIGURE 1.1 Global population growth, 1950–2050

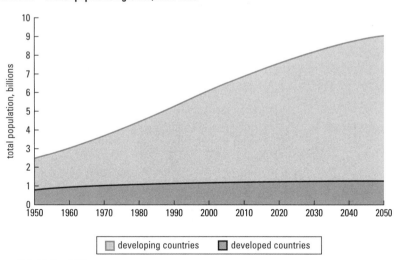

Source: United Nations 2005.

low-income countries are moving from high to low fertility, with significant variations in mortality levels. Projections for the next 50 years generally assume that population growth rates will fall, life expectancies will increase, and fertility rates will decline in all regions. As a result of varying patterns of demographic change, regions around the world will confront health financing challenges of different magnitudes at different times.

The contrasting population age structures for two regions—East Asia and the Pacific and South Asia—illustrate this point (figures 1.2 and 1.3). Overall, the average age of the populations in both the East Asia and the Pacific and the South Asia regions is older in 2025 than in 2005. The population pyramids in the figures indicate that, as fertility rates decline over time, the youngest proportion of the population shrinks, resulting in a more rectangular-shaped age pyramid.

FIGURE 1.2   East Asia and Pacific population pyramids, 2005 and 2025

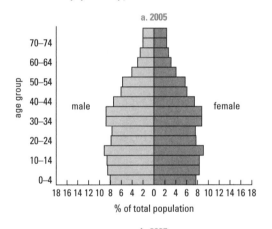

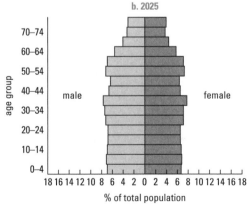

Source: World Bank 2005.

(See figure A1.1 in this chapter's annex for population pyramids for the other World Bank regions.) It is important to remember that changes in the overall size of a population are the aggregate result of changes in the number of persons at different ages.

While developing economies, particularly low-income countries, are still confronting the health financing issues associated with high mortality and high fertility rates, the proportion of aging individuals in all populations will continue to increase as economic, social, and epidemiological advances occur. The future needs of these aging populations must be anticipated, and sustainable health financing schemes must be implemented in the near future to ensure that these populations have their needs met over the long term and that health systems remain functional.

FIGURE 1.3   South Asia population pyramids, 2005 and 2025

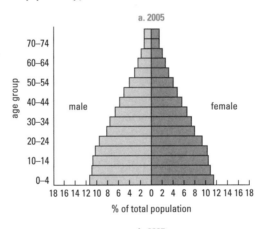

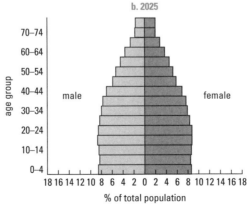

Source: World Bank 2005.

In contrast, developed economies are currently facing the challenges associated with supporting populations that have a large proportion of aging individuals. The costs to the health system posed by this segment of the population can be quite significant, because individuals generate greater health-related costs at the end of life than at any other point in their lifespan. In addition, as fertility rates decline, the proportion of the population that can contribute to health financing schemes that cover the health care costs of the elderly will eventually decrease, resulting in an increasing proportion of the population in retirement relying on a decreasing proportion of the population of working age (for example, an increase in the elderly dependency ratio).

This dynamic poses particular problems for the long term, because fewer resources will be available in social protection systems (such as Social Security) that are designed to provide some financial protection in the future for the segment of the population that is currently middle aged. But in many developing countries it may be counterbalanced by population momentum to some extent, because countries with large proportions of young people will indeed have a sizable proportion of the population entering the working-age ranges for some time to come. That growing workforce, if gainfully employed, is capable of supporting health financing schemes. Lessons learned from high-income countries regarding best practices to support an increasingly aging population structure may prove useful to low- and middle-income countries in the years to come.

For example, the lessons learned by Denmark—a high-income country where the population has a long life expectancy—may prove useful to countries such as Sierra Leone, a low-income country where life expectancy is short. The two countries have dramatically different health financing needs because of the age distribution of deaths in their respective populations (figure 1.4). Most deaths in Denmark's population occur in the "old-old" age group (people age 80 or older). In contrast, most deaths in Sierra Leone's population occur in the under-five age group—indeed, very few deaths occur in the age group that is 80 or older, because few survive to that age. Thus Denmark is faced with the particularly high costs associated with the dying process of the "old-old," whereas Sierra Leone has minimal costs for that group. Furthermore, Denmark's costs are compounded by the capacity of its health system to provide technologically advanced (and expensive) health care services to people in their last years of life. Essentially, health care costs may escalate simply because the Danish health system has the capacity to provide care to the elderly. In contrast, Sierra Leone does not have the health system capacity to provide such care.

The epidemiological transition and health spending

In addition to accommodating changes in population size and structure, countries across the globe are also progressing through an epidemiological transition that has important implications for life expectancy, burden of disease, and (in turn), health financing. The epidemiological transition is the shift in the major causes of

FIGURE 1.4   Age distribution of death in Sierra Leone and Denmark, 2005

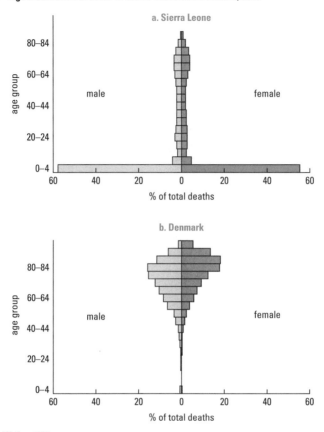

Source: United Nations 2005.

morbidity and mortality—from communicable, maternal, and childhood causes to noncommunicable diseases.

Demographic changes and the epidemiological transition are closely related. As discussed earlier, mortality levels start to decline at the beginning of the demo-graphic transition. This is mainly caused by the reduction in mortality from infectious diseases and maternal and childhood conditions. As the health transition progresses, fertility levels and the burden of communicable diseases decline, and the average age of the population increases. Thus, eventually, there are more elderly people in the population, and they are more susceptible to noncommunicable diseases than younger people. The increase in the number of susceptible individuals at older ages increases the overall incidence and prevalence of noncommunicable diseases, thereby accelerating the epidemiological transition.

Most developing countries are currently confronting a significant challenge because of a continued high burden of communicable diseases. These diseases—particularly malaria, tuberculosis, and HIV/AIDS—pose a serious challenge for public health and health systems in many low-income countries and some middle-income countries. An estimated 80 percent of the deaths due to HIV/AIDS in 2003 occurred in Sub-Saharan Africa, and 90 percent of total deaths due to malaria occurred there as well (WHO 2003; UNAIDS 2003). Furthermore, the incidence of tuberculosis in Sub-Saharan Africa is the highest in the world (WHO 2004).

The staggering burden of disease from these major killers places a heavy burden on already weak and underfinanced health systems in low-income countries. Thirty percent of outpatient clinic visits in Africa are due to malaria-related symptoms, and these symptoms are also major contributors to inpatient deaths (WHO 2003). HIV/AIDS requires testing, counseling, treatment of opportunistic infections, and administration of antiretroviral therapy. Saving lives is of utmost importance and urgency in affected countries, but providing antiretroviral therapy is a long-term and costly undertaking, even if the drugs themselves are funded or subsidized by external sources. As such treatment is rolled out at an increasingly rapid pace, many countries will be faced with the prospect of HIV/AIDS becoming a chronic condition (in addition to a communicable disease), which poses major long-term cost burdens for both the affected individuals and the private or public programs providing support to them.

Tuberculosis is another highly prevalent and expensive disease in low-income countries, even though most of the cost for the treatment is borne by external donors. The most successful method for treating tuberculosis requires an adequate supply of antibiotics as well as intensive participation of health staff to monitor the administration of treatment, which raises both cost and workforce issues. The recent outbreaks of sudden acute respiratory syndrome (SARS), as well as avian influenza in Asia and Europe, are chilling reminders that even the most prescient planning in health systems and health financing may not be enough to counter the global threat of emerging infectious diseases.

The epidemiological transition influences health systems and health financing by affecting population health needs and the type and level of services demanded, and thus the amount and distribution of funds available to pay for them (WHO 2002). As disease burdens shift, health systems need to adapt, expanding or narrowing the scope and scale of services provided and integrating new technologies and approaches as needed.

Figure 1.5 displays the dramatic differences in disease burdens in Sub-Saharan Africa and Europe. Coping with the current burden of communicable diseases, and at the same time laying the groundwork for transforming the health system to deal with the impending noncommunicable disease burden, presents the major

FIGURE 1.5   Global burden of disease, 2002

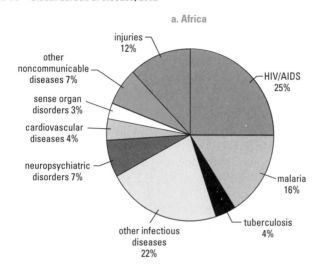

a. Africa

injuries
12%

other
noncommunicable
diseases 7%

sense organ
disorders 3%

cardiovascular
diseases 4%

neuropsychiatric
disorders 7%

other infectious
diseases
22%

tuberculosis
4%

malaria
16%

HIV/AIDS
25%

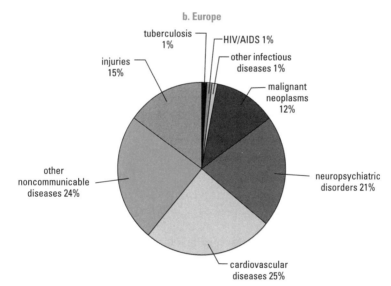

b. Europe

tuberculosis
1%

HIV/AIDS 1%

other infectious
diseases 1%

injuries
15%

malignant
neoplasms
12%

other
noncommunicable
diseases 24%

neuropsychiatric
disorders 21%

cardiovascular
diseases 25%

Source: WHO 2004.

challenge for health policy makers in both African and other developing countries. High-income countries, with both significantly more resources and a more stable but overarching burden posed by noncommunicable diseases, face serious health financing and delivery issues but have far more financial latitude to act.

Implications of demographic and epidemiological transitions for health financing

Although changes in the size and age structure of the population will surely have important consequences for current and future health financing needs, the exact impact is subject to debate. Some researchers have found that health expenditures among an aging population will continue to exert significant pressures on health systems for years to come; others contend that at least in the high-income setting, the aging populations are increasing but healthier, so the effect on health expenditures may not be as serious as anticipated (Olin and Machlin 1999; Fogel 2003; see also chapter 9).

Some low-income countries and many middle-income countries will spend both proportionately and absolutely more on health because of both population increases and higher proportions of the elderly (especially the very elderly). As discussed earlier, the increase in the portion of the elderly population will lead to some increase in overall health expenditures (although the effect will vary by country), given that, on average, health care costs among the elderly are much higher than among other segments of the population (Fogel 2003; Mahal and Berman 2001). As Mahal and Berman point out, "Over time, the share of aggregate health spending accounted for by the elderly can vary depending on their share of the population and whether health spending per person is changing differentially across various age groups" (2001, p. 5). Actuarial estimates using per capita health expenditures in the United States show that a person age 65 to 74 spends, on average, between 3.0 and 4.4 times as much as a person age 35 to 44, and the amount is even higher for someone over 80 (Mays and Lazar 2003; Cutler and Meera 1997; Reinhardt 2000).

Figure 1.6 provides information by region on projected changes in total health spending between 2005 and 2025, as a result of both changes in the numbers of people and changes in the demographic structure of the population—assuming that the base year per capita health spending by age and sex remains unchanged.[3] Alternatively, the figure shows what the spending levels in 2005 would be if each region had its 2025 population structure. For each region, three figures are provided: (1) total effect—changes in total spending as a result of changes in the numbers of people and the age-sex structure, (2) growth effect—changes in total spending due only to changes in the numbers of people, and (3) age-sex structure effect—changes in spending as a result of a person's sex and age bracket.[4]

The figure shows large differences across regions in both the total increases in health spending and the extent to which such increases are the result of changes in population size and age-sex structure. For example, the Middle East and North

FIGURE 1.6   Effects of changes in numbers of people and age-sex structure on health spending by region, 2005–25

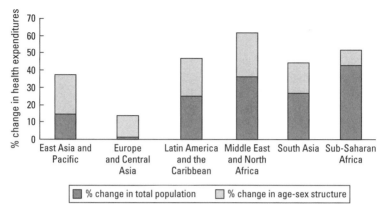

Source: 2000 National Medical Expenditures Survey and HNPStats (Health, Nutrition, and Population database compiled by the World Bank).

Africa, a middle-income region with high population growth rates and relatively long life expectancies, will face a 62 percent increase in health spending over this 20-year period (some 3 percent per year) as a result of population changes alone. Of that total increase, almost three-fifths (37 percentage points) are attributable to increases in population size and the remaining two-fifths (25 percentage points) are due to age-sex structure changes. In contrast, Sub-Saharan Africa, a low-income region characterized by high population growth rates and short life expectancies, will experience a 52 percent increase in health spending, of which 43 percentage points are the result of population growth and only 9 percentage points are the result of age-sex structure changes.

In Europe and Central Asia, a middle-income region with close to zero population growth and long life expectancies, health spending is expected to rise 14 percent overall: 1 percentage point is the result of population growth, and the other 13 percentage points are the result of age-sex structure changes. Latin America and the Caribbean, another middle-income region with moderate population growth and long life expectancies, will experience an overall spending increase of 47 percent, of which 25 percentage points are the result of population growth and 22 percentage points are the result of age-sex structure changes.

East Asia and the Pacific, where population growth is moderate, and South Asia, where it is rapid, also provide interesting contrasts. Life expectancies in East Asia and the Pacific are near the median for developing countries and higher than in South Asia, which, nevertheless, has life expectancies significantly higher than Sub-Saharan Africa. In East Asia and the Pacific, health spending will increase by 37 percent, of which 15 percentage points are the result of population growth and 22 percentage points are the result of changes in the age-sex structure. In South

Asia total spending will increase by 45 percent, of which 27 percentage points are the result of population growth, and 18 percentage points are the result of age-sex structure changes.

Although this analysis is simplistic, it does indicate the orders of magnitude of spending changes that are likely to result as populations grow and age. Excluding Europe and Central Asia, overall increases of 37 percent to 62 percent indicate that governments would need to increase their health spending by two or three percentage points a year just to accommodate demographic changes. These are not insignificant increases, given the relatively low growth rates in GDP expected in several regions highlighted below. They are clearly lower bounds on increases, because they do not take into account critical factors such as the development of new technology, the pace of inflation, or the scope of insurance coverage. Nor do these estimates include the impact of potential new medical crises such as avian flu or the availability of new and expensive drugs to treat malaria. The proportion of the increases due to population increases verses age-sex composition changes also provides policy makers with rudimentary information on changes needed in health delivery systems.

Global distribution of health expenditures

Accurate cross-country comparisons of national health expenditure data are complicated by the fact that many developing countries do not have national health accounts. The following discussion relies on estimates from country-level data compiled by the Organisation for Economic Co-operation and Development (OECD), the World Health Organization (WHO), and the World Bank. Estimates for external resources on health are based on aggregates from the OECD, donor governments, and private foundations.

In analyzing health spending patterns, it is important to distinguish between the sources of health spending and the revenue bases that support these funding sources. National health accounts provide data on sources of health spending, as well as the uses of health spending. Such data give information only on the immediate source of the expenditure, whether from the public sector (e.g., expenditures financed through governmental bodies or social insurance funds), the private sector (e.g., expenditures financed out of pocket and by private insurance), or external sources (e.g., grants or loans from international donors). The mix of these sources has many implications for health systems, particularly in terms of access, equity, efficiency, and financial sustainability.

National health accounts do not provide information on the sources of the government revenues that finance these expenditures (general government tax and nontax revenues, earmarked payroll tax contributions, households, and so on). Revenue source data are critical for understanding the equity of contributions (tax/revenue incidence) and the efficiency and sustainability of the revenue base, whereas the spending information is critical for understanding technical and allocative efficiency, the equity of benefits (benefit incidence), administrative costs, and risk pooling. Expenditure sources and patterns are discussed in this chapter; revenue sources are discussed in chapter 2.

It is clear that low- and middle-income countries bear a disproportionately large share of the global burden of disease compared with high-income countries, yet they spend proportionately very little on health. In 2002 some $3,198 billion (about 10 percent of global GDP) was spent on health care worldwide (World Bank 2005). Yet only about 12 percent of the total was spent in low- and middle-income countries, which account for 84 percent of the global population, 20 percent of global GDP, and 90 percent of the global disease burden (Mathers, Lopez, and Murray 2006). Shares of global GDP and health expenditures are disproportionate by region and income level (figure 1.7).

FIGURE 1.7   Global distribution of GDP and health expenditures in developing countries, 2002

a. Total health expenditures = $351 billion (12% global total)

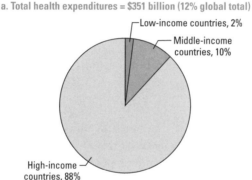

b. Total GDP in developing countries = $6,319 billion (20% global total)

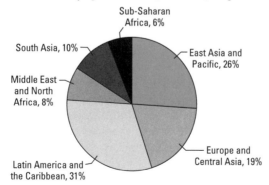

Source: World Bank 2005.

Sources of health spending

Information from several sources about the nature and sources of health spending is essential for developing sound national policies for financing health care. Beyond basic economic indicators such as GDP and GDP per capita, it is helpful to calculate health spending–related measures, including per capita health spending, total health spending as a share of GDP, the public share of total health spending, the percentage of public spending by social security organizations, the private share of total health spending, the percentage of private spending out of pocket, and the share of total health spending through external assistance. For absolute comparisons across countries, amounts should be denominated in U.S. dollars adjusted by standard exchange rates or by purchasing power parities.

Another important element in providing aggregated global and regional information on health spending patterns is the weighting system used to aggregate individual country information to global, regional, and income class levels. Using individual country weights (treating each country the same) provides a measure of the average impact by country. However, weighting by population may also be appropriate, given that some countries have much larger populations than others, and global health policy often focuses on numbers of people in need when calculating external assistance costs. Tables A1.1 and A1.2 in the annex provide health spending information for various components of health expenditure using population and country weights. The following analysis focuses on the population-weighted information. Country-weighted figures are discussed for those components in which there are large differences and in those cases in which country averages may be more meaningful (such as public shares of total health spending and average external assistance by country and region).

High-income countries spent, on average, more than 10 percent of GDP on health in 2002, while middle-income countries and low-income countries spent some 6 percent and 5.3 percent, respectively (annex table A1.1). In exchange rate–based U.S. dollars, per capita total health spending was $26 in South Asia, $32 in Sub-Saharan Africa, $64 in East Asia and the Pacific, $99 in the Middle East and North Africa, $151 in Europe and Central Asia, and $218 in Latin America and the Caribbean. These figures compare with an average per capita health expenditure level in high-income countries of $3,039—an amount more than a hundred times the average spent in all low-income countries ($30). Even after adjusting for differences in costs of living, the differentials are still on the order of 30 times the level in low-income countries (discussed in chapters 6 and 7). The health spending figures in low-income countries fall far short of the amounts needed to provide an essential package of services or to scale up to meet the Millennium Development Goals.

The public share of total health spending provides a measure of how actively governments intervene to ensure the financing of basic public health and personal health services, protect the poor, and facilitate risk pooling through public programs. Public shares increase as countries' incomes increase (annex tables A1.1 and A1.2). Based on population-weighted data, public shares increase from 29 percent in low-income countries to approximately 50 percent in middle-income countries, to 65 percent in high-income countries. The comparable country-weighted figures are 48 percent, approximately 60 percent, and 71 percent, respectively. The key points here are that the bulk of all health spending in low-income countries is private and that, as countries get richer, they cover increasing amounts of health services through the public sector as a result of market failures in private health insurance markets, information asymmetries, and other well-known market failures in the health sector.

Two other important spending trends are apparent from annex tables A1.1 and A1.2. These are the very small share of total health spending derived from social security spending in low-income countries and regions and the importance of out-of-pocket costs in private spending. In Sub-Saharan Africa only 2 percent of all public spending on health (less than 1 percent of total health spending) is made through social insurance institutions, in South Asia it is 8 percent, and for all low-income countries it is 6 percent. Country weighting does not appreciably change this picture. However, for East Asia and the Pacific and middle-income countries, population weighting generally results in significantly higher social security shares.

The importance of out-of-pocket spending in both private and total health spending is a key measure of both the lack of risk pooling (see chapter 2) and the potential inequities in health financing, given poor people's limited ability to pay. Out-of-pocket expenditures are defined as any direct outlay, including gratuities or in-kind contributions, that households make for services and goods from health practitioners, pharmacists, medical supply vendors, and others. Out-of-pocket spending accounts for 93 percent of private spending and more than 60 percent of total health spending in low-income countries (annex table A1.1). In both Sub-Saharan Africa and South Asia, roughly half of all health spending is out of pocket. When countries move up the economic ladder and pursue equity and risk pooling goals increasingly through public financing and the facilitation of private health insurance markets, public shares increase and out-of-pocket shares decrease. In high-income countries, out-of-pocket spending accounts for less than 20 percent of total health spending. Country weighting reduces the out-of-pocket shares somewhat (they account for more than 40 percent of total low-income country health spending), but the story remains the same.

External funds accounted for almost 8 percent (on average) of total health spending in low-income countries in 2002, 18 percent in Sub-Saharan Africa, and 2 percent in South Asia. However, the picture changes appreciably with country weighting, as evidenced by the fact that external assistance accounts for 20 percent of all spending in low-income countries, 19 percent in Sub-Saharan Africa, and 11 percent in South Asia and in East Asia and the Pacific. In 13 Sub-Saharan African countries, external financing accounted for more than 30 percent of overall health spending (Schieber and others forthcoming). External funding is an important and growing source of financing in low-income countries and in Sub-Saharan Africa and South Asia. Given the constraints on domestic resource mobilization in low-income countries, large increases in external assistance are critical for scaling up to reach the Millennium Development Goals (see chapter 2).

There is a clear upward trend between countries' income levels and the levels of public and total health spending as a share of GDP (figure 1.8). However, spending for any given income level varies a great deal, particularly at lower-income levels (Musgrove, Zeramdini, and Carrin 2002). The composition of private health spending also differs across income levels. As incomes increase, both private and out-of-pocket shares of total health spending decrease, and public spending predominates.

Low- and middle-income countries with high levels of out-of-pocket spending have limited opportunities for risk pooling, which hinders allocative efficiency and financial protection efforts.[5] Moreover, low overall spending levels in many low-income countries and some middle-income countries result in limited access to essential services and financial protection, particularly for the poor. As Musgrove (2004) indicates, if GDP is adjusted for basic subsistence needs, poor countries appear to be spending a substantial share of their postsubsistence income on health, reinforcing much of the discussion in the following chapters regarding the need to dedicate additional funds from external financing sources to health.

FIGURE 1.8   Total and public health spending by GDP per capita, 2002

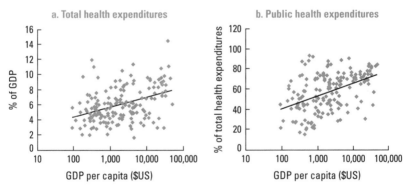

Source: World Bank 2005.

Annex 1.1   Population pyramids and global health expenditures by region and income group

FIGURE A1.1   Population pyramids for World Bank regions

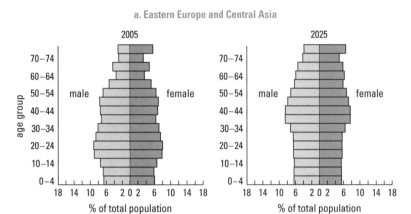

a. Eastern Europe and Central Asia

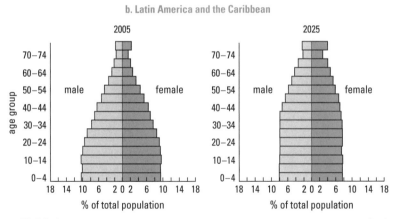

b. Latin America and the Caribbean

Source: World Bank 2005.   *(Continues)*

FIGURE A1.1 Population pyramids for World Bank regions *(Continued)*

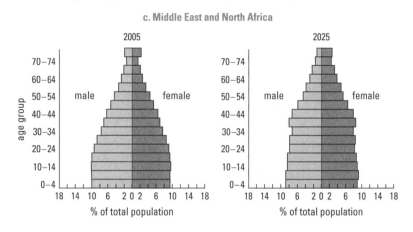

c. Middle East and North Africa

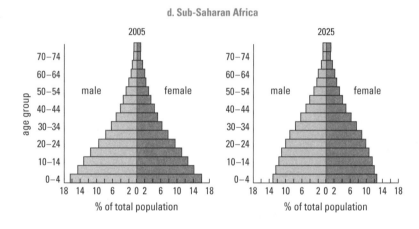

d. Sub-Saharan Africa

TABLE A1.1 Composition of health expenditures in high-, middle-, and low-income countries, population-weighted averages, 2002

	Per capita GDP (current US$)	Per capita GNI (current US$)	Per capita health expenditures (US$)[a]	Per capita health expenditures (international dollar rate)[b]	Total health expenditures (% of GDP)	Public health expenditures (% of total health expenditures)	Social security expenditures (% of total public health expenditures)	Private (% of total health expenditures)	Out-of-pocket (% of private health expenditures)	External (% of total health expenditures)
Regions										
East Asia and the Pacific	1,013.68	999.76	63.66	250.30	5.21	35.29	39.35	64.71	91.86	0.72
Eastern Europe and Central Asia	2,416.54	2,371.17	151.07	459.29	5.93	61.33	41.35	38.67	85.10	1.58
Latin America and the Caribbean	3,284.31	3,182.82	217.85	515.57	7.04	50.27	32.50	49.73	74.28	1.39
Middle East and North Africa	2,153.12	2,105.48	98.92	252.17	4.83	44.92	23.60	55.08	84.77	1.02
South Asia	475.17	471.92	26.04	140.39	5.45	23.66	8.04	76.34	97.08	2.48
Sub-Saharan Africa	487.14	440.72	31.58	119.71	5.32	39.58	1.92	60.42	79.17	17.58
Income levels										
Low-income countries	423.63	408.55	29.52	115.18	5.30	29.14	6.18	70.86	92.84	7.89
Lower-middle-income countries	1,333.33	1,309.93	81.60	304.50	5.60	41.59	35.55	58.41	86.02	0.86
Upper-middle-income countries	5,266.89	5,156.73	309.96	602.33	6.18	56.27	53.43	43.73	82.93	0.43
High-income countries	27,464.45	27,653.55	3,039.30	3,168.54	10.37	65.15	43.95	34.85	55.78	0.03

Sources: World Bank 2005; IMF 2005; WHO 2005.

a. Exchange rate–based U.S. dollars.

b. Purchasing power parity–adjusted U.S. dollars.

TABLE A1.2   Composition of health expenditures in high-, middle-, and low-income countries, country-weighted averages, 2002

	Per capita GDP (current US$)	Per capita GNI (current US$)	Per capita health expenditures (US$)[a]	Per capita health expenditures (international dollar rate)[b]	Total health expenditures (% of GDP)	Public health (% of total health expenditures)	Social security expenditures (% of total public health expenditures)	Private (% of total health expenditures)	Out-of-pocket (% of private health expenditures)	External (% of total health expenditures)
Regions										
East Asia and the Pacific	1,170.04	1,195.70	96.14	198.72	5.86	61.76	8.32	38.24	80.73	11.44
Eastern Europe and Central Asia	2,432.28	2,380.18	152.11	434.02	5.79	61.24	45.06	38.76	94.31	3.42
Latin America and the Caribbean	3,445.66	3,269.69	217.78	431.18	6.62	55.47	26.20	44.53	81.78	3.47
Middle East and North Africa	2,708.87	2,613.70	143.71	290.41	5.29	47.57	15.41	52.43	78.32	2.46
South Asia	767.90	735.86	27.50	95.11	4.81	46.67	8.91	53.32	93.75	11.32
Sub-Saharan Africa	954.93	806.64	47.34	133.07	5.08	51.36	3.17	48.64	79.59	19.44
Income levels										
Low-income countries	452.74	348.29	26.76	82.44	5.18	48.39	4.07	51.61	85.26	19.83
Lower middle-income countries	1,514.00	1,504.44	94.19	282.64	5.89	55.82	21.94	44.18	81.34	4.73
Upper middle-income countries	5,152.12	4,950.51	308.38	578.45	6.10	63.59	34.75	36.41	84.09	1.85
High-income countries	22,794.32	22,918.68	1,921.84	2,258.50	7.94	70.51	36.68	29.48	74.66	0.18

Sources: World Bank 2005; IMF 2005; WHO 2005.

a. Exchange rate–based U.S. dollars.

b. Purchasing power parity–adjusted U.S. dollars.

Endnotes

1. As introduced by Mosley, Bobadilla, and Jamison (1993), the "health transition" encompasses the relationship among demographic, epidemiologic, and health changes that collectively and independently have an impact on the health of a population, the financing of health care, and the development of health systems.

2. According to United Nations medium projections (United Nations 2005) and World Bank projections (World Bank 2005).

3. Because age-sex–specific health spending weights for developing countries are generally not available, U.S. spending weights are used. This may result in overstating the age-sex impact, because the weights reflect the higher levels of technology and resources in the United States, much of it disproportionately focused on the elderly, compared with the levels in developing countries. Nonetheless, much of the health spending in developing countries goes to teaching hospitals in large urban settings and also may disproportionately benefit the rich and elderly.

4. The total effect is calculated by multiplying the number of males and females in each age group by an age-sex–specific spending weight and then dividing the total age-sex weighted spending for 2025 by the total for 2005. The population growth effect is calculated by dividing the projected 2025 total population by the 2005 total population. The age-sex composition effect is calculated as a residual by dividing the total effect by the growth effect. This age-sex effect reflects the changes in the age and sex composition of the population, as well as the interaction of this structural change with changes in the size of the population. Because changes in sex composition are quite small, the results largely reflect age structure changes.

5. For a detailed analysis of country-specific and global health expenditure trends, see Musgrove, Zeramdini, and Carrin (2002).

References

Cutler, D. M., and E. Meera. 1997. *The Medical Costs of the Young and Old: A Forty Year Perspective*. NBER Working Paper 56114. Cambridge, Mass.: National Bureau of Economics Research.

Fogel, R. 2003. "Forecasting the Demand for Health Care in OECD Nations and China." *Contemporary Economic Policy* 21 (1): 1–10.

IMF (International Monetary Fund). 2005. (Statistical Information Management and Analysis (SIMA) Database; accessed July 27.)

Mahal, A., and P. Berman. 2001. "Health Expenditures and the Elderly: A Survey of Issues in Forecasting, Methods Used, and Relevance for Developing Countries." Research Paper 01.23, Harvard Burden of Disease Unit, Cambridge, Mass.

Mathers, C. D., A. D. Lopez, and C. J. L. Murray. Forthcoming. "The Burden of Disease and Mortality by Condition: Data, Methods, and Results for the Year 2001." In A. D. Lopez, C. D. Mathers, M. Ezzati, D. T. Jamison, and C. J. L. Murray, eds., *Global Burden of Disease and Risk Factors*. Washington, D.C.: World Bank; New York: Oxford University Press.

Mays, J., and M. S. Lazar. 2003. "2000 Health Spending Weights Based on United States Medical Expenditure Panel Survey (MEPS)." Unpublished tabulation. Actuarial Research Corporation, Falls Church, Va.

Mosley, W. H., J-L. Bobadilla, and D. T. Jamison. 1993. "The Health Transition: Implications for Health Policy in Developing Countries." In D. T. Jamison, W. H. Mosley, and J-L. Bobadilla, eds., *Disease Control Priorities in Developing Countries*. Washington, D.C.: World Bank; New York: Oxford University Press.

Musgrove, P. 2004. Personal communication with G. Schieber, April.

Musgrove, P., R. Zeramdini, and G. Carrin. 2002. "Basic Patterns in National Health Expenditures." *Bulletin of the World Health Organization* 80 (2): 134–46.

Olin, G. L., and S. R. Machlin. 1999. "Health Care Expenses in the Community Population." Chartbook 11. Agency for Health Care Research and Quality, Rockville, Md.

Reinhardt, U. E. 2000. "Health Care for the Aging Baby Boom: Lessons from Abroad." *Journal of Economic Perspectives* 14 (2): 71–83.

Schieber, G., C. Baeza, D. Kress, and M. Maier. Forthcoming. "Financing Health Systems in the 21st Century." In D. Jamison, J. Berman, A. Meacham, G. Alleyne, M. Claeson, D. Evans, P. Jha, A. Mills, and P. Musgrove, eds., *Disease Control Priorities in Developing Countries*, 2nd ed., Washington, D.C.: World Bank; New York: Oxford University Press.

UNAIDS (The Joint United Nations Programme on HIV/AIDS). 2003. *AIDS Epidemic Update*. Geneva.

United Nations. 2005. *World Population Prospects: 2004 Revision*. New York.

WHO (World Health Organization). 2002. *The World Health Report 2002: Reducing Risks, Saving Lives*. Geneva.

———. 2003. *The Africa Malaria Report 2003*. Geneva.

———. 2004. *Global Tuberculosis Control: Surveillance, Planning, Financing*. Geneva.

———. 2005. *The World Health Report 2005: Making Every Mother and Child Count*. Geneva.

World Bank. 2005. HNPStats. Health, Nutrition and Population database compiled by the World Bank. Washington, DC. http://web.worldbank.org/ WBSITE/EXTERNAL/TOPICS/EXTHEALTHNUTRITIONANDPOPULATION

———. 2005. *World Development Indicators 2005* (CD-ROM). Washington, D.C.

2

Collecting revenue, pooling risk, and purchasing services

Countries need to mobilize sufficient resources to provide essential health services for their populations, reduce inequalities in the ability to pay for those services, and provide financial protection against impoverishment from catastrophic health care costs through explicit policies affecting the three financing functions: collecting revenues, pooling risks, and purchasing goods and services. In managing their health financing functions, countries also need to ensure adequate fiscal space to scale up health spending. Developing countries, particularly low-income countries, face severe challenges in mobilizing sufficient resources to meet even basic service needs. Middle-income countries focus more on providing universal coverage to their populations. Various mechanisms for risk pooling and prepayment are possible for countries at all income levels, but options are heavily constrained by the structure of a country's economy, as well as its financial, institutional, and political capacities.

This chapter contains a discussion of the basic health financing functions of revenue collection, risk pooling, and purchasing. It describes how health financing systems are affected by social, economic, demographic, environmental, external, and political factors.

Developing countries face the following key policy challenges in financing their health systems:

- Raising sufficient and sustainable revenues in an efficient and equitable manner to provide individuals with both essential health services and financial protection against unpredictable catastrophic financial losses caused by illness and injury;
- Managing these revenues in a way that pools health risks equitably and efficiently
- Ensuring the purchase of health services in an allocatively and technically efficient manner;
- Securing the financial sustainability of reforms through the creation of fiscal space by obtaining additional revenues through tax measures or by strengthening tax administration; reducing lower-priority expenditures to make room for

more desirable ones; borrowing resources from domestic or external sources; prudently using their ability to print money (seignorage) to lend it to the government; and receiving grants from outside sources.

Health financing functions: definitions and implications

Health financing involves the basic functions of collecting revenue, pooling resources, and purchasing goods and services (WHO 2000). These functions often involve complex interactions among a range of players in the health sector (figure 2.1). Therefore, policies concerning these functions provide an opportunity to effectuate reforms throughout the health sector.[1]

Revenue collection is the way health systems raise money from households, businesses, and external sources. *Pooling* deals with the accumulation and management of revenues so that members of the pool share collective health risks, thereby protecting individual pool members from large, unpredictable health expenditures. *Prepayment* allows pool members to pay for average expected costs in advance, relieving them of uncertainty and ensuring compensation should a loss occur. Pooling coupled with prepayment enables the establishment of insurance

FIGURE 2.1   Health financing functions

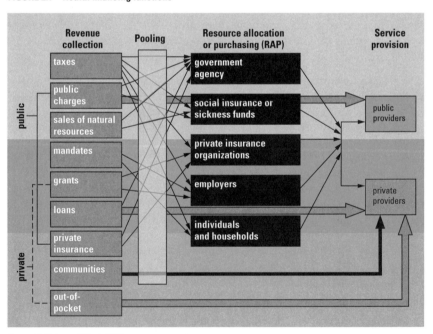

Source: Schieber and Maeda 1997.

and the redistribution of health spending between high- and low-risk individuals (risk subsidies) and high- and low-income individuals (equity subsidies).

By breaking the link between expected health expenditures and ability to pay, prepayment is a critical mechanism for attaining equity objectives. Prepayment in the absence of pooling simply allows for advance purchase or purchase on an installment basis, a useful financial device when dealing with large predictable expenses or expenses that do not correlate with income flows (see the discussion below on medical savings accounts). With neither prepayment nor pooling, the service is simply purchased like any other at the time the consumer demands it, a modality not well suited to many health services on the grounds of equity, predictability, and financial protection. *Purchasing* refers to the mechanisms used to secure services from public and private providers.

How these various functions are arranged has important implications for the way health systems perform, relative to

- Amounts of funds available (currently and in the future) and concomitant levels of essential services and financial protection (the depth and breadth of coverage) for the population;
- Fairness (equity—who bears the tax/revenue burden) with which funds are raised to finance the system;
- Economic efficiency of such revenue-raising efforts in terms of creating distortions or economic losses in the economy (the "excess burden" of taxation);
- Levels of pooling (risk subsidization, insurance) and prepayment (equity subsidization);
- Numbers and types of services purchased and consumed with respect to their effects on health outcomes and costs (the cost-effectiveness and allocative efficiency of services);
- Technical efficiency of service production (the goal being to produce each service at its minimum average cost);
- Financial and physical access to services by the population (including equity in access, benefit incidence).

It is clear from these performance considerations that efficiency and equity are critical aspects of all health financing systems and are relevant for all financing functions. There are important equity considerations regarding financing sources, levels of prepayment and pooling, services provision, provider payment, and physical access to care.[2] There are three broad types of efficiency concerns: efficiency of revenue collection (distortions in the economy that result from various taxes), allocative efficiency (resources being allocated to maximize the welfare of the community by producing the desired health outcomes), and technical efficiency (services being produced at the lowest possible cost).

Complicating this situation are potential equity and efficiency trade-offs (i.e., the least distorting revenue sources may be the least equitable—e.g., a poll tax). Such trade-offs are more problematic in low- and middle-income countries, because, as discussed below, they are far more constrained than high-income countries in their choice of revenue mobilization instruments. The efficiency issues have been dealt with in some detail in various studies (Schieber and Maeda 1997; WHO 2000, 2001; Preker and Langenbrunner 2005), and equity considerations have been receiving increased attention because of the public focus on the Millennium Development Goals and global poverty reduction. Whereas global inequities in need and ability to pay are dealt with in chapter 1 and in the development assistance chapters, the equity aspects of health financing within individual countries are discussed in detail here.

From a broad policy perspective, basic health financing functions are generally embodied in the following three stylized health financing system models:

- *National health service:* compulsory universal coverage, national general revenue financing, and national ownership of health sector inputs;
- *Social insurance:* compulsory universal (or employment group–targeted) coverage under a social security (publicly mandated) system financed by employee and employer contributions to nonprofit insurance funds, with public and private ownership of sector inputs;
- *Private insurance:* employer-based or individual purchase of private health insurance and private ownership of health sector inputs.

Although these stylized models provide a general framework for classifying health systems and financing functions, they are not useful from a detailed policy perspective, because all health systems embody features of the different models. The key health policy issues, as discussed below, are not whether a government uses general revenues versus payroll taxes, but the amounts of revenues raised and the extent to which they are raised in an efficient, equitable, and sustainable manner. Similarly, there is nothing intrinsically good or bad about public versus private ownership and provision. The important issue is whether the systems in place ensure access, equity, and efficiency.

Nevertheless, these models and the various attempts to classify health financing functions in a more detailed manner provide useful information on the linkages with the rest of the health system and macro economy. The models also provide the frameworks for a better understanding of the incentives at play. Bassett (2005) has summarized several of these taxonomies (annex 2.1). Detailed operational assessments of the financing arrangements of national health services and social insurance systems are contained in chapters 3, 7, 8, and 9. The discussions that follow on revenue collection, risk pooling and prepayment, and purchasing elaborate on these basic financing concepts.

Revenue collection and government financing of health services

Governments employ a variety of financial and nonfinancial mechanisms to carry out their functions. Health sector functions entail directly providing services; financing, regulating, and mandating service provision; and providing information (Musgrove 1996).

The key fiscal issues for low- and middle-income countries are for their financing systems, both public and private, to mobilize enough resources to finance basic public and personal health services without resorting to excessive public sector borrowing (and the creation of excessive external debt), to raise revenues equitably and efficiently, and to conform with international standards (Tanzi and Zee 2000). A substantial literature is devoted to the various public and private sources for financing health services and the economic and institutional impacts of using these sources in terms of efficiency, equity, revenue-raising potential, revenue administration, and sustainability (Schieber 1997; Tait 2001; Tanzi and Zee 2000; WHO 2004; World Bank 1993). Efficiency gains are also receiving increased attention as a "revenue" source for financing health services (Hensher 2001). In low-income countries, tax credits are rarely used as a financing source for government spending in health or other sectors (Tanzi and Zee 2000).

From a practical, public finance perspective, all taxes (and indeed, other revenue sources as well) should be judged by the following criteria (IMF and World Bank 2005):

• *Revenue adequacy and stability:* the tax should raise a significant amount of revenue, be relatively stable, and be likely to grow over time.
• *Efficiency:* the tax should minimize economic distortions.
• *Equity:* the tax should treat different income groups fairly.
• *Ease of collection:* the tax should be simple to administer.
• *Political acceptability:* there should be transparency, broad diffusion, and clarity about the uses of the tax to promote acceptability.

Although policy makers must be aware of the potential trade-offs among these criteria, they must also be aware of the underlying institutional and macroeconomic constraints that preclude many less-developed countries from using the most efficient and equitable revenue raising instruments (box 2.1).

Institutional constraints tend to preclude low- and middle-income countries from using the most efficient and equitable revenue-raising instruments. The high level of inequality in most low- and middle-income countries also means that governments face the difficult situation of needing to tax politically powerful and wealthy elites to raise significant revenues in an equitable manner, but being

BOX 2.1 *Institutional realities affecting taxation in low- and middle-income countries*

- Much of the population is widely dispersed in rural areas.
- The bulk of the population is self-employed in small-scale subsistence agriculture and receives income in kind.
- Transactions are difficult to trace.
- High rates of illiteracy, poor accounting standards, and lack of records on expenses limit the use of personal income or profits taxes.
- In urban areas there is a large informal sector of small and transient firms.
- Large firms tend to be government enterprises or extractive industries that are frequently foreign owned.
- Both agricultural products and mineral resources face unstable and unpredictable world prices.
- Dualism (a modern urban sector and a traditional rural sector) and the resulting market segmentation create distortions in terms of both commodity and labor markets, which increase tax burdens.
- There is a greater level of income inequality, which may result in higher tax rates, greater tax avoidance, and higher efficiency losses.
- Trade distortions abound in the form of import tariffs, quotas, export taxes, differential exchange rates, and foreign exchange rationing, resulting in misallocations of resources and inequity.
- The greater importance of state-owned enterprises coupled with nonoptimal user charge structures often results in inefficient public versus private investment decisions.
- Tax administration capacity is quite limited.

Source: Schieber and Maeda 1997, p. 20.

unable to do so easily. As Tanzi and Zee point out, "Tax policy is often the art of the possible rather than the pursuit of the optimal" (2000, p. 4).

Although revenue-raising ability varies by country, in general low-income countries face many more constraints because of their low levels of income, limited overall resources, large informal sectors, and poorly developed administrative structures (box 2.2). However, in general, as a country's income increases, so too does government revenue. Estimates from the IMF (table 2.1) show that in the early 2000s, central governments in low-income countries collected 18 percent of their GDP as revenues, on average, while lower-middle-income countries collected 21 percent, and upper-middle-income countries collected 27 percent. At the top of the income spectrum, high-income countries were collecting 32 percent of GDP as revenues. It is important to keep in mind that, although tax revenues form the bulk of government revenues in all regions and income class groups, other types of government revenues, such as sales of natural resources, are also important revenue sources in certain countries and regions (for example, the Middle East and North Africa).

Available information suggests that most countries actually collect a fairly small portion of their overall and tax revenues as social contributions.[3] Because in principle social insurance schemes are primarily funded through social contributions, their viability and self-sufficiency are highly linked to whether there is

BOX 2.2 *Domestic spending and resource mobilization issues for low-income countries*

Given the calls from the international community for increased investments in health, low-income countries have themselves proposed targets for domestic spending. In the 2001 Abuja Declaration on HIV/AIDS, Tuberculosis, and Other Related Infectious Diseases, African leaders pledged to increase health spending to 15 percent of their government budgets (UNECA 2001; Haines and Cassels 2004). However, obtaining sufficient public revenues to meet such budgetary targets raises difficult political, economic, and equity considerations (Schieber and Maeda 1997; Gupta and others 2004). As shown in table 2.1, the ability of a low-income country to raise enough revenue to meet population health needs and demands is generally quite limited.

Both the Commission on Macroeconomics and Health and the UN Millennium Project suggest that low-income countries might be able to mobilize an additional 1–4 percent of GDP in revenue domestically. However, revenue performance over the past few decades, as Gupta and others point out, has been fairly disappointing, even stagnant in some regions (Gupta and others 2004). In addition, given that revenue-raising ability is closely linked to future economic growth, low-income countries in particular will face difficult challenges unless they can outpace the modest income growth projections forecast in several developing regions.

Source: Authors.

TABLE 2.1   Average central government revenues, early 2000s

	Total revenue as % of GDP	Tax revenue as % of GDP	Social security taxes as % of GDP
Region			
Americas	20.0	16.3	2.3
Sub-Saharan Africa	19.7	15.9	0.3
Eastern Europe and Central Asia	26.7	23.4	8.1
Middle East and North Africa	26.2	17.1	0.8
East Asia and the Pacific	16.6	13.2	0.5
Small Islands (population < 1 million)	32.0	24.5	2.8
Income level			
Low-income countries	17.7	14.5	0.7
Lower-middle-income countries	21.4	16.3	1.4
Upper-middle-income countries	26.9	21.9	4.3
High-income countries	31.9	26.5	7.2

Source: Gupta and others 2004.

adequate capacity in place to both collect revenues and cover current and future benefit liabilities. As seen in table 2.1, even in high-income settings where one would expect social contributions to be significant, this may not be the case when social security taxes reach just over 7 percent of GDP. In the low-income setting, social security contributions make up only 0.7 percent of GDP, but they reach 1.4 percent in lower-middle-income countries and just over 4 percent in upper-middle-income countries.

Even in countries where social insurance schemes exist, the contributions are often relatively low, which helps shed light on why social insurance schemes are often subsidized by general revenue. Thus even though many countries aspire to develop social insurance schemes, they need to consider many factors, including the fact that social contributions alone may not be enough to ensure long-term financial sustainability. Whether there is a greater willingness on the part of individuals to be taxed for payroll contributions, as there is an "earned right" to an earmarked insurance benefit as opposed to general taxes, is a largely hypothetical question worthy of further analysis.

Another important difference between low- and middle-income countries and high-income countries is the greater relative reliance on direct taxes (taxes on income and property, such as personal and corporate income taxes, capital gains, inheritances, death, wealth) by high-income countries. Low- and middle-income countries tend to rely more on indirect taxes, such as consumption taxes both on sales (general sales, value added, and excise taxes) and on factors of production (payroll, land, real estate) (Schieber and Maeda 1997). Developing countries choose the indirect option because of the economic and institutional constraints they face, particularly large rural and informal sectors and weak tax administration (figure 2.2).

FIGURE 2.2   Share of direct and indirect taxes in total revenues in low-, middle-, and high-income countries

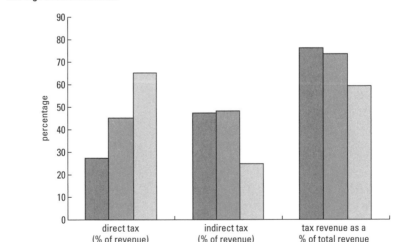

Source: IMF 2004b.

Unfortunately, empirical evidence is quite sparse on the equity and efficiency of government revenue structures in low- and middle-income settings. Thus there is only a limited basis for understanding the effects of excess burdens of taxation, the economic incidence of tax systems, and their implications for equity.

Empirical studies, largely from developed countries, show the importance of not only the type of tax used but also specific features of the tax, including the rates, ceiling, floors, and exemptions (Wagstaff and others 1999; Wagstaff and van Doorslaer 2001). Such features have rather important implications for the revenue-raising potential as well as the equity of the tax system. In a study of the redistributive effects of health care financing arrangements in 12 OECD countries, Wagstaff and others (1999) find that the direct taxes used to finance health care are progressive (that is, the burden of taxes is concentrated on the better off) in all countries.[4] The EQUITAP studies (O'Donnell and others 2005a, 2005b) confirm this result in a survey of 13 Asian territories that span high-, middle-, and low-income countries. The study found that in low- and middle-income countries only the richest households qualify to pay personal income tax and taxes on capital. There is also a great deal of tax evasion in the large informal economy, which tends to increase the progressivity of direct taxes to the extent that the informal sector is skewed toward the lower end of the income distribution. Despite such progressivity, the overall redistribution effect is generally very modest, because of the small share of direct taxes as a financing source for health care (O'Donnell and others 2005a, 2005b).

Indirect taxes, such as sales, value added taxes (VAT), excises, and import taxes, were found to have a more mixed redistributional impact, depending on the specifications of the tax base, rates, exemptions, and exclusions. For example, the study by Wagstaff and others (1999) of certain high-income countries finds that indirect taxes are regressive (the burden of the taxes is concentrated on low-income groups) in all countries in the sample. This is consistent with the notion that indirect taxes are mostly taxes on consumption, and because low-income groups spend more of their income on consumption than high-income groups, their tax payments are also proportionally higher. For the 13 Asian territories, however, O'Donnell and others (2005a, 2005b) find that indirect taxes are slightly progressive, but to a much lesser extent than direct taxes.

The difference in the distributional impact of indirect taxes in high-income countries and in low- and middle-income countries is partly because the tax base is more comprehensive in richer countries than in poorer ones. For example, a sales tax or VAT is often collected only from businesses that meet a minimum turnover threshold. To the extent that the poor buy from businesses that do not meet this criterion (such as market stalls), they are essentially exempt from this tax, which helps to alleviate the regressive character of sales taxes or VATs (Martinez-Vazquez 2004). A similar effect is achieved if goods that are relatively important in the household budget of the poor (such as food products) are exempt from the tax.

The distributional impact of excise taxes depends strongly on the consumption patterns by income group. For example, one study in Madagascar found that car and petrol taxes were strongly progressive, alcohol taxes appear quite progressive in most cases, and even tobacco taxes were reasonably progressive (Gemmell and Morrissey 2005). However, tobacco taxes in other country settings have been found to be regressive, because the poor spend larger shares of their more limited household incomes on tobacco than the rich. However, because the price elasticities of the poor tend to be higher than the nonpoor, an increase in tobacco taxes will result in a larger reduction in their consumption, and hence will be progressive in terms of the reduced tax burden (Jha and Chaloupka 2000; Cnossen 2005).

Thus in low- and middle-income countries, increasing revenue through taxation to finance increased health expenditure does not necessarily result in significant equity implications, if carried out primarily through well-designed indirect taxes, because these taxes can be structured to be generally progressive. Moreover, because both value-added and excise taxes are often associated with a more efficient collection of tax revenue—reflecting their broader base, lower price elasticities, and negative consumption externalities—relying primarily on indirect taxes as revenue sources may be more efficient than using other forms of taxation (Coady, Grosh, and Hoddinot 2004). Such results, however, are heavily country-specific and depend on the exact details concerning the tax base, tax rates, exclusions, exemptions, demand elasticities, and tax administration capabilities. All of these factors are essential determinants of the tax yield, equity, efficiency, and ease of administration.

Risk pooling, financial protection, and equality

The rationales for public intervention in financing health systems are well-known. The issues of public goods, merit goods, externalities, insurance market failures, interdependencies between demand and supply, and consumer ignorance have been well documented (Musgrove 1996). Health financing goals—which include reducing inequality, preventing individuals from falling into poverty as the result of catastrophic medical expenses, and protecting and improving the health status of individuals and populations by ensuring financial access to essential public and personal health services—also provide a strong "public goods" basis for public intervention. Public intervention may be needed because of market failures in private financing and provision (such as information asymmetries) or because of instabilities in insurance markets (such as favorable risk selection by insurers and moral hazard). Indeed, this has been the case with virtually all countries in the OECD, except the United States. In the vast majority of OECD countries, governments have decided to publicly finance or to require private financing (as in Switzerland) for the bulk of health services. Nevertheless, given both low income levels and limits on domestic resource mobilization possibilities in low-income countries and some middle-income countries, these countries face severe challenges in publicly financing essential public and personal health services. They are also often confronted with difficult trade-offs with respect to financing these basic essential services and providing financial protection against catastrophic illness costs.

Ensuring financial protection means that no household contributes or expends so much on health that it falls into and cannot overcome poverty (ILO/STEP 2002). Achieving adequate levels of financial protection and promoting equity in a health financing system require maximizing prepayment for "insurable" health risks (risks associated with large and unpredictable expenses)[5]; achieving the largest possible pooling of health risks within a population, thereby facilitating redistributions among high- and low-risk individuals; ensuring equity in the system through prepayment mechanisms that redistribute costs from low- to high-income individuals; and developing purchasing arrangements that promote efficient and equitable delivery of quality services.

Ensuring financial protection and promoting equity requires a specific government policy focus that ensures contributions are based on ability to pay, prevents individuals from falling into poverty as a result of catastrophic medical expenses, and ensures equitable financial and physical access to services. Health policy makers, advisers, and researchers state that minimizing inequality is an objective of health policy, but government commitment to this goal is often lacking. Thus a special focus on the relationship among different elements of health financing (resource mobilization, pooling, and allocation) and health sector inequalities related to outcomes, outputs, and inputs is clearly warranted, because there are equity implications inherent in all three of the financing functions listed.

One can cluster assessments of inequality in the health sector around three general measures: outcomes, outputs, and inputs. Inequality analyses then can focus on the differential impact of a policy (on collection, pooling, and purchasing) on health outcomes (mortality and morbidity); health outputs (physical services use, financial burden, and expenditure benefits); and more directly on inputs such as direct financial, human, and physical resources. Outcome measures include child and infant mortality, maternal mortality, adult mortality, child stunting, micronutritional deficiencies, and life expectancy by age group, as well as measures that combine mortality and morbidity, such as the concepts of disability-adjusted life years and disability-adjusted life expectancy.

Outputs include service use, financial burden arising from the collection function (tax/revenue incidence), and benefits arising from the pooling and purchasing functions (benefits incidence). A fairly large and growing body of research has focused on the extent to which groups in society differentially use services financed by the public sector. The World Bank recently completed an analysis of more than 50 Demographic and Health Surveys with respect to inequality in both health sector outcomes and outputs (Gwatkin and others 2000). The analysis shows large gaps in both health outcomes and the use of health services between the poorest citizens in a country and their richer counterparts.

Measuring the overall financial benefits and burdens of households and families in accessing health services is somewhat more complex than measuring service use. The simplest element of such policy assessments looks at the direct and indirect out-of-pocket payments for health services and how they apply to different socioeconomic groups. Direct payments include user fees for publicly provided services, payments for drugs and supplies, payments for laboratory services, and insurance premiums and copayments. Indirect out-of-pocket payments include costs of transportation to and from clinics or hospitals and forgone income from taking off from work to seek care.

Unfortunately, there are few studies showing the tax/revenue or benefit incidence (the financial value of the benefits by socioeconomic group) of most health financing systems. A comprehensive evaluation of the equity aspects of a health financing system would look at the tax/revenue incidence, the benefit incidence, and the net incidence (the difference between the financial contributions and the financial benefits). Unfortunately, because of the lack of information on benefit and tax incidence, it is usually difficult to do such an analysis.

One of the critical issues in inequality analyses is the way that different groups in society are identified and grouped. Any measure of socioeconomic status can be used to measure inequality in health outcomes and service use. Income, gender, educational status, occupational categories, residence, ethnicity, tribal affiliation, and social strata affiliation all can and have been used to look at inequalities in the health sector. Most of these measures, but not all, have been used as proxies for the economic status of different groups in the absence of other direct measures of economic well-being. Where detailed household surveys do exist, more direct measures are used, including consumption, expenditures, and more recently, ownership of personal assets and access to societal or community assets.

Some potential equity impacts of health financing policies:

- Different resource-generating mechanisms (user fees with or without retention at the facility level, private health insurance, payroll tax, general tax financing) can have direct impacts on health outcomes by promoting or deterring the use of life-saving preventive or simple curative services for economically vulnerable groups. Different mechanisms can also affect the prevalence of poverty (or change the depth of poverty) by increasing or decreasing the numbers of people falling into poverty because of spending on health needs. Different revenue generation mechanisms have differential incidence impacts by income group.

- The nature of pooling mechanisms can also directly affect health outcomes by influencing who uses lifesaving services. These mechanisms (coupled with prepayment) also determine the differential financial risks faced by low-income groups. Both risk and equity subsidization have important effects on inequality.

- How resources are allocated (geographically, by level, and programmatically) reflects the emphasis policy makers assign to inequalities and the role of the health sector in reducing poverty and achieving equity goals.

A large-scale assessment of the impact of health financing policies in resource generation, pooling, and allocation, especially for developing countries, is seriously lacking and should be a priority for the international community. Box 2.3 provides some guidance on the types of information needed for designing and implementing schemes that favor the poor.

Thus, providing financial protection and promoting equality depend on how health systems arrange the three key health financing functions of revenue collection, risk pooling, and purchasing. Although all health financing functions play an important role in ensuring financial protection and reducing inequality, risk pooling and prepayment (whether through taxes or individual premiums) play the central and often least understood roles.

B O X 2 . 3 *Designing and implementing financing schemes that benefit the poor*

To address the equity concern in health financing strategies, it is useful to ask the following questions during the design of health financing policies.

Are resource-generating options likely to

- increase or decrease the financial access of low-income groups?
- create incentives or disincentives for the poor in seeking care?
- increase or decrease the financial burden on the poor?
- increase the extent or depth of poverty?
- provide a cross-subsidy from the rich to the poor or vice versa?
- improve or reduce the quality of services?

Are risk pooling mechanisms likely to

- increase the number and share of the poor who are covered under pooling arrangements?
- decrease the risk of catastrophic payments for the poor?
- increase access to preventive and simple curative care through pooling?

Are purchasing and resource allocation mechanisms likely to

- increase the number of facilities in areas where the poor live?

- increase mobile facilities that serve the poor?
- take into account population size in different areas?
- take into account health needs (especially of the poor)?
- take into account poverty levels in different regions?
- prioritize programs that serve the poor?
- prioritize programs that address demand generation for the poor?
- prioritize levels of care that serve the poor?
- include innovative demand-side approaches such as conditional cash transfers or vouchers?
- purchase services from providers that serve the poor?
- condition purchasing on incentives for providers to serve the poor?

Source: Yazbeck 2005.

Risk pooling and prepayment

Risk pooling refers to the collection and management of financial resources so that large, unpredictable individual financial risks become predictable and are distributed among all members of the pool. The pooling of financial risks is the core of traditional insurance mechanisms. Whereas pooling ensures predictability and the potential for redistribution across individual health risk categories, prepayment provides various options for financing these risks equitably and efficiently across high- and low-income pool members. Public and private risk pooling arrangements observed today—social health insurance, national health service arrangements, and private insurance—are the result of cultural, economic, and historical decisions about how to organize risk pooling and prepayment, as well as implicit and explicit decisions about income redistribution and social solidarity. Each embodies different means for the creation of risk pools and the financing of such pools through prepaid contributions.[6]

In most low- and middle-income countries, multiple public and limited private arrangements coexist, making system fragmentation the norm rather than the exception. This increases administrative costs, creates potential equity and risk selection problems (for example, when the wealthy are all in one pool), and limits pool sizes. Moreover, health care risks change over an individual's or household's life cycle, but because generally little correlation exists between life-cycle needs and capacity to pay, subsidies are often necessary and are facilitated by risk pooling.

Figure 2.3 represents the evolution of the average cost of financing a given package of health services during the lifetime of an average individual, his or her capacity to pay, and his or her need for subsidies.[7] The dotted line shows the relationship between actual average costs and age. The solid line represents the relationship between the capacity of an individual to pay for the services and the individual's age. To the right of point A, the individual or household would need a subsidy to be able to finance and gain access to the services required without incurring an excess expenditure. It is possible that households or individuals with higher incomes never reach this point. It is also possible that lower-income households or individuals may need a subsidy from the beginning of their lives to access health care services at the levels and in the conditions specified by society as minimally acceptable. In this situation, the individual or household will require subsidization. Risk pooling plays a central role in facilitating such cross-subsidization. Because of economies of scale, risk pooling potentially reduces the average cost of the package, delaying reaching A. In contrast, the absence of a system for spreading risks results in high and unexpected out-of-pocket expenditures for the individual who needs health care services.

Risk pooling and prepayment functions are central to the creation of cross-subsidies between high-risk and low-risk individuals (risk subsidy), as well as between rich and poor (equity subsidy). The larger the pool, the greater the

FIGURE 2.3 Cost of health services, capacity to pay, and need for subsidies over the lifetime of a typical individual

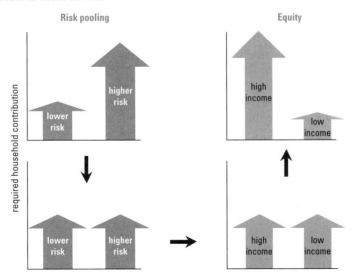

Source: ILO/STEP 2002.

potential for spreading risks and the greater the accuracy in predicting average and total pool costs. Placing all participants in a single pool and requiring contributions according to capacity to pay rather than individual or average pool risk can facilitate cross-subsidization and, depending on the level of pooled resources, can significantly increase financial protection for all pool members (figure 2.4).

FIGURE 2.4 Models of cross-subsidization for pooling risk and increasing equity of household contributions for health services

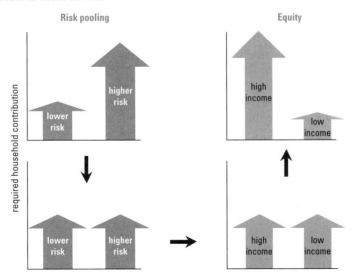

Source: ILO/STEP 2002.

However, spreading risks through insurance schemes is not enough to ensure financial protection, because it can result in low-risk, low-income individuals subsidizing high-income, high-risk members. Furthermore, significant portions of the population may not be able to afford insurance. For this reason, most health care systems are intended not only to spread risk, but also to ensure equity in the financing of health care services through subsidies from high- to low-income individuals. Equity subsidies are the result of such redistribution policies.

There are at least four alternative organizational arrangements for risk pooling and prepayment: ministries of health or national health services, social security organizations, voluntary private health insurance, and community-based health insurance. Each is linked to distinctive instruments for revenue collection (general revenues, payroll taxes, risk-rated premiums, and voluntary contributions) and for purchase of health services. Within these organizational structures, three alternatives often coexist for generating revenues and financing equity subsidies: subsidies within a risk pool, subsidies across different risk pools, and direct public subsidies through transfers from the government. Although medical savings accounts (with or without public subsidization) are also sometimes referred to as a risk pooling mechanism, they do not pool risks across individuals and therefore are far more limited in their scope for predictability and equity subsidization. They are simply intertemporal mechanisms for smoothing health risks over an individual's or household's life cycle.

Subsidies within a risk pool, whether financed through general revenues or through payroll taxes, are prerequisites for pooling risks in traditional national health services and social security systems. The goal of collecting revenues through an income-related or general revenue-based contribution (in contrast to a risk-related contribution, as is generally the case with private insurance) is to generate subsidies from high- to low-income individuals. These systems are effective when payroll contributions are feasible or the general revenue base is sufficient, and a large proportion of the population participates in the same risk pool. However, in a system with multiple competing public or private insurers and a fragmented risk pool, payroll contributions may increase incentives for risk selection. In the case of a national health service or social security system, financial resources might be insufficient or inappropriate for spreading the financial risks or for creating an equity subsidy, particularly if the general revenue or payroll contribution base is regressive.

Subsidies across different risk pools involve the creation of funds, often called solidarity or equalization funds, financed by a portion of contributions to each risk pool. This mechanism is found in systems with multiple insurers—for example, in Argentina, Colombia, Germany, and the Netherlands. A key element of this mechanism's success is the implementation of adequate systems of compensation among different risk and income groups.

Finally, in many OECD countries, direct public transfers funded by general taxation are made to insurers for subsidizing health care for certain groups or for the entire population. Such transfers are also used in some low- and middle-income countries, although at a limited level because of low capacity to collect revenue.

In most low- and middle-income countries, risk pool fragmentation significantly impedes effective risk pooling, while limited revenue-raising capacity precludes the use of broad public subsidies as the main source of finance. Therefore, targeting scarce public subsidies across different risk pooling schemes is probably the most feasible way to finance equity subsidies for the poor and those outside formal pooling arrangements.

However, this method has important transaction costs. Because a significant portion of the population is excluded from the formal sector, the method's use to ensure universal financial protection is limited, particularly in low-income countries. Even if significant subsidies are available from general taxation, the lack of insurance portability restricts the method's effectiveness as a subsidization mechanism among risk pools, because individuals may lose their coverage when they change jobs. Low-income countries and certain middle-income countries will be challenged both to publicly finance essential public and personal health services and to ensure financial protection through equity subsidies. Thus low- and middle-income countries must strive to achieve the best value for publicly financed health services in terms of health outcomes and equity and facilitate effective risk pooling for privately financed services. Providing public financing for cost-effective interventions is one critical aspect of determining which services to finance publicly.

Purchasing

Purchasing, which is sometimes referred to as financing of the supply side, includes the numerous arrangements used by purchasers of health care services to pay medical care providers. A large variety of arrangements exists. Some national health services and social security organizations provide services in publicly owned facilities where staff members are public employees. Sometimes individuals or organizations purchase services through either direct payments or contracting arrangements from public and private providers. Other arrangements combine these approaches.

The framework for resource allocation and purchasing highlighted in table 2.2 provides a taxonomy of the numerous issues surrounding purchasing decisions. Resource allocation and purchasing procedures have important implications for cost, access, quality, and consumer satisfaction. Efficiency gains (both technical and allocative) from purchasing arrangements provide better value for the money and therefore provide a means of obtaining additional "financing" for the health system (Hensher 2001). Although a full discussion of this issue is beyond the scope of this chapter, we note that concomitant reforms in this area have been important in the

TABLE 2.2 Framework for analyzing the policy options for voluntary health insurance

	Key policy options
Policy framework	**Revenue collection mechanisms**
	• Level of prepayment compared with direct out-of-pocket spending
	• Extent to which contributions are compulsory compared with voluntary
	• Degree of progressivity of contributions
	• Subsidies for the poor and buffer against external shocks
	Pooling revenues and sharing risks
	• Size
	• Number
	• Redistribution from rich to poor, healthy to sick, and gainfully employed to inactive
	Resource allocation and purchasing (RAP) arrangement
	• For whom to buy (demand question 1)
	• What to buy, in which form, and what to exclude (supply question 2)
	• From whom to buy—public, private, NGO (supply question 1)
	• How to pay—what payment mechanisms to use (incentive question 2)
	• What price to pay—competitive market price, set prices, subsidized (market question 1)
Institutional environment	• Legal framework
	• Regulatory instruments
	• Administrative procedures
	• Customs and practices
Organizational structures	• Organizational forms (configuration, scale, and scope of insurance funds)
	• Incentive regime (extent of decision rights, market exposure, financial responsibility, accountability, and coverage of social functions)
	• Linkages (extent of horizontal and vertical integration or fragmentation)
Management attributes	• Management levels (stewardship, governance, line management, clinical management)
	• Management skills
	• Management incentives
	• Management tools (financial, resources, health information, behavior)

Source: Preker and Langenbrunner 2005.

financing reforms in many middle-income countries, most high-income countries, and some low-income countries. Preker and Langenbrunner (2005) also document a number of these efforts. Central to these reforms have been the separation of purchasing from provision, money following patients as opposed to historical provider budgets, and the use of incentive-based payment systems. Many of these incentive-based payment systems rely on capitation and managed care, case-based payments to hospitals, and related mechanisms to ensure a more equitable sharing of financial risk between the purchaser and provider.

This issue has taken on increased importance because donors want to be assured that new funding to scale up services in low-income countries is being used efficiently. No one wants to pour money into inefficient health systems. Moreover, the efficiency of a system has important financial implications for long-term fiscal sustainability and for governments to find the "fiscal space" in highly constrained budget settings for large increases in public spending. Indeed, health financing policies (collection, pooling, and purchasing) must be developed in the context of a government's available fiscal space.

Health financing policies and fiscal space to increase health spending

GDP growth is a necessary condition for facilitating domestic resource mobilization, but it is only one of several macroeconomic elements that provide the fiscal space for countries to undertake meritorious investments. In its broadest sense, fiscal space can be defined as the availability of budgetary room that allows a government to provide resources for a desired purpose without any prejudice to the sustainability of a government's financial position (Heller 2005). The issue of fiscal space is at the center of the current debate concerning the purported negative impact of IMF programs that preclude countries from using the increasing amounts of grant funding available for health sector investments and recurrent health expenditures (such as hiring additional health workers). In principle, there are several ways in which a government can create such fiscal space (Heller 2005):

- Additional revenues can be raised through tax measures or strengthened tax administration.
- Lower-priority expenditures can be cut to make room for more desirable ones.
- Resources can be borrowed from either domestic or external sources.
- Governments can use their power of seignorage (that is, having the central bank print money and lend it to the government).
- Governments may also be able to create fiscal space from the receipt of grants from outside sources.

Note that this definition of fiscal space implies that fiscal sustainability—the capacity of a government, at least in the future, to finance its desired expenditure programs as well as service any debt obligations—is a necessary but not sufficient condition for the existence of fiscal space. This suggests that exploitation of fiscal space requires a judgment that the higher expenditure in the short term and any associated future expenditures can be financed from current and future revenues. If financed by debt, the expenditure should be assessed according to its impact on the underlying growth rate or its impact on a country's capacity to generate the revenue needed to service that debt.

The IMF has emphasized its flexibility in allowing for absorption of additional external grant inflows for spending on meritorious programs (IMF 2004a). Yet its guidelines raise three caveats regarding fiscal space and increasing expenditures. First, analysis must take into consideration that higher levels of spending in a sector, even if financed from external grant flows, may have a ripple effect on spending in other sectors that may not have grant financing; this is a concern regarding wages for health workers. Second, increases in expenditures today may need to be limited even if grants are available for financing today, because funds may not be available to cover the implied increased expenditures in the future, when grant financing dries up. Third, changes in accounting rules cannot, by themselves, create additional scope for expenditure on the provision of basic social services or infrastructure.

Certainly, appropriate fiscal analysis at the country level must take into consideration any spillover effects that expenditure decisions in one sector may have on other sectors. The same is true for decisions with effects that carry over several years. Countries must ensure that decisions that are made today and that have expenditure implications in the future also have, under reasonable assumptions, financing mechanisms in the future. This is especially important in health, where commitments regarding coverage of certain health needs may carry expenditure commitments over the next few years as a result of the projected aging of the population and changes in morbidity. This cross-temporal implication of health expenditures must be taken into consideration especially when downsizing expenditures will be politically difficult. This is, for instance, the case for antiretroviral treatment of AIDS patients: donor assistance may be readily available today but is not guaranteed to finance the cohort of AIDS patients for the duration of their lives, and in many low-income countries, the total public sector health budget may not be sufficient to finance such treatments.

It is relevant in this context to note that changes in accounting rules do not produce fiscal space. Recently, there has been a lot of discussion regarding the accounting of grants in IMF programs. Donors have interpreted sector expenditure ceilings resulting from IMF programs as "inflexibility in IMF programs." The fact is that IMF accounting practices measure overall fiscal deficits both with and without grants. Where grants are included, they are accounted for as part of the revenue stream. As mentioned earlier, fiscal space can be generated only by finding additional financing (through taxes, grants, or loans), by reallocating expenditures, or by improving the efficiency of current expenditures. Thus all policies implementing the basic health financing functions must be considered in the context of fiscal space. Although revenue collection activities are very directly related to fiscal space, so are pooling and purchasing policies.

Annex 2.1   Classifications of health financing systems

In the *World Health Report 2000*, the WHO categorizes health systems as having four principle "functions" (stewardship, resource creation, service delivery, and financing) and three principle objectives (health, fair financial contribution, and responsiveness to people's nonmedical expectations). This categorization and the relationships among the seven elements are shown diagrammatically in annex figure A2.1. Financing is a principal system function that comprises collecting, pooling, and purchasing.

The determinants of health financing are indeed a complex amalgam of institutional, demographic, socioeconomic, environmental, external, and political factors. Mossialos and others (2002) have summarized these factors (annex figure A2.2). Demographic profiles, social values, environmental factors, and economic activity are import determinants of both mandated and voluntary health financing, but political structures and external pressures are also particularly important determinants of the nature, scale, and effectiveness of mandated health financing. Political structures will also play some role in determining the nature and effectiveness of voluntary health insurance because such insurance is dependent on government regulation.

Kutzin (2001), Mossialos and Thomson (2002), and Arhin-Tenkorang (2001) have developed more specific frameworks for analyzing health financing and health insurance. Kutzin's framework analyzes policy options in terms of the extent to which the function of health insurance is enhanced. He defines this

FIGURE A2.1   **Relations among functions and objectives of a health system**

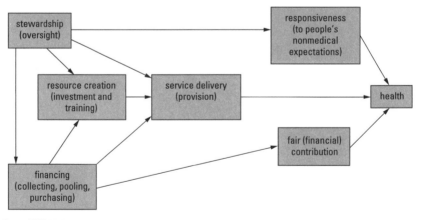

Source: WHO 2000.

FIGURE A2.2 Determinants of health financing

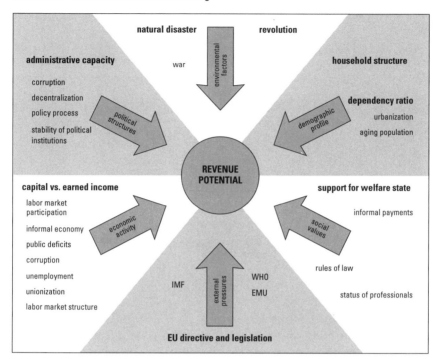

Source: Mossialos and others 2002.

function of health insurance as "access to care with financial risk protection" and attempts to develop a generic framework, unfettered by attachment to any particular organizational form of health insurance, to conceptualize the disaggregated components of health financing sources, resource allocation mechanisms, and associated organizational and institutional arrangements (annex figure A2.3). This framework, which is equally applicable to public and private financing approaches, clarifies the important conceptual distinctions among initial funding sources, contribution mechanisms, collecting organizations, pooling organizations, allocation mechanisms, and purchasing organizations, and it categorizes options under each function (Kutzin 2001).

It is important to note that the collection, pooling, and purchasing functions can be undertaken by different organizations or by one or more organizations in different combinations. For this reason, Kutzin specifically calls for an analysis of how functions are integrated within or separated across organizations (that is, the

FIGURE A2.3 Kutzin's framework of health financing functions

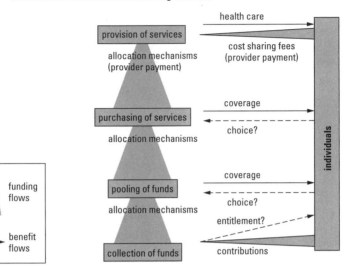

Source: Kutzin 2001.

extent of vertical and horizontal integration). He also highlights the interdependence of regulation and information as key policy tools to enhance the insurance function, and he asserts that it is in the interests of the system for regulatory and informational activities to be implemented for the population as a whole. Kutzin's analysis also highlights the importance of active purchasing, indicating that it is not desirable to simply minimize administrative costs. Administrative costs resulting from effective utilization, management, and provider payment policies can result in substantial reductions in inappropriate benefit payments.

Mossialos and Thomson (2002) have graphically represented Kutzin's main options regarding funding sources, contribution mechanisms, and collecting organizations (annex figure A2.4). Employers might be added to the diagram as an additional collection (and pooling) organization.

Arhin-Tenkorang (2001) has developed a framework based on the evolution of financial protection from community-based insurance through established insurance pools and through insurance pool coordination to universal insurance coverage. This evolution of stages is linked to certain national and donor policies (annex figure A2.5). This alternative framework provides a detailed picture of conceptual issues, basic design issues, and the critical interactions embodied in a health insurance system.

FIGURE A2.4   Funding sources, contribution mechanisms, and collection agents

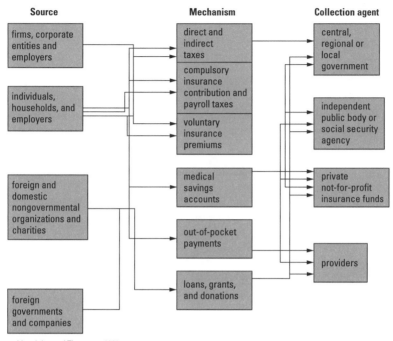

Source: Mossialos and Thompson 2002.

FIGURE A2.5   Stages of financial protection and supporting policies

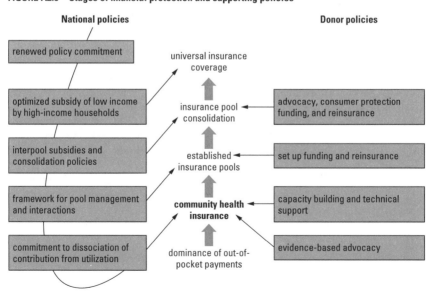

Source: Arhin-Tenkorang 2001.

Endnotes

1. Roberts and others (2004, p. 238) identify five key "control knobs" for health reform: financing, payment, organization, regulation, and persuasion.

2. The concept of equity used in this chapter refers to redistribution and fairness. In our treatment of equity, we also assess inequalities in access, use, and outcomes. The *World Development Report 2006* (World Bank 2005) uses a very broad concept of equity, which is defined in terms of equal opportunity and avoidance of absolute deprivation and which attempts to capture the multidimensional nature of inequality of opportunity.

3. The IMF defines social contribution as "a payment to a social insurance scheme by the insured persons or by other parties on their behalf in order to secure entitlement to the social benefits of the scheme. The contributions may be compulsory or voluntary. A general government unit can pay social contributions on behalf of its employees (an expense) or receive social contributions as the operator of a social insurance scheme (either revenue or the incurrence of a liability)" (2002, p. 20).

4. In some countries, though, the degree of progressivity is lowered by reliance on local income taxes, which are often close to proportional.

5. One function of "insurance" systems is as a prepayment mechanism against large unexpected medical expenses. Although, in theory, prepayment for predictable expenses offers no risk pooling benefits in an insurance sense and can undermine a health insurance system if they are a significant part of covered benefits, individuals in most countries appear to prefer prepayment even for routine services. Although inclusion of prepayments for predictable expenses in the insurance benefit package can perhaps be justified on redistribution grounds, the trade-offs in terms of undermining the insurance function must be considered. Insurance also creates moral hazard, whereby individuals tend to overconsume services for which they do not pay the actual costs at the point of consumption. The richer the benefit package and the more services included on a prepaid basis, the greater the potential for moral hazard in both public and private insurance systems.

6. Although all insurance mechanisms (because of the law of large numbers) provide for better predictability of expenses related to large unpredictable individual risks, private insurers relate individuals' premiums to this average risk and create separate risk categories to avoid the phenomenon of adverse selection (in which the enrollment of sicker-than-average individuals can destabilize premiums). By separating individual contributions from this average cost, public insurance mechanisms (both national health service and social security) can promote much more effective redistribution across high- and low-income individuals, depending on the progressiveness of the payroll contribution and general revenue base of the country. Nonetheless, private health insurance has the advantages of not relying on coercive taxes that distort the economy and providing greater flexibility in choice of insurance than the usual "one size fits all" public system.

7. Capacity to pay is defined as the level of contribution that would keep an individual from being pulled below the poverty line. As the risk of requiring services increases with time, it may reach a level equal to the capacity to pay.

References

Arhin-Tenkorang, D. 2001. "Health Insurance for the Informal Sector in Africa: Design Features, Risk Protection and Resource Mobilization." CMH Working Paper Series WG3:1, Commission on Macroeconomics and Health, Geneva.

Bassett, M. 2005. "Frameworks for Analyzing Health Systems, Health Financing, and the Regulation of Health Insurance." Background paper for Conference on Private Health Insurance in Developing Countries, Wharton Business School, University of Pennsylvania, Philadelphia, March 15–16.

Cnossen, S., ed. 2005. *Theory and Practice of Excise Taxation: Smoking, Drinking, Gambling, Polluting, and Driving.* New York: Oxford University Press.

Coady, D., M. Grosh, and J. Hoddinot. 2004. "Targeting of Transfers in Developing Countries: Review of Lessons and Experience." World Bank, Washington, D.C.

Gemmel, N., and O. Morrissey. 2005. "Distribution and Poverty Impacts of Tax Structure Reform in Developing Countries: How Little We Know." *Development Policy Review* 23 (2): 131–44.

Gupta, S., B. Clements, A. Pivovarsky, and E. Tiongson. 2004. "Foreign Aid and Revenue Response: Does the Composition of Aid Matter?" In S. Gupta, B. Clements, and G. Inchauste, eds., *Helping Countries Develop: The Role of Fiscal Policy.* Washington, D.C.: International Monetary Fund.

Gwatkin, T. D., S. Rutstein, K. Johnson, R. Pande, and A. Wagstaff. 2000. *Socioeconomic Differences in Health, Nutrition, and Population.* Washington, D.C.: World Bank.

Haines, A., and A. Cassels. 2004. "Can the Millennium Development Goals Be Attained?" *British Medical Journal* 329: 394–7.

Heller, P. 2005. "Understanding Fiscal Space." International Monetary Fund, Washington, D.C.

Hensher, M. 2001. "Financing Health Systems through Efficiency Gains." World Health Organization, Geneva.

ILO/STEP (International Labour Organization/Strategies and Tools against Social Exclusion and Poverty). 2002. "Towards Decent Work: Social Protection for Health for All Workers and Their Families." Geneva.

IMF (International Monetary Fund). 2002. "Social Contribution [GFS]." *Government Finance Statistics Manual 2001, Companion Material, Glossary.* Washington, D.C.

———. 2004a. "External Grants and IMF Policies." Washington, D.C.

———. 2004b. "Statistical Information Management and Analysis Database." Washington, D.C.

IMF (International Monetary Fund) and World Bank. 2005. *Financing the Development Agenda.* Washington, D.C.

Jha, P., and F. Chaloupka, eds. 2000. *Tobacco Control in Developing Countries.* New York: Oxford University Press.

Kutzin, J. 2001. "A Descriptive Framework for Country-Level Analysis of Health Care Financing Arrangements." *Health Policy* 56 (3): 171–204.

Martinez-Vasquez, J. 2004. "The Impact of Fiscal Policy on the Poor: Fiscal Incidence Analysis." Andrew Young School of Policy Studies, ISP Working Paper 01-10, International Studies Program, Georgia State University, Atlanta.

Mossialos, E., A. Dixon, J. Figueras, and J. Kutzin, eds. 2002. *Funding Healthcare: Options for Europe.* 4. European Observatory on Health Systems and Policies. Berkshire, U.K.: Open University Press.

Mossialos, E., and S. Thomson. 2002. "Voluntary Health Insurance in the European Union: A Critical Assessment." *International Journal of Health Services* 32 (1): 19–88.

Musgrove, P. 1996. "Public and Private Roles in Health: Theory and Financing Patterns." Discussion Paper 339, World Bank, Washington, D.C.

O'Donnell, O., E. van Doorslaer, R. Rannan-Eliya, A. Somanathan, S. Adhikari, B. Akkazieva, and others. 2005a. "Who Pays for Health Care in Asia?" EQUITAP Working Paper 1, Erasmus University, Rotterdam and Institute for Policy Studies, Colombo.

O'Donnell, O., E. van Doorslaer, R. Rannan-Eliya, A. Somanathan, S. Adhikari, D. Harbianto, and others. 2005b. "Who Benefits from Public Spending on Health Care in Asia?" EQUITAP Working Paper 3, Erasmus University, Rotterdam and Institute for Policy Studies, Colombo, Sri Lanka.

Preker, A. S., and J. Langenbrunner. 2005. "Spending Wisely: Buying Health Services for the Poor." World Bank, Washington, D.C.

Roberts, M. J., W. Hsiao, P. Berman, and M. Reich. 2004. *Getting Health Reform Right: A Guide to Improving Performance and Equity.* New York: Oxford University Press.

Schieber, G. 1997. *Innovations and Health Care Financing.* Discussion Paper 365, World Bank, Washington, D.C.

Schieber, G., and A. Maeda. 1997. "A Curmudgeon's Guide to Financing Health in Developing Countries." In G. Schieber, ed., "Innovations in Health Care Financing." Discussion Paper 365, World Bank, Washington, D.C.

Tait, A. 2001. "Mobilization of Domestic Resources for Health through Taxation: A Summary Survey." Background Paper 14 for Working Group Three of the Commission on Macroeconomics and Health, World Health Organization, Geneva.

Tanzi, V., and H. H. Zee. 2000. "Tax Policy for Emerging Markets: Developing Countries." IMF Working Paper, International Monetary Fund, Washington, D.C.

UNECA (United Nations Economic Commission for Africa). 2001. *Abuja Declaration on HIV/AIDS, Tuberculosis, and Other Related Infectious Diseases.* Addis Ababa.

Wagstaff, A., and E. van Doorslaer. 2001. "What Makes the Personal Income Tax Progressive? A Comparative Analysis for Fifteen OECD Countries." *International Tax and Public Finance* 8 (3): 299–315.

Wagstaff, A., E. van Doorslaer, H. van der Burg, S. Calonge, T. Christiansen, G. Citoni, and others. 1999. "Redistributive Effect, Progressivity, and Differential Tax Treatment: Personal Income Taxes in Twelve OECD Countries." *Journal of Public Economics* 72 (1): 73–98.

WHO (World Health Organization). 2000. *World Health Report 2000: Health Systems—Improving Performance.* Geneva.

———. 2001. *Report of the Commission on Macroeconomics and Health: Investing in Health for Economic Development.* Geneva.

———. 2004. *Poverty Reduction Strategy Papers: Their Significance for Health—Second Synthesis Report.* Geneva.

World Bank. 1993. *World Development Report 1993: Investing in Health.* New York: Oxford University Press.

———. 2005. *World Development Report 2006: Equity and Development.* New York: Oxford University Press.

Yazbeck, A. 2005. Personal communication. April 9.

3

Risk pooling mechanisms

Four types of health insurance are widely used to pool risks, foster prepayment, raise revenues, and purchase services: state-based systems funded by the government and operated through ministries of health or national health services, social health insurance, community-based health insurance, and voluntary health insurance. The four approaches differ in important aspects that can affect their performance in countries with different income levels, employment structures, health needs, and administrative capacities. This chapter defines each approach, evaluates its strengths and weaknesses, and assesses its relevance and feasibility for low- and middle-income countries. None of these approaches is found to be inherently good or bad. Rather, the policy maker's challenge is to create viable "pathways" for the development of health insurance in a country—pathways that steadily improve financial protection through risk pooling and prepayment, increase the quality and effectiveness of health services, improve outcome indicators and equity, and do so in an affordable, equitable, and sustainable manner.

In considering the four prominent risk pooling systems used in connection with the provision of health insurance, policy makers worldwide need to be pragmatic to ensure that the development of health financing is well aligned with broader, country-specific economic, institutional, and cultural development. Therefore, both a general understanding of financing mechanisms and more specific methods for evaluating them at the country level are important. This chapter examines each of the four types of risk pooling mechanisms in detail and describes frameworks for the government regulation of voluntary health insurance systems. The principal conclusions about the appropriateness of each risk pooling system for developing countries are summarized here and discussed in detail in later sections:

- *State-funded systems.* The advantages of state-funded health care systems explain why they are the most widespread form of health financing. They provide universal access to coverage, can rely on many different financing resources, and can be relatively simple to manage. However, since they must compete annually for a share of the state budget, they may receive insufficient and unstable resources. In many countries, the publicly financed health delivery system has been found to be inefficient, like many other publicly managed services. Furthermore, state-funded systems tend to benefit the rich more than the poor, particularly in developing countries. Therefore, to successfully implement a state-funded system in low- and middle-income countries, conditions must be established to raise sufficient resources for health (through sustained economic growth, a competent tax administration, and a consensus within the population in favor of taxation). Sound institutions must also be in place to make the system work. In addition, specific efforts must be made to target the poor while preserving the universal character of the system—in other words, to avoid making it "a poor system for poor people" (Mossialos and Dixon 2002).

- *Social health insurance.* Social health insurance can be an effective way to raise additional resources for health and to reach universal coverage. In particular, by making the financing of health care more transparent and stable, social health insurance may encourage the population to contribute more to the health coverage system. But these objectives can be reached at different speeds, depending on the political and socioeconomic characteristics of each country. For many low-income countries, particularly those with stagnant economies and ever growing proportions of workers in the informal sector, these objectives may be unrealistic in the foreseeable future. Therefore, before implementing a social health insurance scheme, a government should examine its suitability for the country's socioeconomic and political conditions and assess potential problems to determine whether they can be overcome or reduced to the degree needed to ensure that the advantages of social health insurance outweigh its potential drawbacks. This preparatory work may lead to the conclusion that it is appropriate to proceed with the reform, but it can also lead to a decision to postpone reform until the necessary preconditions are satisfied. Experience also shows that, in its initial stage of development, social health insurance has a tendency to divert resources from the poorer segment of the population to the richer segment. Consequently, countries considering establishment of a social health insurance system should be aware of this side effect and include mechanisms to protect the poor within their system framework. Finally, social health insurance can induce cost escalation, as observed in many countries of the OECD. Therefore, governments wishing to implement social health insurance schemes must design appropriate mechanisms to contain costs.
- *Community-based health insurance.* These schemes provide financial protection for people who otherwise would have no access to health coverage, and they can result in some degree of resource mobilization. Nonetheless, because most community-based systems are small and often barely financially viable, they are not particularly effective in reaching the poorest segments of the population. Community-based health insurance can be established in settings with informal labor markets and limited institutional capacity, but a strong sense of local community solidarity is a prerequisite. The intervention of governments—

through subsidies, technical assistance, and initiatives to link community-based health insurance schemes with more formal health financing—is important to improve the efficiency and sustainability of such schemes. What emerges from the literature on community-based health insurance is that it is "better than nothing" in low-income settings where the implementation of any kind of collective financing scheme is problematic. But community-based health insurance is not likely to be the solution to all health care financing problems in low-income countries and should be regarded more "as a complement to—not a substitute for—strong government involvement in health care financing" (Preker and others 2004, p. 41). The most challenging and promising issues include how to design community-based health insurance schemes to ensure the best possible compatibility with larger systems and how to make these small schemes evolve toward more comprehensive and sophisticated health financing systems.

- *Voluntary health insurance.* Voluntary systems require a certain level of commercial institutional capacity and can benefit from (but not necessarily depend on) a similar level of public sector institutional capacity. Unlike social health insurance (which is harder to develop, widen, or sustain when national social solidarity is low, government institutional capacity is weak, and labor markets are informal), voluntary systems do not rely as much on local or national social solidarity and stable formal labor markets, although those conditions certainly help. However, such systems, unless subsidized by the government, can benefit only those citizens or businesses with the ability to pay. Moreover, these systems may be prone to certain types of market failures in addition to equity challenges (Tapay and Colombo 2004). They must therefore be developed cautiously and with an appropriate regulatory framework.

State-funded health care systems

State-funded systems are suitable for most countries that have the administrative and economic capacity to raise taxes, establish an efficient network of providers, and the capacity to target the poor. State-funded health care systems constitute the most widespread health financing mechanism around the world. General government revenues represent the main source of health care expenditures in 106 of 191 countries belonging to the WHO (Savedoff 2004b). In high-income countries, two-thirds of public health expenditures are funded by general revenues; in middle-income countries, almost three-quarters; and in low-income countries, virtually all public health expenditures come from general revenue (WHO 2004; see chapter 2, table 2.1).

Most health specialists claim that these systems originate from the Beveridge report published in 1942, and they are often called "Beveridgean systems" (Beveridge 1942). Indeed, although that report actually recommended funding health care through defined contributions—not general taxation[1]—the National Health

Service Act of 1946, largely inspired by Beveridge's work, established the provision of tax-funded services in Britain, free of charge, for the prevention, diagnosis, and treatment of disease. The British national health system thus emerged as the model for government-funded health systems, even though similar arrangements already had existed in the Soviet Union (1918) and New Zealand (1938).

In theory, a national health service system is a universal pooling arrangement under which the entire population has access to publicly provided services financed through general revenues. In practice, except for some OECD countries, national health service systems usually coexist with one or more of the other risk pooling arrangements. In most low- and middle-income countries, ministries of health act as national health services for substantial segments of the population, while other mechanisms, such as community-based health insurance (in low-income countries) and social health insurance provide coverage for other segments of the population. Such fragmentation tends to increase administrative costs and limits the efficiency and equity of the risk pooling arrangements. However, for clarity, this section concentrates on the main characteristics of the "pure" form of general revenue–funded systems. It defines national health service systems (box 3.1), examines their main strengths and weaknesses, and assesses the key factors necessary to ensure their development and effectiveness in developing countries.

Economic impact, equity, and simplicity of financing modalities depend on actual revenue sources used by the government. In theory, pure national health services perform well because they pool the risks of the entire population and are financed through the government budget, which "prepays" the costs of care. But it is very difficult to give a general opinion on the equity, efficiency, and sustainability of these general revenue–based systems because financing depends on the mix of general and specific taxes, other public revenue sources, and the types of external assistance received. As discussed in chapter 2, although broadly based general taxes (such as income and sales) in theory perform better in terms of revenue raising, efficiency, and equity than earmarked taxes or out-of-pocket payments, the specific institutional characteristics of developing country economies generally preclude the most effective use of such broad-based revenue sources.

Strengths of state-funded health care systems

The main strengths of state-funded health care systems are a direct consequence of their organizational principles.

Comprehensive coverage of the population. Given their noncontributory nature, national health service systems are easy to extend to all citizens, including workers in the informal sector. The comprehensiveness of coverage prevents risk selection problems and makes state-funded systems theoretically the most equitable form of health financing. Inclusion of all citizens in one pool makes the systems

---

BOX 3.1 *What is a national health service system?*

National health service systems are characterized by three main features: their funding comes primarily from general revenues, they provide medical coverage to the whole population, and they usually deliver health care through a network of public providers.

Financing from general revenues
Most of the time, national health service systems receive budget allocations from the national government. Therefore, the origin of their resources is the same as the budget in general. Resources include mainly general (as opposed to earmarked) taxes, other public revenues from sales of natural resources, sales of government assets, and public tolls (for instance, tolls for use of the Suez Canal) but also include borrowing and grant assistance. In many countries, however, central government revenues are complemented by earmarked taxes or funds from local authorities. In England, for instance, for fiscal 2005, it is estimated that 74 percent of the resources of the National Health Service will come from general taxation and 20 percent from "national insurance contributions" (earmarked taxes); the rest will come from miscellaneous sources (U.K. Department of Health 2005).

Universal coverage
In principle, tax-financed systems cover every citizen, regardless of individual health status, occupation, or income. In other words, in national health service systems, health care coverage is considered an attribute of citizenship.

Public health delivery system
Even though there is no automatic connection between the source of financing of health services and the way they are delivered, many general revenue–funded systems rely mainly on public providers. In these countries, the ministry of health heads a large network of public providers organized as a national health service. Facilities are owned by the government, and health personnel are public employees. However, some countries reimburse or contract with private providers. Although an examination of the advantages and disadvantages of public provision is outside the scope of this analysis (see World Bank 2004), the key issue is not the type or ownership of providers, but rather how to ensure that whatever approach is used results in efficient and equitable purchasing arrangements that promote allocative and technical efficiency and guarantee access to covered persons.

Source: Authors.

---

potentially very effective in managing risk because of "the law of large numbers." This law increases their financial viability compared with fragmented systems.

Large scope for raising resources. Contrary to social health insurance systems, which are financed mainly by payroll contributions, national health service systems can rely on a very broad revenue base of tax and nontax sources. Consequently, the financial burden may be spread over a larger share of the population. Unlike many social health insurance systems, in which the burden is concentrated on formal sector workers, who may represent a small part of the population (especially in low- and middle-income countries), national health systems may resort to value-added taxes, sales taxes, or imports taxes, which affect the whole population (Savedoff 2004b). In fact, state-funded systems are much more often developed in those low- and middle-income countries where the informal sector represents a significant share of the population.

A simple mode of governance and a potential for administrative efficiency and cost control. Most national health service systems are integrated systems in which responsibilities are clearly organized in a hierarchical way. This organization makes governance much simpler than in less coordinated arrangements involving multiple players. There is a hierarchical chain of command and control that goes directly from the head of state or the parliament to the ministry of health and to local authorities in some cases. Where public providers are used, there is a direct line of authority between the providers and the overseeing financing authority. The simplicity of governance provides the opportunity to organize the health care system more efficiently and with lower transaction costs. For this reason, in many developing countries, state-funded systems allowed the implementation of successful public health programs. However, in certain countries where the central government shares its responsibilities with local authorities, the decision schemes are not very clear and coordination problems arise. With the recent emphasis on decentralization reforms in many countries that have national health service systems (discussed in chapter 6), this situation is developing. Ultimately, state-funded systems are also very exposed to political pressure, which limits their capacity to make purely rational decisions (discussed below).

As single pool organizations, state-funded systems can also benefit from economies of scale, which makes them potentially more efficient than fragmented systems. Furthermore, despite a large diversity of cases, national health systems seem to control health expenditures more effectively than other arrangements. This control may stem from the fact that they "combine in one authority both the incentive and the capacity to contain costs to a greater extent than is possible with any of the other financing mechanisms" (Evans 2002, p. 45). Of course, this is true only if cost control is a priority for the government. The extent of this advantage depends on the structure of health service provision. Certain inefficiencies may accompany this approach, such as a bloated provider structure and limited managerial authority or capacity on the part of the ministry of health. In the 1970s, many tax-financed health systems in OECD countries were among the most costly. But since 1990, control of health expenditures has become one of the main issues for high-income countries and, for the most part, the only systems that have been able to reduce the share of GDP spent on health care were those financed through general revenues (Evans 2002). These issues are discussed further in chapter 9.

Weaknesses of state-funded health care systems

Unstable funding. Since national health service systems are financed from the general budget, the amount of funding available depends on the outcome of annual budget discussions and is vulnerable to changes in political priorities or external shocks (such as military conflict that requires additional defense spending).

Ministries of health have to compete with other sectors for the same resources, which is not the case when health care is financed through earmarked taxes or contributions. Although this process theoretically might allow the population to express financing priorities, it explains why complaints of underfunding and poor quality are common in tax-based systems, particularly in contrast with social or private health insurance, where the major health system debates often focus on containing costs (Savedoff 2004b). This problem is even more acute in low-income countries where the tax base is very small. On the basis of an analysis of national health accounts data, the Commission on Macroeconomics and Health found that the portion of total general government expenditures devoted to health was almost always less than 10 percent in developing countries (WHO 2002). The amount allocated to the health sector also reflects the traditionally weaker institutional power of the ministry of health within the government, particularly in relation to the ministry of finance (Mossialos and Dixon 2002).

Disproportionate benefits for the rich. National health service systems are supposed to provide free health care to the whole population. They seek to ensure equal access to health care for all citizens irrespective of their income. But the reality is somewhat different. In many low- and middle-income countries, health services tend to be used mainly by urban high- and middle-income households. Benefit incidence analyses in seven African countries that rely mainly on state-financed medical care showed this pattern clearly (Castro-Leal and others 1999). In all these countries, the poorest 20 percent receives a significantly smaller amount of public subsidy than the richest 20 percent. With the exception of one country where the rich use private care, the share allocated to the richest 20 percent is far more than 20 percent (between 24 and 48 percent), while the share received by the poorest 20 percent is systematically lower than 20 percent (between 4 and 17 percent).

Several factors explain this phenomenon. First, the poor tend to use fewer health services when they are ill than the rich, mainly because they face problems of access (health services are often far away from where they live) and high opportunity costs for the working time they lose (Castro-Leal and others 1999). In some cases, user charges imposed by the government to complement public resources also limit their access to health care. Second, there is a disproportionate use of costly hospital services by the rich, while the poor use mainly less costly local primary care facilities (WHO 2000). Third, country studies show that local health services often do not satisfy the population (for reasons such as unreliable staff and unavailable drugs). Thus, the people living in remote areas without access to urban hospitals have to pay more accessible, but uncovered, practitioners with their own resources (WHO 2002). Finally, health professionals serving those with public coverage sometimes charge their patients illicit fees ("informal charges"), which automatically exclude the poor (box 3.2), or use publicly funded facilities to

---

BOX 3.2   *Informal payments to health care providers in Azerbaijan*

Earning only 28 percent of the average salary in the country, Azerbaijani health care providers often try to find complementary resources. Direct payments by patients represented 57 percent of total health expenditures in 2001. Some of these payments are formal user charges introduced in 1998 for listed services in government-funded health facilities. But they also include a significant amount of informal fees, including charges for drugs and medical supplies, fees for visiting patients, direct unofficial payments to doctors and other health care staff for services provided, and fees for positions obtained in medical institutions.

The 2003 World Bank Poverty Assessment estimated that unofficial charges for childbirth vary from $100 to $150 in smaller towns to $300 to $700 in Baku hospitals, up to 14 times the average monthly salary (World Bank 2005). Altogether, informal fees are estimated to constitute 20 percent of all health expenditures, creating important problems of access to health care for the poor. Yet they are seen more as a means to complement insufficient government funding than as a form of corruption.

Source: Holley, Akhundov, and Nolte 2004.

---

provide care to private patients. This pattern is facilitated by the inability of many governments to control the activity of public hospitals (WHO 2000).

Potential inefficiency in health care delivery. In countries with a long history of national health service systems, there have been recurrent criticisms about the systems' lack of efficiency. These criticisms are reinforced by the fact that in many countries users cannot access alternative providers. The main criticisms concern aging infrastructure, unresponsive staff, inability to downsize or reorient priorities, abuse of monopoly power, obsolete medical technology compared with the private sector, and waiting lists for nonemergency treatments. Notably, however, many of these criticisms focus on provision rather than on financing.

In the past two decades, many reforms have focused on improving the efficiency of the system mainly through decentralization and the introduction of internal markets (which includes purchasing/provider splits; provider payment reform; and diverse forms of hospital autonomy, including privatization) (Enthoven 1985). This phenomenon also reflects a general decline of the role of the state all over the world through "the transformation from centrally planned to market-oriented economies, reduced state intervention in national economies, fewer government controls, and more decentralization" (WHO 2000, p. xiv).

Perhaps the most ambitious and symbolic reform might be the one initiated in Britain in March 2000 with the publication of the "NHS Plan." Aimed at improving the efficiency of the system and increasing devolution while raising resources allocated to the National Health Survey (NHS) system, this plan is still being implemented. However, there have been significant restrictions to the full implementation and functioning of such reforms in many countries (for example, Ukraine and Portugal). This is often because it can be difficult for public providers to adjust their organization in the absence of major reforms to public sector management, particularly personnel management (for example, the challenge posed by rigid civil services statutes). More generally, it is linked to the difficulty of reforming long-standing organizations.

Sensitivity to political pressure. Tax-financed health systems are highly exposed to political pressure. Because the government is directly responsible for the system, it cannot ignore pressures from the public, unions representing health care professionals, or local officials defending the interests of their constituencies. This situation may lead to irrational and inefficient decisions and prevent needed reforms, such as hospital closures or mergers and staff reductions, from being implemented.

Feasibility of state-funded health care systems in developing countries

Revenue-raising capacity. The ability of a country to raise revenues primarily depends on its economic situation, which affects its potential to levy taxes and thereby generate revenue (see chapter 2). This is why revenue-raising capacity is directly correlated with income, even though there are important regional variations. In particular, as shown in chapter 2, countries with important oil or gas revenues (such as those in the Middle East and North Africa region) or with centralized revenue-raising systems created under socialism have higher ratios of revenue to GDP. In contrast, countries in East Asia and the Pacific or Latin America and the Caribbean have low ratios, which may be caused by ineffective tax administration or preferences for individual rather than government responsibility (Schieber and Maeda 1997).

As discussed in chapter 2, while low-income countries might be able to mobilize an additional 1–4 percent of GDP in revenue domestically, revenue performance over the past few decades has been fairly disappointing—even stagnant in some regions. Given that future economic growth projections are also modest, low-income countries in particular will face difficult challenges in mobilizing additional government revenues. Therefore, raising additional resources for health through domestic resource mobilization efforts constitutes a real challenge for developing countries: they have to improve their tax administration while improving growth and building consensus in favor of the acceptability of taxation within the population, particularly the elite.

Quality of governance and institutions. The crucial importance of strong tax administration has already been emphasized. The quality of a country's institutions also plays a key role in determining the effectiveness of health spending, as shown in chapters 5 and 6. Research has shown that additional government spending on health has little significant impact on the key health indicators for the Millennium Development Goals in countries with poor governance (as measured by the World Bank's mechanism for evaluating a country's institutions—the Country Policy and Institutional Assessment) (Wagstaff and Claeson 2004). Therefore, it is crucial for low- and middle-income countries to be able to rely on solid and competent institutions to ensure the quality of state-funded health systems.

Ability to target the poor while maintaining the universality of the system. It is essential, particularly in developing countries, to ensure equal access to health care. As health benefits often accrue more to the better off, specific measures must be implemented to improve the targeting of spending to the poor. First, budget reallocations toward primary care would improve the situation, but only if the quality of local health services is improved at the same time. However, targeting the poor must not lead to a situation in which the system does not meet the needs of the middle- and high-income population. Otherwise, this population may increasingly rely on privately funded providers and refuse to support the publicly financed system. Such a flight from public services may have negative consequences for the whole system. Indeed, the "coalition supporting tax financing may begin to weaken" (Evans 2002, p. 51). In this respect, a key challenge for national health systems is to make sure that publicly funded facilities provide good quality services, so that the wealthier segments of the population continue to use them.

Social health insurance

Social health insurance is distinguished from general revenue-funded systems by the presence of independent or quasi-independent insurance funds, a reliance on compulsory earmarked payroll contributions, and a clear link between these contributions and a set of defined rights for the insured population. Social health insurance systems have been established in more than 60 countries, beginning with Germany at the end of the nineteenth century. Twenty-seven have reached universal coverage through social health insurance (Carrin and James 2004). Social health insurance is particularly widespread among OECD countries, but is also in use in developing countries, mainly in Latin America (Argentina, Bolivia, Brazil, Chile, Colombia, Costa Rica, the Dominican Republic, Ecuador, Peru, Uruguay, República Bolivariana de Venezuela, and others) and to a lesser extent in other parts of the world (Algeria, Kenya, Lebanon, and Tunisia). Today, many low- and middle-income countries have instituted, or are considering starting, social health insurance systems (Bosnia and Herzegovina, China, Croatia, Estonia, Ghana, Hungary, Indonesia, the Kyrgyz Republic, Macedonia, Moldova, Morocco, Nigeria, the Philippines, Poland, the Russian Federation, Serbia, Slovenia, Tanzania, and Vietnam).

Very often, policy makers view social health insurance as an effective way to raise additional resources for health and as a means for decreasing the financing burden of health care coverage (Carrin 2002). There is also a strong presumption that individuals may be more willing to be taxed (pay payroll taxes) if there is a specific individual entitlement that accompanies the tax (a benefit tax). In some cases, especially in countries that experienced communist rule, social health insurance provides an opportunity to reduce the role of the state or to build democratic and participatory institutions (as in China, Estonia, and Hungary). Finally, countries that used to have national health service systems or "Beveridgean" systems may experiment with social health insurance as a way to improve the efficiency of the health care system by "outsourcing" health insurance coverage (as in Jamaica, Kenya, and Malaysia).

Many donors, especially in Europe, tend to support governments that wish to implement social health insurance, because of their long and positive experience with such systems in their own countries. However, there is no consensus on the merits of social health insurance. Some researchers think it can be introduced successfully only in countries with suitable characteristics and that, in most developing countries, instead of improving the situation, it can increase the problems of governing the health system (Savedoff 2004a).

To help resolve this debate, it is necessary to focus on the definition of social health insurance (box 3.3), its weaknesses and strengths, and the economic, administrative, and political feasibility of its implementation in low- and middle-income countries.

Main technical features of social health insurance

Financing mainly through employee and employer payroll contributions. In most countries, the financing of social health insurance is mainly based on payroll contributions made by employers and employees. However, there are big differences among countries relating to the absence or existence of a contribution ceiling, the distribution of employer and employee contributions, the uniformity of the rate, and the receipt of other types of resources (Normand and Busse 2002).

General taxation often remains an important source of income for the health care systems in social health insurance countries. Indeed, contributions may not be sufficient to attain universal coverage, because the number of people to be covered is greater than the number that can actually contribute to the system. Therefore, government subsidies through general taxation are often needed (Carrin and James 2004). In some countries, such as Armenia and Lithuania, social insurance funds were even created entirely from transfers of general revenues.

External aid and earmarked taxes are other sources of funding often used to subsidize social health insurance. In some countries, earmarked taxes are targeted

BOX 3.3 *What is social health insurance?*

Defining social health insurance is not an easy task. For some authors, it includes any insurance scheme that is not for profit. For others, it refers exclusively to Bismarckian systems[1] (Savedoff 2004a). Therefore, the best way to understand social health insurance might be to adopt a pragmatic approach and concentrate on the most common principles and features of existing social health insurance systems. This attempt to define social health insurance more precisely will necessarily be vulnerable to criticism because these features are very seldom present together and because wide differences can be observed in the organization of health financing systems identified as "social health insurance." Some even use the vocabulary of health insurance, yet have developed many similarities with government-funded systems (Normand and Busse 2002). However, it does not seem possible to use a more "scientific" method.

This discussion focuses on four underlying principles. Technical features that give concrete expression to these principles are discussed in the text.

First, in social health insurance systems, membership is publicly mandated for a designated population. Usually, most countries go through two important steps—which may take several decades—from existing employer-based insurance schemes to compulsory schemes for specific employment groups (such as civil servants or industrial workers) before they progressively extend social health insurance to the whole population (Carrin and James 2004). This "incremental" process has been observed both in countries that have long used social health insurance as a way to provide universal coverage, such as Germany, and in those that have done so more recently, such as the Republic of Korea (Bärnighausen and Sauerborn 2002).

Second, there is a direct link between the payment of contributions to finance the system and the receipt of medical care benefits, even though there are exceptions to that rule (the contributions of people with insufficient income may be financed by the government so that these people can be included in the system). Only contributors have the right to access specific items of care. This is different from national health service systems where care is supplied to the entire population, but only if the necessary resources are available. In social health insurance countries, at least in principle, "there is a public commitment to take and give under prescribed conditions stipulated by laws and regulations" (Ron, Abel-Smith, and Tamburi 1990).

Third, the concept of social solidarity is essential in every social health insurance system. The application of this concept implies a high level of cross-subsidization across the system, between rich and poor, low-risk and high-risk people, and individuals and families.

Fourth, the management of social health insurance involves some degree of autonomy from the government, often through quasi-independent organizations in charge of the system.

[1]Defined as "a system of national social security and health insurance introduced into the nineteenth century German empire under the then Chancellor Bismarck. This system is a legally mandatory system for the majority or the whole population to obtain health insurance with a designated (statutory) third-party payer through nonrisk related contributions which are kept separate from taxes or other legally mandated payments" (European Observatory on Health Systems and Policies 2005).

Source: Authors.

to products that harm people's health (for example, tobacco, alcohol) to reduce their consumption.

Management by nonprofit insurance funds. In most social health insurance schemes, the state defines the main characteristics of the system: the conditions of affiliation, the content of the benefit package, and the way contributions are calculated and collected (Busse, Saltman, and Dubois 2004). However, most social health insurance systems are managed by sickness funds that are set apart from the government, at least to some degree.

The sickness funds are usually nonprofit institutions supervised by the government. Their role and organization are established by the state. However, they enjoy a degree of managerial freedom and are often run by a board, some members of which are elected. The board usually includes the main stakeholders. Sickness funds often directly collect contributions even though, in some cases, resources are first collected by the state and then redistributed to the existing funds. Social health insurance funds finance health services provided either in their own facilities or by private or public providers. For private and public providers, the funds either directly cover all or part of the costs of the providers or cover them indirectly by reimbursing the insured population, and the relationships between the providers and the funds are often governed by contracts. These contracts may specify the prices of covered services, terms regarding the quality of care, and payment schedules, among other elements.

Depending on the country, there might be several funds (as in Argentina, Chile, Colombia, France, Germany, Japan, the Netherlands, and Russia) or a single one (as in Estonia and Hungary). Assignment of beneficiaries to a particular fund may be based on employment (as in Argentina, Bolivia, and Mexico), geography or age (as in Japan), or individual choice (as in Chile, Colombia, and Germany). Very often, the number of funds does not proceed from a deliberate choice but can be explained by history. As a result, it is often impossible to eradicate or merge existing local or employment-based funds when a broader social health insurance scheme is implemented.

In existing systems, there is usually a progressive evolution toward fewer funds in order to achieve better risk pooling and economies of scale. Having fewer funds reduces administrative costs and spreads risk over a larger membership, although there is a trade-off between efficiency and client choice, which would be fostered by more competing funds (Bärnighausen and Sauerborn 2002). Moreover, when several funds survive, financial mechanisms are often implemented to compensate for the differences in their incomes and standardized expenditures (as in France). Finally, if several funds are allowed to compete, the administrative costs of the system are generally higher because of the costs involved in efforts to attract clients.

Existence of a benefits package. Social health insurance systems usually fully or partially cover a defined benefits package for all members. This benefits package is more or less comprehensive, depending on the resources of the system.

Apart from these few common characteristics, social health insurance systems often vary greatly in their structure and scope. This is particularly true regarding the delivery of health care and the patient-provider relationship. In Western European countries, social health insurance systems generally provide care by contracting with public and private providers, and people benefit from individual choice of providers and freedom of access, although some countries have implemented gatekeeper systems. In contrast, in many developing countries, sickness funds provide care to the insured population through their own providers (as in the Arab Republic of Egypt, India, Islamic Republic of Iran, Jordan, Turkey, and a number of Latin American countries) and beneficiary choice of providers is restricted.

Strengths of social health insurance

The performance of social health insurance can be assessed according to the WHO's characterization of the purpose of health financing schemes: "to make funding available, as well as to set the right financial incentives for providers, to ensure that all individuals have access to effective public health and personal health care" (WHO 2000, p. 95). Because social health insurance is primarily a way of raising resources, it is also necessary to consider the fairness of financial contributions and the system's impact on the economy. Using these different evaluative criteria, the advantages and drawbacks of social health insurance are described below.

More resources for the health care system. Social health insurance is often viewed as an easy and effective way to raise resources to improve health. Indeed, social contributions are supposed to be easier to collect than general taxes because the employer can deduct them from salaries. More important, citizens may be more willing to pay their contributions because the destination of the money is visible, specific, and related to a vital need. Finally, in situations when there is no room for an increase in government spending for health, countries may want to look for a more diverse revenue base specifically earmarked for the health sector. This is what happened in most Eastern European countries in the late 1980s and early 1990s when they had to cut real spending for health in the first years of the transition: 17 of them have introduced payroll contributions, 10 as a predominant mechanism of financing and 7 as a complementary resource to general tax revenues and out-of-pocket payments. However, the results of this policy have been somewhat disappointing (see below).

Less dependence on budget negotiations than state-funded systems. Systems financed through earmarked payroll taxes are less subject to yearly budgetary negotiations than funds coming from general taxation. Therefore, they are regarded as a more stable source of income. But, financing social health insurance through contributions alone may not generate sufficient resources, especially if policy makers wish to cover more of the population than those who have contributed through payroll contributions. Indeed, the unemployed, the retired, students, and the poor also need coverage. Thus, in many social health insurance systems, contributions are supplemented by government subsidies financed through general taxation. Moreover, in some countries, governments offer guarantees for the social health insurance funds' debt (as in France). Finally, most social health insurance systems are funded on a pay-as-you-go basis. As a result of the demographic transition, large contingent liabilities for future retirees are accumulating in many systems, particularly in developing countries, raising serious questions about their long-term solvency.

High redistributive dimension. Existing social health insurance systems usually are highly redistributive, with cross-subsidies from high-income to low-income participants (especially if there is no ceiling on the income subject to contributions), from high-risk to low-risk participants (individual health risks have no impact on the level of contributions), from young to old, and from individuals to families (usually, dependants of a contributing person are covered with no increase in the contributions paid).

There is no clear conclusion regarding the relative progressivity of social contributions versus general revenue financing. However, some studies seem to show that social contributions are less progressive or, at best, as progressive (Normand and Busse 2002). Obviously, in countries with income ceilings, the progressivity is limited.

Strong support by the population. Countries with a long history of social health insurance tend to display a striking, very strong, almost emotional attachment to it. The reasons for this phenomenon lie mainly in the fact that social health insurance systems are perceived to be privately funded and delivered (which gives the patient the status of a customer), managed by the participants themselves, and (most important), very stable in organizational and financial terms. Social health insurance is also viewed as a way of fostering solidarity and empowering citizens through participation (Saltman 2004).

Whatever the reasons, this phenomenon cannot be denied and may explain part of the appeal of social health insurance for countries seeking to implement a new health financing system. Moreover, in many of these countries, when governments have failed to provide good coverage to the population, social health insurance is seen as a last resort solution. But social health insurance also has major drawbacks and, to be successfully implemented, it is best if countries meet the set of preconditions discussed later.

Weaknesses of social health insurance

Possible exclusion of the poor. Most countries start implementing social health insurance for a limited part of the population. Very often, it first covers civil servants and big private firms' employees. In the earlier stages, the poorer segments of the population (most informal sector workers, unemployed people) are often left without coverage or are covered by the state, even though governments generally contend that universal coverage is the ultimate goal of the reform. However, there is a risk that the system may never move beyond the initial narrow base of formal sector workers and that, instead of improving the situation of the poorer groups, it may increase inequities (Conn and Walford 1998).

First, it is usually very difficult and expensive to add informal sector workers to the covered population. They tend to live in remote areas and not fully understand the benefits they can get from being part of the system, and their income is very difficult to assess. Second, public subsidies to the health infrastructure are often needed to supplement the resources coming from contributions. This phenomenon diverts money to the insured population that could otherwise be used to finance services for the poor. Third, in most developing countries, tax administration is weak, making it difficult to collect taxes from rural and informal sector employees.

Negative economic impact of payroll contributions. Although in theory and in the long run, a tax on wages would be shifted onto employees, in countries where product and labor markets are not very competitive, employers may not be able to reduce wages to compensate for an increase in payroll contributions in the short run. Therefore, social security contributions may increase labor costs and, in turn, lead to higher unemployment. They may also reduce the competitiveness of the country and deter investments, thus slowing down the growth of the economy. Further, if the government is a major employer, payroll contributions will significantly increase public expenditures.

Even in developed countries, such as France, social contributions have been blamed for the high level of unemployment. This led to a major reform of the financing of the social health insurance system, which was intended to reduce the weight of payroll-based deductions by transforming employees' contributions into a tax on all sources of income (salaries, social benefits, capital gains, gambling income).

Complex and expensive to manage. These systems involve many different players, complex interactions, and complicated tasks—all of which must be managed. Among other functions, sickness funds must often negotiate contracts with providers and set up appropriate monitoring mechanisms. They must reimburse the expenses of the insured population efficiently and control its consumption behavior to avoid abuse. They also have the responsibility to manage substantial amounts of money, which involves investing reserves when they exist and ensuring the long-run solvency of the fund. The government must establish effective supervision rules to avoid fraud and foster efficiency. Finally, new collecting mechanisms must be created for social contributions.

Therefore, in social health insurance systems, administrative costs are higher than in national health service schemes. Where these tasks have not been properly managed, the implementation of social health insurance has not been very successful. This is the case in many Latin American counties, where weak regulation and inefficient health institutions have hindered the development of social health insurance.

Escalating costs. Social health insurance, like national health service systems, can generate an excess demand for health services, because the costs of the services are heavily subsidized (a moral hazard). It can also lead to excessive provision of services when a fee-for-service payment method is applied without appropriate regulatory tools. Moreover, it is often easier to increase social contributions, which are generally well accepted by the population, than to reduce benefits, because people feel they have paid for their benefits. Finally, the management of sickness funds by people representing diverse interests (members of trade unions or employers organizations, civil servants, local authorities) makes it very difficult to take radical measures. These tendencies have been observed in countries with a long history of social health insurance. For all these reasons, countries with social health insurance systems usually spend more on health than those with national health systems (see chapter 9).

Poor coverage for chronic diseases and preventive care. Fee-for-service provider payment methods and freedom of access to health care services—often attributes of such schemes—make social health insurance a very efficient system for meeting health needs that can be provided by an individual provider during a single consultation. Conversely, it is not the best system for chronic diseases, which require the intervention of several professionals and strong coordination among them. Nor is it ideal for preventive care, such as immunizations and screenings, because the links between public health services run by the government, private providers, and sickness funds are often too weak to facilitate adequate cooperation (McKee, Delnoij, and Brand 2004).

Feasibility of social health insurance in developing countries

As this list of strengths and weaknesses demonstrates, social health insurance is neither a good nor bad system in itself. In fact, the success of its implementation in a given country depends on the presence of a series of preconditions and governments' abilities to influence them.

Level of income. A variety of countries started implementing social health insurance when their GNP was in the lower-middle-income range, and they had strong economic growth during the transition period leading to universal coverage (Carrin and James 2004). Indeed, it is easy to absorb new contributions in a prosperous economy. In countries where growth is very slow or nonexistent, it might be better to wait, because social health insurance will not be able to mobilize additional resources. Korea is a good example of rapid implementation of social health insurance thanks to a booming economy. During the main phase of extension

(1977–89), the average annual growth rate of GDP per capita was 13.3 percent. Therefore, universal coverage was achieved only 26 years after the creation of the first voluntary health insurance fund in 1965 (Bärnighausen and Sauerborn 2002). Conversely, many Latin American and Caribbean countries have not had rapid enough economic growth to allow them to affiliate the majority of the population. In Bolivia, for instance, less than 10 percent of the population is covered through social health insurance, despite the system being founded in the 1930s.

Size of the informal sector. Where the informal sector is large, the payroll base for contributions is very narrow, providing limited ability to raise significant resources for health care. In contrast, countries where the formal sector is dominant are able to register workers much more easily. This is particularly true in countries with a high proportion of industrial workers, because most companies in this sector will have a formal payroll system from which contributions can be paid. It is also the case when the state sector is the main employer, although this situation might not be stable in countries where the economy is in transition between a state-run system and a market-led one. Because employment in the public sector tends to decrease while informal private employment grows, the market transition often has a negative impact on the collection of revenue (Ensor 1999). On the whole, far from decreasing, the informal sector is still growing in developing countries (ILO 2005). Finally, although it is always difficult to assess and levy taxes on the income of self-employed workers, it is even more difficult to do so with respect to people working in agriculture, because their income might be very uneven over the year and from one year to another (Normand and Weber 1994).

Distribution of the population. Successful experiences seem to be associated with growing urbanization and increased population density, because these evolutions facilitate the registration of social health insurance members and the collection of contributions (Ensor 1999; Carrin and James 2004). Conversely, case studies show that countries where the rural population is preponderant have seen much slower implementation of social health insurance.

A very interesting study confirms the importance of the first three preconditions described above. A group of low- and middle-income countries were ranked according to a composite index of four variables: population density, percentage of the population urbanized, percentage of the workforce in industry, and per capita income. A high ranking implies that social health insurance is relatively easy to implement. The study shows that in most of the countries on top of the list coverage is actually very high: Argentina, Brazil, and Korea, among others (Ensor 1999).

Margin to increase labor costs. It is necessary to assess the extent to which increased wages due to payroll contributions affect the competitiveness of a given economy. In some cases, they may represent an excessive burden and negatively affect growth and employment. They may also harm the labor market by increasing tax evasion and reducing the size of the formal sector. Furthermore, in many countries, salaries are already a major source of taxation (income tax, unemployment insurance contributions), and this burden limits the potential to impose significant new payroll taxes (Normand and Weber 1994).

Administrative capacity. Social health insurance systems require skilled administrative staff, particularly to run health insurance funds and to regulate and supervise their activity. Sometimes, it is possible to utilize people formerly employed in private health insurance companies, or "mutuelles." In any case, it is essential to determine whether the capacity to run these systems exists before establishing them (box 3.4).

Good-quality health care infrastructure. The quality of the health services available to the insured population is critical to the success of social health insurance systems. Social health insurance gives the insured population a right to access these services. Yet the successful implementation of a social health insurance scheme depends on the effective availability of services. The best-designed social health insurance system remains an empty shell if a country does not

---

BOX 3.4 *The impact of poor management and supervision on the implementation of social health insurance*

Kenya has the oldest insurance scheme in Africa. Theoretically, its National Hospital Insurance Fund (NHIF), established in 1966, is supposed to pay for hospital stays, treatment, and drugs for the whole population. But the reality is completely different. Often, the NHIF covers only board and lodging expenses, and patients have to pay all the other costs of treatment themselves. And a mere 7 percent of the population is insured. The main reason for the failure of the system is the lack of trust people have in the NHIF. It is seen as one of the most corrupt institutions in the country, and more than half of its budget is spent on administrative costs.

Similar problems occurred in Armenia and Kazakhstan, where health financing was moved off budget and out of the control of the treasury system before other accountability measures were developed. The lack of accountability and clearly defined financial flows rapidly led to suspicions of corruption, which were soon confirmed. In Kazakhstan millions of dollars of revenues disappeared from the health insurance system during its brief existence, and the director of the federal fund was under investigation for fraud and eventually fled the country. In Armenia site visits revealed that no government funds had reached most health care facilities for more than nine months after the State Health Agency was established as an autonomous off-budget fund and became responsible for allocating government health care funds and purchasing services.

Sources: GTZ 2004 and Langenbrunner 2005.

have the infrastructure to provide the health services included in the benefits package. In turn, the existence of good-quality infrastructure will encourage the population to join the system and support it.

In countries where the facilities available to the insured population are inadequate, those who can afford it prefer to pay out of pocket or to buy private health insurance to gain access to better services. Over the long term, this phenomenon may endanger the whole system. For example, in countries where an insured person is covered only if he or she uses facilities managed by the sickness funds, the person is encouraged to join a second system. This is the origin of the so-called *doble affiliación* that is common in many Latin American countries, including the Dominican Republic (Savedoff 2005). It also happens in countries where social health insurance gives access only to public providers. In Tunisia, for instance, many private sector employees who are covered by a social health insurance scheme, which gives them only the right to be treated in public facilities, voluntarily get private insurance to be able to resort to private providers.

Existence of a consensus in favor of social health insurance. The successful implementation of social health insurance depends to a large extent on the existence of a broad consensus among the main stakeholders to comply with the scheme's rules. Indeed, the society as a whole may place a limit on the degree of equity it is ready to accept or fund. For instance, when all contributions are pooled and the benefit package is universal, differences in contributions between groups may turn out to be so large that they are no longer acceptable to many people. If the same benefits are granted to everyone, it may bring an end to the health care privileges of the elite. Consequently, they may resist the implementation of social health insurance. Thus, the acceptability or sustainability of the social health insurance scheme may be jeopardized, as a significant part of the population may be unwilling to accept this important implicit redistribution.

Political stability and political rights. The political context of a country also plays a fundamental role in the successful implementation of social health insurance. Indeed, without a high level of political rights, it is doubtful that the government will get the support needed for expanding social health insurance. The government might also lack incentives for improving the living conditions of the population through health care reform.

Therefore, the feasibility of the implementation of social health insurance systems depends on a set of country-specific socioeconomic and political factors, principally the rate of economic growth, the extent of the formal sector, the geographic distribution of the population, the extent of urbanization, the possibility of increasing labor costs, the administrative capacity of the system, the quality of the health care infrastructure, the level of solidarity, the support of the main stakeholders, and the stability of the political context. If some or most of these preconditions are missing, the establishment of social health insurance will likely face obstacles and may be disappointing. In particular, hopes that it will help to raise additional resources for health might be dashed. In that respect, the experience of many Eastern European countries in the 1990s and early part of this decade is particularly revealing (box 3.5).

A model used in a recent paper also shows the importance of some of the preconditions discussed here to the successful expansion of health coverage. It indicates that four variables go far toward explaining the ability of a country to

---

BOX 3.5 *Failure of payroll contributions to increase health funding in Eastern Europe*

Contrary to the expectation that payroll contributions would increase overall levels of funding for health care, the diversified tax base often failed to bring about additional revenues. This phenomenon has several explanations.

First, employers often failed to comply with payroll tax requirements. In general, the countries of Eastern Europe and especially those of the former Soviet Union have faced considerable difficulty in collecting payroll taxes for health. Some countries, such as the Czech Republic, Estonia, and Hungary, have structural characteristics that increase the likelihood of successful introduction of a payroll tax, including relatively higher per capita income and a large percentage of the population living in urban areas and working in the formal sector. Ensor (1999) noted that registration was initially made easier because of the large number of employees in the government sector or the number of large state enterprises in many countries, such as Kazakhstan. But there have been major challenges in many countries. A significant economic burden was created by new health and social insurance taxes (totaling 44 percent in Hungary). The region as a whole has traditionally suffered from much higher payroll taxes than other regions.

Some countries had less developed regulatory and administrative capacity to raise revenues, a large proportion of unemployed or self-employed workers, and weak tax collection systems, as in Albania and Romania. Other countries—Kazakhstan, Kyrgyzstan, Russia,

and even Estonia—have reported similar problems of collection caused by tax avoidance by labor and small businesses. Also contributing to the problem were the weakness of collection mechanisms, the high debt of enterprises, and the large populations outside the system, particularly farmers and the unemployed. Low levels of compliance may have been further exacerbated by the frequent absence of a link between contribution and benefit. The historical legacy of the socialist era meant that all citizens of many countries had a constitutional right to health care, and this right was generally retained in the transition period. Premium collection only resulted in 9 to 52 percent of expected revenues in different oblasts in Kazakhstan in 1996 and only 40 percent on average in 1998. Consequently, the new social health insurance system became discredited and was canceled at the end of 1999.

A final major factor was the overall weak macroeconomic context. Many countries experienced negative growth in the 1990s. Despite introducing social health insurance, these countries continued to rely on general taxation as the main source of funding for health care. Finally, the countries that have moved furthest toward reliance on earmarked contributions (accounting for more than 60 percent of total expenditure on health) are also those with the highest levels of per capita GDP.

Source: Langenbrunner 2005.

expand population health coverage:[2] a good level of income per capita, a well edu-
cated workforce, low income inequalities (a sign that redistribution is well
accepted), and a high level of political rights (Carrin and James 2003).

In any case, given the complexity of social health insurance, every country willing to implement such a scheme may have to go through a long transition period.
In eight social health insurance countries where sufficient information was available, the average length of the transition between the passage of the first law
related to health insurance and the passage of the law implementing universal
coverage was 70 years (Carrin and James 2004). The length of this transition phase
depends on the preconditions described above.

It is beneficial for countries to have a number of these preconditions already in
place, but a government can help foster the development of some of them. Thus,
the context is fundamental, but political will and appropriate decisions can compensate for an unfavorable initial situation, at least to some degree.

Capacity of the government to expand social health insurance

Ability to extend the system.   One of the biggest challenges faced by social health
insurance in developing countries is extending coverage from its original narrow
base of formal urban and modern rural sectors to the entire population. Governments play a decisive part in the success or failure of this undertaking.

First, it is essential that institutions and policy makers design a realistic and
progressive scenario of extension and stick to it. The scenario must be realistic,
because if initial promises are not kept the government might lose the support of
the population, which may endanger the whole process. In that respect, it is fundamental to carry out very solid actuarial studies before implementing the system.
It is also very important to be as transparent as possible to gain the trust of the
main stakeholders.

The expansion should be progressive, not only because expansion over time
helps address the fundamental question of financial sustainability, but also because
social health insurance is essentially complex and requires time to understand and
fully implement. Starting with a limited share of the population will allow administrators of the system to gain the necessary experience before extending it either
on a geographical basis or from employees of big firms to workers in smaller firms,
as was done in Korea (Ron, Abel-Smith, and Tamburi 1990).

Second, the government's choice of method to develop social health insurance
is critical. It must be as transparent and participative as possible to gather the support of the population. The government must also insist on the advantages of the
system by pointing out its benefits for specific groups of the population in order
to build consensus (Normand and Weber 1994).

Third, the government must find ways to encourage informal workers to join. It
must show them that social health insurance will improve their access to care.

Indeed, at the beginning, the payment of regular contributions may not be a readily understood concept. People may wonder why they have to pay when they are not sick (ILO and ISSA 1999). In that sense, it is essential to design an attractive (and financially sustainable) package, but also to make health services available for informal sector workers, who may not have ready access to care. It is also very important to market the reform and communicate its advantages. Innovative techniques may also be used to collect the contributions of informal sector workers: assessment of their income on the basis of property, payment of flat-rate or minimum contributions, and involvement of local networks to reach informal workers (such as bus drivers' organizations, fishing cooperatives, church organizations, and village communities in Kenya, and village cooperatives in the Philippines). Finally, a more "coercive" approach can be used by requiring people to pay the full costs of health services if they do not contribute to the social health insurance. In Costa Rica this method significantly reduced tax evasion (MSH 2000). Voluntary enrollment is not advisable because it presents the risk of adverse selection.

Fourth, the government may need to subsidize the extension of social health insurance to the poor (box 3.6). Indeed, the people initially covered are often reluctant to extend social health insurance, because this will mean a high level of cross-subsidization between them and the newly insured. Therefore, countries such as Chile, Colombia, Costa Rica, and the Philippines have subsidized the poor

---

BOX 3.6 *Government subsidies to extend social health insurance to the disadvantaged*

The 1993 health sector reform in Colombia is a good example of a successful government initiative to extend social health insurance to the poor. The reform reorganized health care finances from supply-side subsidies for public hospitals to a managed competition model with demand-side subsidies for the poor. It set up a scheme for poor individuals with subsidized premiums provided through an equity fund. The equity fund receives resources from the budget and part of the resources generated from the payroll tax for the contributory scheme. The equity fund subsidizes insurance premiums for poor individuals identified on the basis of a proxy-means test. The subsidized basic package was supplemented by public hospitals with the existing supply subsidies. Eventually all of the supply subsidies are to be phased out and replaced by an expanded benefits package to the poor.

As a result of the reform, Colombia increased the share of its population that is financially protected from health shocks from 23 percent in 1993 to 62 percent a decade later. More than 11 million poor participants benefited from the insurance. Child mortality rates fell from 44 per 1,000 births to 15 per 1,000 among the insured. Now, this reform has to face the bigger challenge of its financial sustainability, largely because it remains incomplete. Subsidies to public hospitals continue and add to the fiscal cost of the equity fund. The government also had to cover the deficits of the previous social insurance system, which was badly affected by the obligation to compete with private insurers.

Sources: Escobar 2005; Escobar and Panapoulou 2002; Cataneda 2003.

so that they can be integrated into the system, either by paying money to the insurance funds directly or by paying part of the premiums for the poor, informal, and self-employed workers joining the system.

Ability to contain costs. Because social health insurance is often associated with high costs, it is fundamental for the institutions running the system to contain costs, particularly by controlling adverse selection and moral hazard–induced behaviors on the part of providers and patients. A varied set of tools can be used to reach this goal: performance-related provider payments, expenditure caps, risk-adjusted capitation arrangements, well-designed contractual agreements between providers and health insurance funds, and good monitoring of the system, among others. Although this section does not discuss these techniques, it is nonetheless important to stress that cost containment is a key element in the success or failure of social health insurance systems.

Community-based health insurance

Community-based health insurance schemes have existed all over the world for centuries. They have served as the building blocks for the creation of social health insurance systems in countries such as Germany, Japan, and Korea.

But today in low-income countries, community-based health insurance plays an increasing role in providing medical coverage to populations without access to other forms of formal medical protection, such as social health insurance or private insurance. Community-based health insurance is part of an overall health financing strategy in a number of countries, given the high out-of-pocket financing of care, the uncertainty surrounding anticipated financial flows from donors, the large rural and informal sector populations, and the weak capacity of governments to raise taxes. Community-based health insurance is found throughout the world, but it is particularly prevalent in Sub-Saharan Africa: in West Africa alone, the number of community-based health insurance schemes grew from 199 in 2000 to 585 in 2003 (Bennett, Kelley, and Silvers 2004). Many community-based health insurance schemes have also developed in Asia in China, India, Nepal, and the Philippines, and in Latin America in Argentina, Colombia, Ecuador, and Mexico.

Therefore, with interest in cost recovery fading as a mechanism to mobilize resources for health in low-income countries, the attention of the global community has turned increasingly to community-based health insurance for resource mobilization and allocative efficiency. Another factor contributing to the rise in interest in community-based health insurance pertains to financial protection.

Community-based health insurance schemes are sometimes referred to as health insurance for the informal sector, mutual health organizations, or microinsurance schemes. They can be broadly defined as not-for-profit prepayment plans[3] for health care, with community control and voluntary membership. They generally spread risk from the healthy to the sick, but if premiums are based on income, there can also be risk sharing from the better off to the poor. However, there is a large variety of community-based health insurance schemes. They are quite heterogeneous in populations covered, services offered, regulation, management, and objectives. It can be difficult to compare the community organized and managed *mutuelles de santé* prevalent in francophone West Africa with some of the hospital-run and organized community financing schemes common in East Africa.[4] Moreover, some of the plans are closely associated with government health care financing policies (Rwanda, Tanzania), whereas in West Africa, most of the plans are set up, run, and managed by the community. This section focuses on the definition of community-based health insurance (box 3.7), before describing its main weaknesses and strengths.

BOX 3.7 *What is community-based health insurance?*

Community-based health insurance schemes are highly diverse and defy efforts to arrive at a single, widely applicable definition. Based on a substantial analysis of the existing literature on community-based health insurance, however, Jakab and Krishnan (2004) identify three features common to most existing schemes:

- *Affiliation is based on community membership, and the community is strongly involved in managing the system.* The term "community" refers to a group of people who share common characteristics. This broad definition covers various situations. Members of community-based health insurance schemes can be linked by geographic proximity or by the same profession, religion, ethnicity, or any "other kind of affiliation that facilitates their cooperation for financial protection" (Jakab and Krishnan 2004). In community-based health insurance schemes, affiliation is based on community membership, although all members of the community may not be part of the scheme, particularly if they are too poor to pay the premiums. Members of the community also participate in the management of the scheme: designing the rules and collecting, pooling, and allocating resources. But this participation does not mean that community-based health insurance schemes

are owned by the community. The ILO/STEP study shows that communities are the legal owner of the schemes in only 9 percent of the 128 cases reviewed (ILO and STEP 2002). The main owners are central or local governments (44 percent), NGOs outside the community (25 percent), and hospitals (11 percent) (ILO and STEP 2002).

- *Beneficiaries are excluded from other kinds of health coverage.* Community-based health insurance schemes regroup poor people excluded from other forms of financing methods. For example, they may be excluded from social health insurance because they work in the informal sector, from government-funded services because these services are not accessible, or from private health insurance because they cannot pay the premiums.

- *Members share a set of social values.* Most schemes convey deeply rooted values and principles, such as voluntary affiliation, participation, and solidarity. Often, these schemes have existed for a long time as traditional forms of solidarity of the poor. The design of community-based health insurance schemes, in particular the rules governing the collection of resources and the benefits, generally reflects these principles.

The various forms of community-based health insurance

Community-based health insurance schemes differ widely in size, organization, objectives, and management. The following classifications convey some of the diversity of these arrangements:

- Atim (1998) divides mutual health organizations in West and Central Africa on the basis of two dimensions: their ownership (traditional clan or ethnic social network, social movement or association type, comanaged provider, or community scheme) and their geographical and socioprofessional criteria (rural/ urban or profession/enterprise/association/trade union).

- Another typology by Bennett, Creese, and Monash (1998) is based on the nature of the risks covered. They distinguish "type 1" schemes covering high-cost, low-frequency events and "type 2" schemes covering low-cost, high-frequency risks.

- Based on a study of community-based health insurance schemes in several Asian countries, Hsiao (2001) identifies five types of schemes: schemes involving direct government subsidy to the individuals (such as the Thai Health Card), cooperative health care in which financing and provision are integrated at village and subdistrict levels, community-sponsored third-party insurance, provider-sponsored prepayment (free access to specific providers in exchange for monthly premiums), and producer or consumer cooperatives (such as the Grameen Bank, which functions as an insurer and a provider for its members and nonmembers living in the same operational area).

- Based on a wide review of nearly three dozen case studies, Jakab and Krishnan (2004) classify schemes in four categories: community cost sharing (resource mobilization through out-of-pocket payments, but the community is involved in fixing user fees, allocating resources, developing exemption criteria, and managing the scheme); community prepayment or mutual health organizations (prepayment, risk sharing, strong involvement of the community in the design and management of the scheme); provider-based health insurance (schemes centered on a single hospital—often started by the providers, prepayment, risk sharing, coverage of catastrophic risks, community role more supervisory than strategic); and government or social health insurance support for the community scheme (schemes attached to social health insurance systems or government-funded programs, active participation of the community in the management of the system, but significant financial contributions of the government or social health insurance funds).

Strengths of community-based health insurance

Precisely assessing the overall impact of community-based health insurance schemes is very difficult because "in most cases, community-financing arrangements are not registered," and therefore "centrally maintained data do not exist" (Jakab and Krishnan 2004, p. 69). However, the literature suggests the following conclusions.

Better access to health care for low-income people. Jakab and Krishnan (2004) reviewed more than 45 published and unpublished reports on the experience of community-based health insurance and evaluated the schemes along three main dimensions: resource mobilization, financial protection, and access by the poor. The authors find good evidence that community financing arrangements make a positive contribution to the financing of health care in low-income settings. The variation in ability to raise resources is attributed to the low income of the contributing population. Financial protection provided by the plans is found to be significant, both through reductions in out-of-pocket spending and through increased use of health care resources. Regarding access by the poor, the authors find that community-based health insurance "extends coverage to a large number of people who would otherwise not have financial protection" (p. 75).

Ekman (2004), however, is a bit less categorical. He applies a systematic as opposed to a narrative review to assess the impact of community-based health insurance. Schemes' results are evaluated on the basis of the following criteria: resource mobilization, quality of care, provider efficiency, moral hazard, financial protection, out-of-pocket spending, and access to care. He finds that "[o]verall, the evidence base is limited in scope and questionable in quality. There is strong evidence that community-based health insurance provides some financial protection by reducing out-of-pocket spending. There is evidence of moderate strength that such schemes improve cost-recovery" (p. 249).

Useful as a component of a health financing system involving other instruments. Community-based health insurance schemes may complete or fill the gaps of other health financing schemes (social health insurance or government financing), or they may be a first step toward a larger-scale system. When they start to operate, most community-based health insurance schemes are independent from governments or social health insurance systems. Very often, they were created precisely because these institutions were unable to provide medical protection to the population. But as they develop, community-based schemes must coordinate with other existing financing instruments in the interest of the population. More important, a way to overcome the limits of community-based health insurance might be to consider it not as the answer to all the health financing needs of a country, but as part of a solution involving other financing mechanisms.

Community-based health insurance may be very useful to supplement other forms of medical coverage. Indeed, as previously discussed, community-based schemes cannot provide medical coverage to the whole population. But they can help meet the needs of specific categories of people, such as the rural middle class and informal workers (Bennett, Kelley, and Silvers 2004). For this reason, in many countries governments try to launch community-based health insurance schemes (as in Rwanda) or use existing ones to extend health coverage to certain populations. For instance, in Tanzania, the Community Health Fund targets informal workers, while workers in the formal sector are covered through a new social health insurance scheme (Bennett, Kelley, and Silvers 2004). A similar strategy is used in Ghana. Community-based health insurance may also cover all or part of the user fees people have to pay in government-funded health care facilities or cover services that are not covered in the benefit package offered by the government or social health insurance. In some cases, they may also finance access to private providers (Bennett, Kelley, and Silvers 2004).

Governments may use community-based health insurance to extend coverage funded by larger financing instruments, such as social health insurance. In this respect, a very interesting development is under way in the Philippines, where the government is using existing community schemes to develop the national health insurance system (box 3.8).

The ILO/STEP study sums up these elements by claiming that "the very significant prevalence of CBHOs[5] as 'entry points', with significant pooling outside the scheme and important presence of direct and indirect subsidies (. . .) suggest that more than searching for impact of CBHOs as isolated self standing organizational arrangement, its impact and importance should be evaluated as a potential strategy to link the community with (. . .) other alternative organizational arrangements for extending social protection in health" (ILO and STEP 2002, p. 50).

BOX 3.8 *The use of community-based health insurance to extend social health insurance to the informal sector in the Philippines*

The Philippine Health Insurance Corporation (commonly known as PhilHealth) was created in 1995 by the Philippine government. The aim was to reach universal coverage within 15 years. However, 10 years later, formal sector workers still account for two-thirds of the members of the scheme, although about half of all workers make their living in the informal sector.

Therefore, to accelerate the expansion of PhilHealth to the informal sector, the PhilHealth Organized Groups Interface (POGI) was launched in June 2003. In this program, local and regional community-based health insurance schemes can be accredited and rated and then become POGI partner organizations

representing PhilHealth in their communities. According to their financial and managerial skills, the community-based schemes are delegated more or less extensive responsibilities, ranging from the marketing of social health insurance in the community to the collection of contributions, for which they receive financial incentives.

This initiative is currently being tested in 12 communities in two provinces. Even in this pilot phase, positive results have been observed. The boards of two community-based health insurance schemes have decided to mandate that their members join PhilHealth.

Source: GTZ 2004.

Weaknesses of community-based health insurance

Limited protection for members. The ability of community-based health insurance schemes to raise significant resources is limited by the low overall income of the community. Therefore, such schemes usually have to complement their basic resources with user fees, government subsidies, and donor assistance.

Furthermore, the protection they can provide is, most of the time, hindered by the small size of the pool. Even though the size varies widely (from several dozen members to several millions), most schemes are very small. Based on 85 cases, the ILO/STEP study finds that 22 percent of the schemes have fewer than 100 members, almost 70 percent have fewer than 2,000 members, and 83 percent have fewer than 10,000 members (ILO and STEP 2002).

Moreover, effective population coverage within a given community is very limited: about 10 percent of the targeted population on average, according to Ekman (2004), and 8.2 percent according to Waelkens and Criel (2004), based on data available for 103 schemes in Sub-Saharan Africa. The main reasons so many people choose not to participate are that they do not understand the need for health insurance or they do not trust the managers of the scheme. Hsiao (2001) finds that, because membership is voluntary, people will tend to join a scheme if they expect the benefits to be higher than the costs and if the community has a high level of social cohesion. He also argues that trust in the managers of the scheme is essential to explain the willingness of community members to join.

As a result of limited resources, small size, and scanty coverage, most community-based health insurance schemes are not very effective, as demonstrated in the comprehensive review recently completed by the ILO (ILO and STEP 2002). The outcome variables for the evaluation are health status, utilization, and financial protection.[6] The authors find "no evidence from the documents reviewed that CBHOs positively impact health status or at least the utilization of services and financial protection for their members and/or for society at large, particularly the poor" (p. 49).

Sustainability is questionable. The small size of the pool makes many community-based health insurance schemes vulnerable to failure.[7] Indeed, the realization of one single large risk might lead them to bankruptcy. Moreover, most schemes are especially subject to covariant risks, because in a limited geographical area, an individual's health is not independent from the health of his or her neighbors, especially when an epidemic or a natural disaster occurs (Tabor 2005). This is the reason researchers increasingly focus on reinsurance (Dror and Preker 2004). Reinsurance would pool the risks of several schemes, thus granting them greater financial stability. However, today, there is "very limited experience with and capacity to undertake reinsurance" (Bennett, Kelley, and Silvers 2004, p. 14).

The financial stability of community-based health insurance schemes is also affected by problems of adverse selection inherent in voluntary prepayment schemes. Bennett, Creese, and Monash (1998) found that benefit packages were very seldom defined precisely. The tendency was to include all services that could be delivered by the facilities participating in the scheme. This broad approach made it easier for people with preexisting conditions to join, thus creating severe adverse selection issues.

The viability of community-based health insurance is very often jeopardized by the limited management skills available at the community level. Given their small size, most community-based health insurance schemes are fragile "by construction." However, it is necessary to qualify this conclusion, given that many schemes do not bear the financial risk. In the ILO and STEP study of 136 cases for which information is available, the financial risk was supported by central or local governments (and in a few cases by NGOs) in 66 percent of the cases (ILO and STEP 2002).

Limited benefit to the poorer part of the population.   On the issue of financial protection, Ekman (2004) finds that community-based health insurance works for those who enroll, but that the enrollees tend to be relatively well off. He finds that "there is strong evidence that such programs do provide effective protection to the members of the schemes by significantly reducing the level of out of pocket payment for care," but that "the findings suggest that most schemes fail to cover the least well off groups in the catchments areas" (p. 252). Bennet, Creese, and Monash (1998), based on a review of 82 nonprofit insurance schemes for people outside formal employment in developing countries, also found that very few schemes were able to reach the very poor without the support of subsidies from governments or other partners.

Preker and others (2004) agree that the poor do not have access to such plans. They attribute this phenomenon mainly to lack of affordability. Indeed, even very small premiums may be too expensive for the very poor. Moreover, payments in kind are rarely accepted because of the difficulty of managing them, which represents a barrier for cash-poor people (Bennett, Kelley, and Silvers 2004). Finally, the pro-poor orientation of community-based health insurance schemes is often thwarted by the fact that most are financed through regressive flat-rate contributions. Therefore, the report of the Commission on Macroeconomics and Health calls for increased support for community-based health insurance and for the establishment of a cofinancing scheme that would complement premiums paid by individuals toward their health insurance with government or donor funding (WHO 2001).

Nonfinancial reasons have also been put forward to explain the incapacity of the poor to benefit from community-based health insurance. These include providers' attitudes toward the poor and the lack of geographic proximity of services (Bennett, Kelley, and Silvers 2004).

Limited effect on the delivery of care. Some authors argue that community-based health insurance improves the quality of health services by contracting with health providers, thus prompting them to improve their services (Tabor 2005). Based on a review of numerous schemes in Africa and Asia, Hsiao (2001) finds that community-based health insurance does not have a significant impact on the level of resources for health, but he argues that it is a way to better organize health spending to purchase cheaper and better services and goods.

However, most studies based on an extensive analysis of the literature on community-based health insurance tend to contradict this finding. According to Ekman (2004), there is weak or no evidence that schemes have an effect on the quality of care or the efficiency with which care is produced. This finding is somewhat confirmed by the ILO and STEP study, which finds that only a minority of schemes (16 percent of the 62 cases for which information is available) negotiate the quality and costs of services with providers. Most simply purchase services at market prices (ILO and STEP 2002).

In conclusion, community-based health insurance schemes face very difficult issues that affect both their effectiveness and their sustainability. Solutions to these difficulties are not easy. In their comprehensive review of the literature on community-based health insurance, Jakab and Krishnan (2004) identified many cumulative conditions necessary to ensure the success of a scheme: the ability to prevent adverse selection, accommodate an irregular revenue stream of membership, prevent fraud, and accommodate the poorest; good management with strong community involvement; organizational linkages between the scheme and providers (which enable the community to negotiate preferential rates); and the steady availability of donor support and government funding. Hsiao (2001) also stresses that an appropriate intervention of the government may be necessary to ensure the success of a scheme. In particular, governments may subsidize premiums for the poorer part of the community, thus facilitating their participation both by decreasing the cost of premiums and by making the gains attached to participation in the scheme more visible (as with the Thai Health Card). Government funding may also reinforce the impact of community-based health insurance, either by financing some of the health care providers contracted by the scheme or by subsidizing the scheme directly, as in Tanzania, where insurance contributions are matched by subsidies from the government.

Voluntary health insurance

"Private" or "voluntary" health insurance is a health financing model that is particularly prevalent in high-income countries as a supplement to publicly financed coverage (box 3.9). In practice, private or voluntary health insurance arrangements encompass a wide spectrum of voluntary financing mechanisms (that is, mechanisms not mandated by the government) and diverse relationships with public and private health sector inputs. Recent analysis in this area includes work by the OECD (OECD 2004) and WHO (Sekhri and Savedoff 2005), as well as work by researchers at the London School of Economics (Mossialos and Thomson 2002). This section seeks to define and distinguish voluntary and private health insurance from each other and related mechanisms, summarize some strengths and weaknesses of voluntary health insurance, and examine its desirability and feasibility in low- and middle-income countries.

Core competencies of carriers

Bowie and Adams (2005) have identified 11 generic commercial competencies that voluntary health insurers require if they are to develop and sustain a market position: define and develop products, price products, sell products, collect premiums, administer claims, manage risks, manage external relations, provide relevant service and information to customers and suppliers, utilize communications and information technology, manage (operationally), and govern (strategically). Some of these skills differ from those needed to manage a public or social health insurance system—particularly in product development, pricing, and sales.

BOX 3.9 *What is voluntary health insurance?*

"Private health insurance" has been defined in various ways, including health insurance providing economically private goods (personal health services rather than public health services), health insurance provided by private (for-profit) organizations, and health insurance characterized by premiums not based on income, in contrast to tax-based or social security contributions (OECD 2004). Voluntary health insurance is defined as any health insurance that is paid for by voluntary contributions. Voluntary health insurance can thus be distinguished from national health service systems and social insurance financing models, which are both characterized by mandated payments. The level of compulsion is important, because it often determines the breadth of the risk pool and may also indicate the importance policy makers assign to coverage. The analysis in this book focuses on the level of compulsion as a key distinguishing factor and examines voluntary health insurance schemes.

In reality, most private health insurance markets are voluntary. For example, Switzerland is alone among OECD member countries in mandating the purchase of private health insurance (by individuals). Uruguay requires persons in certain income bands ($600–$1,800 annually) to purchase private coverage, and Saudi Arabia is in the process of introducing compulsory private health insurance for expatriates (Sekhri, Savedoff, and Tripathi 2005).

When analyzing and evaluating voluntary health insurance, it is important to identify the functions or roles that such insurance plays in a particular country context—that is, whether the voluntary scheme is a primary or additional source of health care funding. The taxonomy of private health insurance functions developed by the OECD breaks down voluntary health insurance functions as follows: (a) the main source of health coverage for a population or subpopulation (primary), (b) coverage of the same services or benefits as the public system (duplicate) (although the providers and timely access to, quality, and amenities of the services may vary), (c) coverage of cost sharing under the public system (complementary), or (d) coverage of services uncovered by the public system (supplementary) (OECD 2004). This division of functions facilitates meaningful comparisons across systems.

Source: Authors.

Voluntary health insurance carriers must also manage various risks, several of which also differ from those faced by publicly funded programs. Bowie and Adams (2005) analyzed voluntary health insurance as sets of income, expenditure, asset, and liability risks. Additional work by Bassett (2005) has highlighted sets of contextual, policy, and regulatory risks; commercial risks; market structure risks; and behavioral risks. A revised version of this analysis is presented in table A3.1. Some risks arise from the country and economic context of particular markets and are higher in poorer economies with less stable market, policy, competitive, and regulatory contexts. Others arise from the particular market structure of private and voluntary health insurance markets and the potential behavior of competitors and other stakeholders (such as relative bargaining power of buyers and sellers).

Strengths of voluntary health insurance

Even in high-income countries, it is very difficult to draw generic, empirically based, policy lessons from the experience of voluntary health insurance. The systemwide impact of voluntary health insurance appears to be influenced by a variety of factors, including its functions, the nature and extent of mandated financing, and the extent to which there are binding (and relatively inelastic) constraints on key inputs (such as the number of doctors practicing in a country).

In examining the strengths of voluntary health insurance markets, this section considers both its historical and potential performance. In its study of OECD countries' markets for private health insurance, the OECD concluded that, on balance, private insurance makes the following contributions (OECD 2004)[8]:

- Affords financial protection (compared with out-of-pocket expenditure)
- Enhances access to health services (when mandated financing is incomplete)
- Increases service capacity and promotes innovation
- Helps finance health care services not covered publicly, in the case of supplementary private health insurance.

An alternative approach is to consider the "potential" of voluntary health insurance as a set of financing functions—collection, allocation, pooling, claims administration, and purchasing (of benefits)—that can be (following Kutzin 2001) "integrated within or separated across" (p. 198) both public and private organizations. In these circumstances, the performance of voluntary health insurance can be considered not only in terms of the competence and efficiency with which each financing function is undertaken, but also in terms of the synergies that can be obtained through "vertical integration" (process or ownership) between insurers and providers and through "horizontal integration" with other insurance, financial, or social protection products.

Over the past decade some health insurance companies, particularly in the United States, have been exploring different models of vertical integration, including "staff model" and "contracting" managed care organizations and "preferred provider organizations." Similarly, in other country markets, various combinations of financial products are bundled to reduce marketing and administrative costs. It is, for example, worth noting that in Thailand the great majority of voluntary health insurance is sold as a supplement to life insurance (Pitayarangsarit and Tangcharoensathien 2002).

Kutzin has stressed the benefits that might arise from health insurers' development of an "active purchasing function" in terms of quality assurance (and enhancement) and cost control (and reduction) (Evans 2002, p. 183). To date such benefits have (in the private/voluntary health insurance market) been largely confined to vertically integrated not-for-profit insurers such as Kaiser Permanente in the United States. These types of arrangements often incorporate the providers within their health plan by ownership, salary arrangements, or contracts and are thus able to exert more influence over the quality and quantity of the health care services they cover and finance.

Another benefit of private/voluntary health insurance, often overlooked, is its role in the accumulation of capital and the development of financial markets. Private and voluntary health insurance organizations typically hold between 10 percent and 30 percent of annual premiums in reserves (for future liabilities and shocks)—in cash, bonds, stocks, property, and other investment instruments. Cumulatively, therefore, insurance markets can make a significant contribution to a country's overall savings rate.

Weaknesses of voluntary health insurance

The OECD work concludes that private health insurance markets have generally posed these challenges:

- They have not reduced certain financial barriers to access (such as affordability and price volatility).
- They have increased differential access to health care in some countries (but decreased it in others).
- They have not served as an impetus to quality improvement, with some exceptions.
- They have removed very little cost pressure from public health financing systems.
- They have increased total health expenditure in several OECD countries.
- They have not been able to achieve value-based competition.
- They have generally incurred high administrative costs.

The OECD notes that "there is a complex interplay between competition in health care insurance and delivery markets. . . . Providers' market power in the context of competing insurers affects the extent to which the PHI [private health insurance] market can be expected to promote efficiency and the provision of high-quality care. More competition across insurers does not necessarily result in lower cost if the V/PHI [voluntary/private health insurance] is fragmented in its relationships with providers" (OECD 2004). Although a large market share might enhance an insurer's bargaining clout with providers, this same large share might hinder competition. The OECD also quotes research by Nichols and others (2004) that suggests the importance of an additional contextual factor: "vibrant price and quality competition amongst providers has been identified as a necessary prerequisite of competitive health insurance markets."

Several of the drawbacks of voluntary health insurance markets arise from the related risks of adverse selection and cream skimming. Adverse selection has been defined as "a situation," often resulting from asymmetric information, in which "individuals are able to purchase insurance at rates that are below actuarially fair rates" or as "a process that occurs when individuals with different expected losses are charged the same premium, whereby those with low expected losses drop out of the insurance pool, leaving only individuals with high expected losses" (European Observatory on Health Systems and Policies 2005, citing World Bank 2000 and Witter 1997). The danger of such behavior in a voluntary health insurance market is that it will tend to drive other potential customers out of the market. Adverse selection can be ameliorated by "full underwriting" (that is, prior clinical examination of the insured life's health status), targeted benefit exclusions, and waiting periods prior to benefit entitlement. Yet all of these mechanisms have equity implications (restricting access to, or raising costs for, sicker individuals) and tend to depress demand.

Where adverse selection is present (or perceived as a risk), voluntary health insurance carriers may be tempted to cream skim, that is, to seek to enroll only so-called good risks and avoid enrolling customers whose profile suggests that they may pose the risk of adverse selection. Adverse selection and cream skimming are both behaviors that limit the scope of voluntary health insurance and may undercut the potential for meaningful competition among carriers. Certain regulatory provisions can combat such activity. These include open enrollment provisions, which require insurers to accept all applicants at specified times in the year or throughout the year, and community rating, which prohibits or limits the consideration of health status factors in setting premiums. Yet insurers may resist these regulations on the grounds that they may reduce consumers' motivation to purchase insurance before they need medical services, thereby increasing adverse selection. Hence, governments will need to balance concerns about cream skimming with legitimate concerns about adverse selection. Table 3.1 details some of the regulatory interventions used in voluntary health insurance markets and highlights some of the problems they seek to address.

Relevance of voluntary health insurance in developing countries

Is voluntary health insurance relevant for low- or middle-income countries? The answer may depend on how willing a country's political leaders and policy makers

TABLE 3.1   Instruments to regulate health financing mechanisms not funded by governments in high-, low-, and middle-income countries

Purpose of regulation	High-income countries	Low- and middle-income countries
Establish basic conditions for market exchange		
Solvency of insurance plans	Establish adequate minimum capital and surplus standards	Modest regulation of private health insurance with weak enforcement Huge profits usually made by companies that are able to obtain a license to sell.
	Limit investment options	
	Establish financial reporting requirements	
	Establish standards for long-term actuarial soundness for both private and social insurance	
Sales and marketing practices	Advertising Disclosure of commission rates, limit maximum sales and marketing expenses	Some regulations but weak enforcement
	Content and form of insurance policy	
Perfect when market can't do equitable distribution		
Risk pooling	Require insurance to set premiums on a communitywide basis	Similar laws for social insurance, but weak enforcement
	Compel eligible households to enroll in social insurance plans	
Equity in financing and benefits	Premium based on a percentage of wages in social insurance	Similar
Correct market failures		
Risk selection	Require open enrollment; prohibit medical underwriting	Social insurance is usually regulated, but not private insurance
	Establish risk-adjusted premiums	
	Reinsure high-risk individuals by transferring funds retrospectively from insurers with lower average risks to those with higher risks	
	Require insurance to set premiums on a communitywide basis	
Adverse selection	Disclosure by enrollee of medical history and condition	Very few regulations
Monopolistic pricing	Require minimum loss ratio: that is, pay a minimum percentage of premiums for health service benefits	Very few countries regulate
Correct unacceptable market results		
Free-rider	Compel all eligible people to enroll in social insurance	Same, but less effective enforcement
Cost-effectiveness	Regulate benefit package of compulsory insurance	Similar

Source: Roberts 2004.

are to trade broad equity goals for limited (but better) access for some to personal health services on the basis of ability and willingness to pay. Voluntary health insurance can, in principle, increase financial protection and access to health services for those willing and able to pay. One of the necessary conditions for demand for voluntary health insurance—high levels of out-of-pocket expenses—exists in many low- and middle-income countries (Xu and others 2003). However, as Sekhri and Savedoff (2005) have illustrated, voluntary health insurance represents more than 15 percent of private health expenditures in only a minority of low- and middle-income countries.

Several factors explain at least some of the reasons for the relatively small contribution of voluntary health insurance in out-of-pocket health spending in low- and middle-income countries. First, some out-of-pocket expenditures go to "informal" (illegal) payments to obtain access to notionally prepaid national health service systems or social insurance health services. Second, some go to legal copayments at the point of use to gain access to the same services. Third, some are spent on health care services and pharmaceuticals from providers and suppliers of doubtful technical quality. Multinational health insurers are therefore often reluctant to establish a presence in such markets. Fourth, in some low- and middle-income countries the population willing and able to pay is not sufficiently geographically concentrated to make it practicable to sell or administer voluntary health insurance. Finally, in some low- and middle-income countries, formal financial service sectors in general and insurance markets in particular are still in their infancy, and people are wary of investing in a product of uncertain personal benefit.

In these contexts, it could be challenging to establish an organization with the whole range of competencies required to administer a full-fledged voluntary health insurance scheme. Actuarial and accounting skills are in particularly short supply. Furthermore, many insurers are hesitant to enter a market without an established regulatory system because the rules of the game are unclear. Governments therefore need to invest in the establishment of a regulatory infrastructure to encourage the development of the market and a fair, competitive landscape.

In some low- and middle-income countries, policy makers might seek to constrain the allowed roles or performance of voluntary health insurance because of concerns that such a financing mechanism would either diminish support for alternative (mandated) health financing mechanisms or that voluntary health insurance would capture a disproportionately large proportion of the available human resources (such as doctors and nurses). The elasticity of the supply of clinical personnel will affect the potential risk in this area.

Feasibility of voluntary health insurance in developing countries

Is voluntary health insurance a feasible health financing mechanism in low- and middle-income countries? Should policy makers be encouraged to develop the role of voluntary health insurance in countries where there are significant and intractable gaps in effective population coverage or technical capacity in mandated health financing schemes?

In low-income countries, only a minority of the population is likely to be willing and able to afford unsubsidized voluntary health insurance. This constraint at least partly explains why voluntary health insurance entities have limited presence in many developing countries. In Accra, Ghana, for example, there is just one small private health insurance business (run by a medically qualified entrepreneur) aimed at middle-class professionals working in the city's financial sector (Atim and others 2001). Nonetheless, even in low-income countries, some voluntary health insurance presence does exist. A WHO report identified 38 countries where private health insurance contributed more than 5 percent of total health expenditures. Nearly half of these are in low- and lower-middle-income countries (Sekhri, Savedoff, and Tripathi 2005).

In middle-income countries with large literate and mobile urban populations, voluntary health insurance becomes a more plausible instrument as either a primary or additional source of health financing. In fact, in some countries, such as Brazil, Chile, Namibia, South Africa, and Zimbabwe, private health insurance contributes more than 20 percent to total health spending (Sekhri, Savedoff, and Tripathi 2005).

Employer-based or affinity group insurance schemes are likely to raise fewer challenges (and to be more financially stable) than individual subscription schemes, which tend to attract a disproportionate number of high-risk subscribers—the problem of adverse selection. Risk-rated premiums, medical examination before contract, and waiting or qualifying periods are reliable and well-tested market mechanisms for controlling adverse selection, but they do not address access concerns and may not be the most appropriate solutions in all cases.

Among the documented market failures of voluntary health insurance markets, some of the most problematic for policy makers in developing countries are those that worsen inequalities in care and access for the poor (Sekhri, Savedoff, and Tripathi 2005). Concerns about the equity effects of voluntary health insurance can be addressed through a variety of policy instruments, including tapered premium subsidies from public funds, limits on allowed functions or roles for such coverage within the health system, controls on access to public service providers, and regulation of the issuance of insurance products, as well as their content and price. Private health insurance is also often associated with high administrative costs, although the extent and nature of these costs vary by country, type of insurance, and insurer (OECD 2004). These costs can include billing, medical underwriting (where permitted), agents' commissions, distribution, marketing, and other expenses. Fraud and abuse may become a concern, as it has sometimes in public coverage programs, and regulatory systems must also have provisions to prohibit false claims. Therefore, policy makers wishing to establish or encourage a voluntary health insurance market will need to anticipate the overall impact of voluntary health insurance on the demand for and supply of health services and address any anticipated bottlenecks. Policy makers will also need to establish effective mechanisms for regulating voluntary health insurance and related markets.

Regulatory frameworks for voluntary health insurance

This section provides an overview of frameworks for regulating voluntary health insurance when insurance is provided through competing nongovernment carriers. It identifies key regulatory questions and describes some experience with regulation in developed and developing countries.

The term "regulation" can be used narrowly to mean the instruments by which governments implement legislative requirements. It can also be used in a broader sense to "include the full range of legal instruments by which governing institutions, at all levels of government, impose obligations or constraints on private sector behavior. Constitutions, parliamentary laws, subordinate legislation, decrees, orders, norms, licenses, plans, codes, and even some forms of administrative guidance can all be considered 'regulation'" (OECD 1995, p. 20). This section discusses regulation in its broader sense.

Regulation of voluntary health insurance encompasses principles of both health care and financial regulation. Roberts (2004) cites the following four fundamental objectives of health care regulation; these broad objectives encompass many of the key goals behind the regulation of voluntary health insurance markets:

1. To ensure that market exchanges and transactions are done honestly and openly;
2. To rectify market failures;
3. To deal with the unequal distribution of income and variations in health needs (differences in endowments);
4. To constrain market results on ethical grounds (organ sales).

In simple terms, objectives 1 and 2 can be regarded as the financial or market-related objectives, and 3 and 4, as the equity objectives of health care regulation. Yet, in some cases, market failures within voluntary health insurance markets result in inequitable access to coverage; thus, the consequences of market failures are not limited to financial issues. Some regulators of voluntary health insurance markets focus on the financial pieces of regulation, but it is recommended that policy makers consider the equity and health care challenges that can arise within voluntary health insurance markets and make explicit decisions with respect to whether and to what extent they wish to tackle them through regulation.

The structure of regulation. The traditional approach to regulation has been institutional; that is, it has assigned separate regulatory agencies to each category of institution or sector (or both). This approach is coming under pressure for three reasons. First, regulatory frameworks within market economies tend to have at least three tiers: the general framework of civil and criminal law, sector-specific regulation, and the regulation of private firms (competition, advertising, consumer protection, and so on) (Jones 1994). Second, some financial and health care suppliers (known as conglomerates) are integrating both horizontally into related markets and vertically up and down the supply chain (as when health insurers purchase hospitals), posing challenges to this traditional model. Third, as cited by Carmichael and Pomerleano (2002, p. 40), there is legitimate concern about "regulatory arbitrage"—the attempt to select institutional forms to exploit (and gain competitive and financial advantages from) differences in regulation that apply to institutionally distinct suppliers operating in a single market.

Countries tend to employ various regulatory models in their oversight of voluntary health insurance markets. Private health insurers are often regulated, at least in part, by the same regulator as other lines of insurance, particularly in the area of plan solvency. The OECD study on private health insurance found that there was a trend among OECD countries to regulate according to entities' activities and functions, rather than by the type of entity (for-profit, not-for-profit) (OECD 2004). This trend probably stems from the potential for entities to otherwise exploit institutionally based regulation. These regulators are often, although not always, located within the ministry of finance or a similar agency. In addition, health care regulators often play a role in the regulation of voluntary health insurance, as is the case in Mexico and the Netherlands. In some cases, as in Australia, Ireland, and some U.S. states, the health authorities are the main regulators of such insurance, generally with support from financial regulators relating to the financial aspects of the market and carriers (OECD 2004, table 3.17). Uruguay has divided its regulatory responsibilities for voluntary health insurance between two agencies: the Ministry of Public Health monitors the operations of nonprofit institutions, whereas the Ministry of Economy and Finance oversees for-profit insurers.

In general, voluntary health insurance markets are rarely under the sole control of a single oversight body. A full range of issues, including competition, antitrust, consumer protection, and advertising, touch on the activities of voluntary health insurance carriers. Hence, it is likely that multiple players will be involved in regulation. However, the extent to which the health system issues are actively addressed by regulation varies greatly across countries and is a product of resources, expertise, and governmental priorities, among other factors.

Regulatory "backing" and implementation The effectiveness of a regulator is determined by its ability to address its regulatory objectives in a timely and cost-effective manner. Regulators require high-level political support, legislative backing (including powers of enforcement), adequate funding, and a strong skills base (Carmichael and Pomerleano 2002). Only then can they effectively implement regulations.

Roberts has used his analysis of the objectives of health care regulation to develop a specific tabulation of instruments used in both high-income and low- and middle-income countries to regulate financing mechanisms that are not funded by the government (table 3.1). Many of Roberts' regulatory instruments are designed to address the unequal distribution of income and the variations in health needs and the resulting consequences of such redistributive instruments (such as increased adverse selection). He also identifies measures that can help correct market failures common in voluntary health insurance markets, such as risk selection, adverse selection, and problematic pricing mechanisms, all of which also have equity and distributive effects.

Table 3.1 includes many key features of voluntary health insurance regulatory frameworks and indicates that, in Roberts' review, many key protections are not in place or are weakly enforced in low- and middle-income countries. The scope and content of voluntary health insurance regulatory frameworks in developing countries is still not well understood and could benefit from further research and analysis.

In contrast, developed countries tend to have more advanced voluntary health insurance regulatory frameworks, although they do not always touch on the full range of issues highlighted in Roberts' analysis. The OECD examined the scope and type of private health insurance regulations found in OECD countries. It found that the scope of regulation varied significantly and, in European countries, was limited by European Union insurance directives. As a general matter, the role played by such insurance within the nation's health coverage system had a significant impact on the depth and breadth of government involvement in this sector. Areas addressed under some countries' private health insurance regulatory frameworks include the following (OECD 2004):

- Access to coverage
- Adverse selection
- Benefits package
- Premiums and price regulation
- Disclosure
- Tax or other fiscal incentives or subsidies to purchase
- Prudential and financial requirements
- Regulation of consumer complaints or inquiries

The imposition of access and premium requirements has been most controversial in markets where health insurance products are marketed through individuals, rather than employers, because the potential for adverse selection, for "premium spirals" (whereby lower-risk persons drop out in response to premium prices, initiating a downward spiral of enrollment and an upward spiral of premium costs), and for persons to opportunistically purchase cover (when they foresee a need for a medical service) are particularly high. Heated debates have surrounded the extent to which premium and access standards may hinder broad purchase of coverage and increase costs in a voluntary market where such standards tend to protect those of higher risk. However, in the absence of such standards or voluntary industry practices that favor broad nondiscriminatory issuance of policies, it is difficult to ensure that voluntary health insurance products can be purchased by higher-risk individuals at an affordable cost. This issue is one of the key dilemmas facing regulators of private health insurance markets.

Nonetheless, some have argued that many types of regulations on voluntary health insurance contracts diminish the efficiency of such markets. Zwiefel, Krey, and Tagli (forthcoming) find that some measures used in OECD countries, such as imposed premiums, obligations to provide certain products or benefits, and product approval, have effects that tend to run counter to proper market incentives and competition. Zwiefel, Krey and Tagli favor a focus on capital and liquidity requirements, information disclosure requirements to regulators and consumers, and standard accounting and auditing requirements. However, they indicate that a mandatory risk adjustment scheme among insurers can complement premium regulation and help avoid cream skimming by insurers. This approach has been controversial in certain markets, where the industry has argued it is anticompetitive. The relative competitive and efficiency merits of many voluntary health insurance regulations are often the subject of differing viewpoints and may depend on the particular traits of the insurance and health care markets in which they are implemented, as well as on the goals of policy makers and regulators.

A fundamental policy decision with major implications for the scope and nature of the regulatory task is whether to impose redistributive goals on voluntary health insurance and, if so, whether the redistribution is to occur between known high risks and low risks, between rich and poor, or between dependent and workingage populations. The imposition of related standards—such as standards for access or premiums—may have consequences for the profile of likely purchasers, as well as for the financial health of the plans. These consequences need to be considered and an effort made to counter their potential negative effects through particular instruments within the regulatory scheme.

Ultimately, the balance between mandated and voluntary health financing mechanisms and the gradient of redistribution (and other constraints) in each segment must be a matter of sovereign decision making by individual governments on the basis of their revenue-raising ability, the population's willingness to purchase voluntary health insurance, and the country's regulatory capacity, among other factors. In low- and middle-income countries, salient concerns also include whether limited public funding for health should be devoted to voluntary health insurance schemes that often cover the comparatively better off, or whether such resources are better spent on direct financial support for services for the poorest and most vulnerable populations.

Annex 3.1   The four types of financial risk in voluntary/private health insurance

TABLE A3.1   Selected risks in voluntary/private health insurance

Sources of risk	Financial risk type			
Contextual, policy, and regulatory risks	Income risk	Expenditure risk	Asset risk	Liability risk
Public policy risks				
Poor economy—low and unstable growth	risk increases	*	risk increases	*
High and unstable burden of disease	*	risk increases	*	risk increases
Demography—dependent population increasing	risk increases	risk increases	*	*
Unclear or unstable public policy context and allowed roles	risk increases	risk increases	*	*
Unstable or heavy regulation	*	risk increases	*	risk increases
Low control over composition of benefit package	risk increases	risk increases	*	*
Low control over price of benefit package and/or low loading	risk increases	*	*	risk increases
Market structure risks				
Low concentration of supply	risk increases	*	*	*
Degree of competitor horizontal integration	risk increases	*	*	*
Degree of competitor vertical integration	*	risk increases	*	*
Behavioral risks				
Abuse and fraud	risk increases	risk increases	risk increases	risk increases
Moral hazard	risk increases	risk increases	*	risk increases
Adverse selection	risk increases	risk increases	*	risk increases
Commercial risks				
Low risk aversion	risk increases	*	*	*
High diversity of preferences	risk increases	*	*	*
Low pool size	risk increases	*	*	*
Low control over utilization	*	risk increases	*	*
Low control over provider payments	*	risk increases	*	risk increases
Low density of provision	risk increases	*	*	*
High density of provision	*	risk increases	*	*
Barriers to exit	*	risk increases	risk increases	risk increases
Threat of new entrants	risk increases	*	*	*
Threat of substitute products	risk increases	*	*	*
Bargaining power—suppliers	*	risk increases	*	*
Bargaining power—buyers	risk increases	*	*	*

Source: Authors.

Note: * denotes no impact.

The categorization of selected risks in voluntary/private health insurance by their source and financial type (table A3.1) aims to help insurers, policy makers, and regulators profile the existing or likely risks under different conditions.

For the sources of risk, one evaluative framework proposes five main elements: public policy, demand, market structure, behavior, and performance (Mossialos and Thomson 2002). The public policy, market structure, and behavior categories are used here. The fourth source of risk in the table, "commercial risks," comprise the risks that insurance carriers assume from consumers, service providers, and competitors. The bottom five commercial risks—barriers to exit and so on—are from "five competitive forces" (Porter 1980).

For the financial risks borne by voluntary/private health insurance, Bowie and Adams (2005) categorize such risks according to their major accounting categories: income, expenditure, and assets and liabilities. Income risks reduce the likely income of a voluntary/public health insurance scheme. Expenditure risks increase such schemes' likely expenditures in the present financial year. Liabilities refer to the expenditure risks such schemes face in future financial years. All financial risks can, indirectly and cumulatively, become risks to the assets of a scheme. Table A3.1 highlights only risks that are "direct" risks to scheme assets.

Assets can be divided into three major categories: cash, investment assets, and other assets. The key features of "investment assets" are their security, return, and liquidity. "Other assets" are often held in property or in businesses that support or complement the core insurance businesses. An example of "other assets" held by voluntary/private health insurers in developing countries includes an ownership or "controlling" interest in a piece of the pharmaceutical supply chain—to ensure the reliable, efficient, and quality-assured supply of this key health care resource funded by such voluntary/private health insurance carriers.

Liabilities can also be divided into three main categories: outstanding claims, unearned income, and unexpired risk. Unearned income refers to premiums received for future time periods. Unexpired risk is a provision for any anticipated difference between the expected costs of future claims and the unearned premium reserve, when the latter is not expected to cover all liabilities (for example, tough winter months in temperate climates).

Endnotes

1. Beveridge wrote, "Benefit in return for contributions, rather than free allowance from the State, is what the people of Britain desire."

2. The model is applied to 149 countries using general taxation financing, social health insurance, or a mixed system, with no differences in terms of results for each type of system.

3. Based on 238 cases for which data were available, the ILO and STEP study (2002) found that 94 percent of the schemes had prepayment mechanisms.

4. Examples include the Chagoria Hospital plan in Kenya, Kisiizi in Uganda, and the Evangelican Lutheran Church of Tanzania plan.

5. CBHOs, or community-based health organizations, is the term used by the ILO and STEP report for community-based health insurances.

6. Another dimension, dignity, was proposed for the evaluation, but insufficient evidence was found to make a determination.

7. This section is based mainly on a theoretical analysis of community-based health insurance. Indeed, very little empirical evidence exists on the longevity of community-based health insurance schemes, because most are very recent and because the literature focuses mostly on surviving schemes (ILO and STEP 2002).

8. All following quotations in this section are taken from OECD 2004, p. 94–167. A synopsis of the longer OECD work is found in Tapay and Colombo (2004).

References

Atim, C. 1998. *The Contribution of Mutual Organizations to Financing, Delivery, and Access to Health Care: Synthesis and Research in Nine West and Central African Countries.* Bethesda, Md.: Abt Associates Inc., Partnerships for Health Reform Project.

Atim, C., S. Grey, P. Apoya, S. Anie, and M. Aikins. 2001. *A Survey of Health Financing Schemes in Ghana.* Bethesda, Md.: Abt Associates.

Bärnighausen, T., and R. Sauerborn. 2002. "One Hundred and Eighteen Years of the German Health Insurance System: Are There Any Lessons for Middle- and Low-Income Countries?" *Social Science and Medicine* 54 (10): 1559–87.

Bassett, M. 2005. "Voluntary Health Insurance in Development." Paper presented at the Conference on Private Health Insurance in Developing Countries, Wharton Business School, University of Pennsylvania, March 15–16, Philadelphia [http://hc.wharton .upenn.edu/impactconference/presentations.html].

Bennett, S., A. Creese, and R. Monash. 1998. *Health Insurance Schemes for People Outside Formal Sector Employment.* Discussion of Analysis, Research, and Assessment, Paper 16. Geneva: World Health Organization.

Bennett, S., A. G. Kelley, and B. Silvers. 2004. *21 Questions on CBHF: An Overview of Community-Based Health Financing.* Bethesda, Md.: Abt Associates, Inc., Partnerships for Health Reform Project.

Beveridge, W. 1942. *Social Insurance and Allied Service.* London: His Majesty's Stationery Office.

Bowie, R., and G. Adams. 2005. "Financial and Management Practice in a Voluntary Medical Insurance Company in the Developed World." Background paper for the Conference on Private Health Insurance in Developing Countries, Wharton Business School, University of Pennsylvania, March 15–16, Philadelphia.

Busse, R., R. Saltman, and H. Dubois. 2004. "Organization and Financing of Social Health Insurance: Current Status and Recent Policy Development." In R. B. Saltman, R. Busse, and J. Figueras, eds., *Social Health Insurance Systems in Western Europe.* European Observatory on Health Systems and Policies. Berkshire, U.K.: Open University Press.

Carmichael, J., and M. Pomerleano. 2002. *The Development and Regulation of Non-Bank Financial Institutions.* Washington, D.C.: World Bank.

Carrin, G. 2002. "Social Health Insurance in Developing Countries: A Continuing Challenge." *International Social Security Review* 55 (2): 57–69.

Carrin, G., and C. James. 2003. "Determinants of Achieving Universal Coverage of Health Care: An Empirical Analysis." In Martine Audibert, Jacky Mathonnat, and Eric De Roodenbeke, eds., *Le financement de la santé dans les pays d'Afrique et d'Asie à faible revenu.* Paris: Karthala.

————. 2004. "Social Health Insurance as a Pathway to Universal Coverage: Key Design Features in the Transition Period." Health Financing Technical Paper, World Health Organization, Geneva.

Castro-Leal, F., J. Dayton, L. Demery, and K. Mehra. 1999. "Public Social Spending in Africa: Do the Poor Benefit?" *The World Bank Research Observer* 14 (1): 49–72.

Cataneda, T. 2003. "Targeting Social Spending to the Poor with Proxy-Means Testing: Columbia's SISBEN System." World Bank, Washington, D.C.

Conn, C. P., and V. Walford. 1998. *An Introduction to Health Insurance for Low-Income Countries.* London: U.K. Department for International Development.

Dror, D., and A. Preker. 2004. *Social Re-Insurance: A New Approach to Sustainable Community Health Financing.* Geneva: World Bank. International Labour Organization; Washington, D.C.: World Bank.

Ekman, B. 2004. "Community-Based Health Insurance in Low-Income Countries: A Systematic Review of the Evidence." *Health Policy and Planning* 19 (5): 249–70.

Ensor, T. 1999. "Developing Health Insurance in Transitional Asia." *Social Science and Medicine* 48 (7): 871–9.

Enthoven, A. C. 1985. *Reflections on the Management of the National Health Service: An American Looks at Incentives to Efficiency in Health Services Management in the U.K.* London: Nuffield Provincial Hospitals Trust.

Escobar, M-L. 2005. "The Columbia Health Sector and the Poor." World Bank, Washington, D.C.

Escobar, M-L., and P. Panapoulou. 2002. "Health." In M. M. Giugale, O. Lafourcade, and C. Luff, eds., *Columbia: The Economic Foundations for Peace.* Washington, D.C.: World Bank.

European Observatory on Health Systems and Policies. 2005. "Glossary." www.euro.who. int/observatory/glossary/toppage.

Evans, R. G. 2002. "Funding Health Care: Taxation and the Alternatives." In E. Mossialos, A. Dixon, J. Figueras, and J. Kutzin, eds., *Funding Health Care: Options for Europe.* Buckingham: Open University Press.

GTZ (Deutsche Gesellschaft für Technische Zusammenarbeit). 2004. *Social Health Insurance—Systems of Solidarity: Experiences from German Development Cooperation.* Eschborn, Germany.

Holley, J., O. Akhundov, and E. Nolte. 2004. *Health Care Systems in Transition: Azerbaijan.* World Health Organization Regional Office for Europe on behalf of the European Observatory on Health Systems and Policies, Copenhagen.

Hsiao, W. 2001. "Unmet Health Needs of Two Billion: Is Community Financing a Solution?" Health, Nutrition, and Population Discussion Paper, World Bank, Washington, D.C.

ILO (International Labour Office). 2005. *Global Employment Trends.* Geneva.

ILO and ISSA (International Social Security Association). 1999. *Social Health Insurance.* Geneva.

ILO and STEP (Strategies and Tools against Exclusion and Poverty). 2002. "Extending Social Protection in Health through Community-Based Health Organizations." Discussion Paper, Geneva.

Jakab, M., and C. Krishnan. 2004. "Review of the Strengths and Weaknesses of Community Financing." In A. Preker and G. Carrin, eds., *Health Financing for Poor People: Resource Mobilization and Risk Sharing.* World Bank, Washington, D.C.

Jones, B. 1994. *Politics U.K.* New York: Harvester Wheatsheaf.

Kutzin, J. 2001. "A Descriptive Framework for Country-Level Analysis of Health Care Financing Arrangements." *Health Policy* 56 (3): 171–204.

Langenbrunner, J. 2005. "Health Care Financing and Purchasing in ECA: An Overview of Issues and Reforms." Unpublished paper, World Bank, Washington, D.C.

McKee, M., D. Delnoij, and H. Brand. 2004. "Prevention and Public Health in Social Health Insurance Systems." In R. B. Saltman, R. Busse, and J. Figueras, eds., *Social Health Insurance Systems in Western Europe.* European Observatory on Health Systems and Policies. Berkshire, U.K.: Open University Press.

Mossialos, E., and A. Dixon. 2002. "Funding Health Care in Europe: Weighing Up the Options." In E. Mossialos, A. Dixon, J. Figueras, and J. Kutzin, eds., *Funding Health Care: Options for Europe.* European Observatory on Health Systems and Policies. Berkshire, U.K.: Open University Press.

Mossialos, E., and S. Thomson. 2002. "Voluntary Health Insurance in the European Union." Report prepared for the Directorate General for Employment and Social Affairs of the European Commission, Brussels.

MSH (Management Sciences for Health). 2000. *Social Insurance Assessment Tool.* Boston, Mass.

Nichols, L. M., P. Ginsburg, R. Berenson, J. Christianson, and R. Hurley. 2004. "Are Market Forces Strong Enough to Deliver Efficient Health Care Systems? Confidence Is Waning." *Health Affairs* 23 (2): 8–21.

Normand, C., and R. Busse. 2002. "Social Health Insurance Financing." In E. Mossialos, A. Dixon, J. Figueras, and J. Kutzin, eds., *Funding Health Care: Options for Europe.* European Observatory on Health Systems and Policies. Berkshire, U.K.: Open University Press.

Normand, C., and C. Weber. 1994. *Social Health Insurance: A Guidebook for Planning.* Geneva: World Health Organization and International Labour Office.

OECD (Organisation for Economic Co-operation and Development). 1995. *Recommendation of the Council of the OECD on Improving the Quality of Government Regulation.* Basel, Switzerland.

————. 2004. *Private Health Insurance in OECD Countries.* N. Tapay and F. Colombo, co-authors. Paris.

Pitayarangsarit, S., and V. Tangcharoensathien. 2002. "Private Health Insurance." In P. Pramualratana and S. Wisbulpolprasert, eds., *Health Insurance Systems in Thailand.* Nonthaburi, Thailand: Health Systems Research Institute.

Porter, M. E. 1980. *Competitive Strategy: Techniques for Analyzing Industries and Competitors.* New York: Free Press.

Preker, A., G. Carrin, D. Dro, M. Jakab, W. Hsiao, and D. Arhin-Tenkorang. 2004. "Rich-Poor Differences in Health Care Financing." In A. Preker and G. Carrin, eds., *Health Financing for Poor People: Resource Mobilization and Risk Sharing.* Washington, D.C.: World Bank.

Roberts, M. J. 2004. *Getting Health Reform Right: A Guide to Improving Performance and Equity.* New York: Oxford University Press.

Ron, A., B. Abel-Smith, and G. Tamburi. 1990. *Health Insurance in Developing Countries: The Social Security Approach.* Geneva: International Labour Office.

Saltman, R. B. 2004. "Social Health Insurance in Perspective: The Challenge of Sustaining Stability." In R. B. Saltman, R. Busse, and J. Figueras, eds., *Social Health Insurance Systems in Western Europe.* European Observatory on Health Systems and Policies. Berkshire, U.K.: Open University Press.

Savedoff, W. D. 2004a. "Is There a Case for Social Insurance?" *Health Policy and Planning* 19 (3): 183–84.

———. 2004b. "Tax-Based Financing for Health Systems: Options and Experiences." Health Financing Policy Issue Paper, World Health Organization, Geneva.

———. 2005. "Mandatory Health Insurance in Developing Countries: Overview, Framework, and Research Program." Health, Nutrition and Population Team, World Bank, Washington, D.C.

Schieber, G., and A. Maeda. 1997. "A Curmudgeon's Guide to Financing Health in Developing Countries." In G. Schieber, ed., "Innovations in Health Care Financing." Discussion Paper 365, World Bank, Washington, D.C.

Sekhri, N., and W. Savedoff. 2005. "Private Health Insurance: Implications for Developing Countries." *Bulletin for the World Health Organization* 83 (2): 127–34.

Sekhri, N., W. Savedoff, and S. Tripathi. 2005. "Regulating Private Insurance to Serve the Public Interest: Policy Issues for Developing Countries." World Health Organization, Geneva.

Tabor, S. 2005. "Community-Based Health Insurance and Social Protection Policy." Social Protection Discussion Paper Series, World Bank, Washington, D.C.

Tapay, N., and F. Colombo. 2004. "Private Health Insurance in OECD Countries: The Benefits and Costs for Individuals and Health Systems." In *Towards High Performing Health Systems-Policy Studies.* Paris: Organisation for Economic Co-operation and Development.

U.K. Department of Health. 2005. *Departmental Report 2005.* London: Her Majesty's Stationery Office.

Waelkens, M-P., and C. Criel. 2004. "Les mutuelles de santé en Afrique sub-saharienne. Etat des lieux et réflexions sur un agenda de recherche." Health, Nutrition, and Population, Discussion Paper, World Bank, Washington, D.C.

Wagstaff, A., and M. Claeson. 2004. *The Millennium Development Goals for Health: Rising to the Challenges.* Washington, D.C.: World Bank.

WHO (World Health Organization). 2000. *The World Health Report 2000: Health Systems: Improving Performance.* Geneva.

————. 2001. *Report of the Commission on Macroeconomics and Health: Investing in Health for Economic Development.* Geneva.

————. 2002. *Mobilization of Domestic Resources for Health. Report of the Commission on Macroeconomics and Health: Investing in Health for Economic Development.* Geneva.

————. 2004. *The World Health Report 2004: Changing History.* Geneva.

Witter, S. 1997. (cited in European Observatory on Health Systems and Policies 2005)

World Bank. 2000. (cited in European Observatory on Health Systems and Policies 2005)

World Bank. 2004. *World Development Report 2004.* Washington, D.C.

————. 2005. *Azerbaijan Republic Poverty Assessment. Vol II: The Main Report.* Washington, D.C.

Xu, K., D. B. Evans, K. Kawabata, R. Zaramdini, J. Klavus, and C. J. L. Murray. 2003. "Household Catastrophic Health Expenditure: A Multicountry Analysis." *Lancet* 362 (9378): 111–7.

Zweifel, P., B. Krey, and M. Tagli. Forthcoming. *Private Voluntary Health Insurance in Developing Countries: Supply.* Health, Nutrition, and Population, Discussion Paper, World Bank, Washington, D.C. [http://hc.wharton.upenn.edu/impactconference/presentations.html].

4

External assistance for health

Donor countries, international organizations, and development agencies will need to commit billions of dollars of additional external assistance to enable low-income countries to reach the Millennium Development Goals. Yet, recent increases in such assistance have fallen short of commitments, and even the funds that have been made available have posed problems for recipient countries. Timing is often unpredictable, exchange rates are volatile, loan and grant maturity periods are too short, and aid is not well aligned with the country's own budget processes and health priorities. For additional assistance to be effective, donors must be willing to make more flexible, long-term commitments that are integrated with the recipient's development goals, and recipient countries must work to increase their accountability and absorptive capacity.

External assistance for health, in the form of development assistance specifically for health interventions (referred to as health aid), and overall official development assistance are important components of health financing, particularly in low-income countries. Massive increases in health aid are needed for countries to reach the Millennium Development Goals. The global estimates of what it would cost to achieve the health Millennium Development Goals range from an additional $25 billion to $70 billion a year, much of which must come in the form of aid. This chapter reviews the recent trends in development assistance broadly, as well as private financial flows to low- and middle-income countries. With regard to aid specifically for health interventions, it assesses the increasing diversity of donors, programs, and resources. It also examines the effectiveness and sustainability of aid from the perspective of donors and recipients—particularly the need for donors to make their commitments predictable and fungible within the recipient country's budget and for recipients to increase their capacity to absorb and be accountable for additional funds.

Official development assistance reached $70 billion in 2003, barely higher in real terms than in 1992. Recent increases are largely due to increases in health aid, which has grown through the increasing presence of global partnerships, such as the Global Fund to Fight AIDS, Tuberculosis, and Malaria and the Global Alliance for Vaccines and Immunization, as well as private foundations. Despite the increases, total official development assistance is only at about 0.25 percent of gross national income in Organisation for Economic Co-operation and Development (OECD) countries, far short of the 0.7 percent those nations set as a goal at an international conference in Monterrey, Mexico, in 2002.

Although health aid increased to more than $10 billion in 2003 from $2.6 billion in 1990, estimates indicate that between three and seven times that much would be needed to reach the Millennium Development Goals for health. It is unclear whether the commitments will be met in terms of amount and duration required, at least in the short run. Meanwhile, recipient countries face budget constraints, and expectations of large amounts of additional official development assistance may be preventing them from making the difficult choices needed in resource-constrained environments.

Official development assistance in general, and health aid in particular, have been criticized for unpredictability of funding; proliferation of disease- and intervention-specific programs, which are often not integrated into any particular country's on-going programs; large numbers of new actors and donors; inflexibility of aid for dealing with sudden problems and crises; and lack of accountability of donors for the absence of results and progress. These problems reduce the impact of donor funding in achieving economic growth and health improvements, which is explored in detail in the next chapter.

The problems identified with aid lead to the following conclusions and recommendations:

- The flow of aid can be volatile for many reasons, including exchange rate fluctuations, political and budgetary decisions by donors, administrative delays on the donor's side, problems of absorptive capacity in the recipient country, and noncompliance with agreed conditionalities. Thus, there can be no single instrument or solution to the volatility issue; rather, the problem must be solved by tackling each source of volatility.

- Fiscal sustainability requires consideration of the fiscal contingencies generated by the volatility of donor funding. It should also motivate appropriate accountability by donors and improved capacity to use domestic resources to finance the increased expenditures initially funded by donors.

- The maturity of donor commitments must be long, in many cases more than 20 years, depending on the magnitude of the increased expenditures and the recipient country's ability to raise additional domestic revenues.

- Donor funding should increasingly be provided through budget support and aligned with increases in domestic resources over the program period.

- On the recipient side, there must be efforts to improve public expenditure management, governance, and accountability. Health plans must align with the country's broader poverty reduction strategy, medium-term expenditure framework, and monitoring and evaluation systems. Chapter 7 develops these issues further.

- Private capital flows from foreign direct investment and workers' remittances, which amount to some $250 billion each year, have been largely overlooked as a source of health financing, especially in middle-income countries. If the Millennium Development Goals are to be reached, official development assistance, particularly technical assistance, should emphasize the need for appropriate policies and institutions to attract foreign direct investment to both middle- and low-income countries, as well as effective mechanisms for using workers' remittances. The emphasis on grant financing, although important, should not divert attention from these other fundamental private sources of sustainable financing for development.

Trends in official development assistance

The current international development architecture responsible for the financing and management of official development assistance is a complicated structure including the International Monetary Fund (IMF), the World Bank, more than 20 regional development banks, some 40 bilateral development agencies, the United Nations family of organizations, thousands of large and small nongovernmental organizations, and numerous private foundations. As never before in its 50-year history, the international development system is now bringing together the state, the private sector, and civil society in complex interactions that will determine the success or failure of future development efforts. Harmonization is necessary for success in achieving the Millennium Development Goals. However, the increasing number of players in the development scene makes such harmonization increasingly difficult (Sagasti, Bezanson, and Prada 2005).

The Asian financial crisis of 1997, the Russian crisis of 1997–2000, the more recent Argentine debt default, the impact of HIV/AIDS across the world but especially in Africa, and the global public health scares of new diseases such as SARS and avian flu have led to a realization of the need to revamp international aid in a global world and to reverse the decline of official development assistance. This perception was strongly reinforced by the terrorist attacks in September 2001, which have increased global awareness of the need to deal with inequality to increase the world's security. Actions to create a new global partnership are reflected in the UN's Millennium Development Goals of 2000, the "Monterrey Consensus" on financial development and the Johannesburg Summit on Sustainable Development in 2002, and the New Partnership for Africa's Development. These renewed efforts to revamp international development have also been reflected in the recent increases in official development assistance.

After declining about 25 percent in real terms over the 1990s, official development assistance started to recuperate in 1998, reaching $70 billion in 2003—barely higher in real terms than in 1992 (figure 4.1).[1] Official development assistance to developing countries increased in real terms by 7 percent in 2002 and

FIGURE 4.1   **Actual and projected official development assistance, 1990–2010**

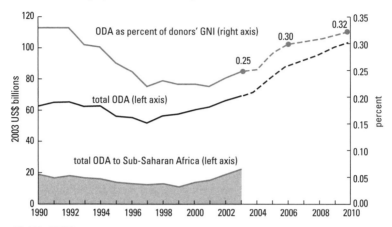

Source: World Bank 2005b.
Note: Dashed lines indicate projections of official development assistance (ODA) based on commitments made by members of OECD's Development Assistance Committee following the 2002 UN conference in Monterrey, Mexico.

by 3.9 percent in 2003.[2] As a percentage of gross national income in OECD countries, assistance declined from 0.34 percent in 1992 to 0.22 percent in 2001 before increasing slightly in 2003 to 0.25 percent.

The increases in official development assistance over the past five years have not been directed toward financing efforts to reach the Millennium Development Goals, but rather have concentrated mostly on debt relief, emergency and disaster relief, technical cooperation, and administrative overhead. Of the total nominal increase between 2001 and 2003, 66 percent went to debt relief and technical cooperation (World Bank 2005b).

Sub-Saharan Africa offers a unique example of the importance of official development assistance (figure 4.2). While this region historically received approximately 20 percent of total official assistance, countries in this region received 54 percent of the total increase in such assistance between 2001 and 2003. Official development assistance is the main source of external finance in Sub-Saharan Africa, representing more than 55 percent of total external flows of about $41 billion that these countries received in 2003. Foreign direct investment represented another 25 percent of the total long-term flows, remittances 15 percent, and other private flows 5 percent. In other regions, where foreign direct investment and remittances account for the bulk of external financial flows, official development assistance accounts for only 9 percent of such flows.

Two trends in official development assistance need special review because of their importance for the health sector: promises to provide more official development assistance and find new sources of finance and mechanisms for disbursing official development assistance.

FIGURE 4.2   Long-term capital flows to Sub-Saharan Africa and the rest of the developing countries, 2003

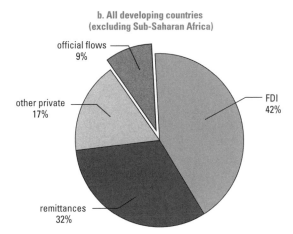

a. Sub-Saharan Africa

official flows
55%

other private
5%

remittances
15%

FDI
25%

b. All developing countries
(excluding Sub-Saharan Africa)

official flows
9%

other private
17%

remittances
32%

FDI
42%

Source: World Bank 2005b.

Promises of more aid and new financing methods

Many countries are struggling to meet the promises they made to increase official development assistance. For example, of all OECD countries, only five (Denmark, Luxemburg, the Netherlands, Norway, and Sweden) have reached or passed the goal established at Monterrey of 0.7 percent of gross national income. Moreover, countries in the European Community are facing difficulties living up to the much less ambitious commitment of 0.33 percent to be reached by 2006. The large fiscal deficits of several donor countries and the relatively slow growth of official development assistance in real terms create room for doubt regarding the firmness of the promises for more aid to developing countries.[3]

Yet, more recently at the July 2005 meeting of the Group of Eight (G-8) nations in Gleneagles, Scotland, the G-8 promised that aid for all developing countries will increase by around $50 billion a year by 2010, of which at least $25 billion extra a year would go to Africa (G-8 2005). France, Germany, Italy, the United Kingdom, and the European Union all reconfirmed their commitments to reach a 0.7 percent ratio by 2015. The United States proposed to double aid to Sub-Saharan Africa between 2004 and 2010 but specified no commitment to aid as a percentage of gross national income. Similarly, Japan committed to increase its official development assistance volume by $10 billion in aggregate, including a $5 billion Health and Development Initiative, over the next five years. Simultaneously, the G-8 agreed to a proposal to cancel 100 percent of outstanding debts of eligible heavily indebted poor countries to the International Monetary Fund, International Development Association, and African Development Bank and to provide additional resources to ensure that the financing capacities of the international financial institutes are not reduced. However, no specific mechanism or dates (other than before 2010) were provided for the increased funding.

To finance donor commitments of additional assistance, several innovative financing mechanisms have been proposed.

Airline ticket taxation. In June 2005, an international donors conference in Berlin proposed a "solidarity contribution levied on plane tickets . . . to combat hunger and poverty and finance global sustainable development, inter alia, health programs including the fight against HIV/AIDS and other pandemics" (World Bank 2005a, p. 5). The levy would apply to plane tickets issued to passengers departing from airports located in participating countries. Passengers in transit would be exempted. Airline companies would collect the tax, and rates would be country specific. Initial estimates were that the tax would yield €10 billion annually (about $12 billion) on a €5 tax on all plane tickets worldwide with a €20 surcharge on business and first class tickets.

An international finance facility. The United Kingdom's proposal to create an international finance facility (IFF) is based on the notions of frontloading aid (spending money now for critical development investments to reach the Millennium Development Goals) and using off-budget donor commitments (in response to fiscal constraints facing donors that have pledged to increase official development assistance).[4] A pilot facility of the IFF targeted to immunizations is under way. That facility would raise frontloaded, reliable funding over a number of years to expand global immunization efforts to help achieve the Millennium Development Goal on child mortality by accelerating production of new and existing vaccines and strengthening capacity to deliver vaccines.

The Tobin tax. The Tobin tax dates from an idea proposed in the 1970s to curb speculative currency flows. The tax would be levied on currency transactions collected on a national or market basis. Applying the tax proceeds to development financing is a new wrinkle to the long-standing idea of a tax to reduce potentially destabilizing hot currency flows. The annualized global foreign exchange market turnover is estimated at $300 trillion. After adjusting for various sources of leakage, it is estimated that a reasonable tax rate of one or two basis points would raise from $15 billion to $28 billion annually.[5]

Taxes on global "bads." Perhaps the earliest example of a proposal to tax a global bad is the proposed global carbon tax. A more recent initiative was advocated by President Jacques Chirac of France to fund development by taxing global arms sales. The basic idea is straight from the principles of public finance: levy a tax on the production of activities associated with negative externalities (carbon emissions or arms sales). The tax revenues can be used to promote a social good (development), while the increased price as a result of the tax reduces the offending behavior, increasing societal welfare. Estimates for the amount of resources that could be raised from a tax on hydrocarbon fuels according to their carbon content vary, but revenues from high-income countries alone could raise $60 billion.

IMF gold sales. A number of proposals have been advanced to fund development through gold sales by the International Monetary Fund (Sagasti, Bezanson, and Prada 2005). The rationale is that the gold held by the IMF is valued at the price prevailing at the creation of the Bretton Woods Institutions, $30 an ounce, although the current market price is much higher. The simplest proposal calls for the IMF to slowly sell gold in the international market in amounts too small relative to total market volume to have an appreciable impact on price. Critics have argued that this would destabilize global gold and financial markets. Another approach is for the IMF to use an "off-market" sale, an approach that has been used only in exceptional circumstances.

Creation of new special drawing rights. The special drawing right (SDR) is an international reserve asset created by the IMF in 1969 to supplement the official reserves of member countries. SDRs are allocated to member countries in proportion to their IMF quotas. The SDR is not a claim on the IMF but is potentially a claim on the convertible currencies of IMF members. Countries holding SDRs can exchange them against currencies of other members. SDRs were introduced under the Bretton Woods fixed exchange rate system because gold and U.S. dollars were not sufficient to support the expansion of world trade. With the shift to floating exchange rates, the need for SDRs as a reserve asset has declined. Today, the stock of SDRs outstanding is approximately SDR 21 billion (approximately $32 billion). Of late, there have been calls for the IMF to issue new SDRs, with donor countries making voluntary donations of their SDR allocations to fund development. Estimates of the revenue-raising potential vary from $25 billion to $30 billion.

How to proceed. As proposed by the World Bank and IMF, any new mechanism to finance development or to comply with official development assistance commitments must be assessed on the basis of five criteria: revenue adequacy, efficiency, equity, ease of collection, and minimum required coalition size (World Bank and IMF 2005). Regardless of the merits of each proposal, reaching agreement among donor countries is likely to be a long and tenuous process with questionable likelihood of success.

As previously discussed, more official development assistance is certainly necessary, especially for low-income countries, and more effort to provide such funding is certainly welcome. However, overly ambitious goals and promises regarding official development assistance may create unreasonable expectations in recipient countries, which may postpone the difficult choices needed in a resource constrained environment. Donor countries should certainly provide adequate support of development efforts, and they should also recognize that recipient countries would benefit from realistic commitments, which would allow them to improve planning and make rational choices.

Mechanisms for disbursement

Official development assistance can be provided in many ways. How the resources are disbursed determines whether they can be used to finance recurrent expenditures, how much the recipient country can allocate to the uses it considers most deserving, what mechanisms will be used to make the resources available to the final beneficiary, and even whether the resources will ever reach the country they are supposed to benefit.

Depending on how it is provided, donor assistance may not be recorded in the recipient country's balance of payments; may be recorded in the balance of payments but not in the government's budget ("off budget"); may be recorded on budget, but be earmarked for a particular purpose or project; or may be provided as general budget support, essentially free of restrictions regarding the expenditures it finances. Assistance not recorded in the balance of payments refers largely to technical assistance (for instance, foreign consultants) contracted and paid for by donors outside the beneficiary country. Off-budget funding (support that is reflected in the balance of payments and not in the government's budget) is for projects implemented directly by donors through nongovernmental organizations or through contracting directly with providers, by-passing the government's public expenditure management. On-budget but earmarked funding refers to funding that is provided for a particular project or purpose, such as for building health facilities or purchasing certain drugs. General budget support is assistance that is provided through the government's budget and that governments allocate as they see fit. General budget support essentially is provided to finance gaps in financing the government's overall program.

A recent analysis of 14 countries that have developed World Bank poverty reduction strategies (Foster 2005a) shows that, although budget support is increasing as a share of donor support, on average less than 20 percent of donor disbursements are provided as general budget support. On average, for every $1 disbursed by donors to these 14 countries, the study estimates the following distribution:

Not recorded in balance of payments	$0.30
Recorded in balance of payments but not in government budget	$0.20
Earmarked to specific projects recorded in budget	$0.30
General budget support	$0.20

Off-budget funding has been particularly prevalent in the health sector. In Uganda off-budget spending is estimated to be more than 50 percent of total health spending. In Tanzania off-budget spending was estimated to represent more than 46 percent of health spending in 2000. Although some of the off-budget spending is domestically funded, through, for example, user fees, it is largely donor funded. In part, donors encourage this behavior to be able to account for the direct impact of their resources (Wagstaff and Claeson 2004). Several countries are uncomfortable with this approach. In 2004 the Uganda Ministry of Finance was reported as having decided to cap new project aid commitments that are outside the budget (*New Vision*, Uganda, August 20, 2004). In India, an immunization program promoted by Global Alliance for Vaccines and Immunization was not implemented because the government believed it was not sustainable financially without continued, long-term, predictable grant support (Lele, Ridker, and Upadhyay forthcoming).

Donors may also decide to provide their assistance though the budget but request that the funding be earmarked. Earmarking tends to increase the rigidities of government budgets and, as with off-budget funding, may not lead to increases in overall government spending as recipient countries decide to divert their own domestic resources to other uses. This diversion is called fungibility and is analyzed in detail in a later section.

Trends in private financial flows

Discussions about official development assistance and the Millennium Development Goals have largely concentrated on low-income countries and direct donor aid, overshadowing talk about the needs of middle-income countries and the potential of private flows. However, private flows to developing countries are critical to achieving tangible improvements in health outcomes and to reaching the Millennium Development Goals. Private capital flows to developing countries reached an annual net average of $169 billion between 2000 and 2003 (World Bank 2004b), close to three times the size of official development assistance over the same period. The source of this financing is mostly foreign direct investment.[6] Although the explosive growth in foreign direct investment that took place in the 1990s was accompanied by new policies, such as protection of property rights and clear rules regarding pricing, several issues about foreign direct investment that are more relevant now should be noted.

A large part of foreign direct investment during the 1990s came about as a result of privatizations of public enterprises, which cannot be repeated. Second, foreign direct investment has been concentrated in a few countries and in the energy, minerals, and telecommunications sectors.[7] Third, there is some recent disenchantment in Latin America (Argentina and Bolivia) with foreign direct investment, especially when it is associated with contentious privatizations in the water, petroleum, and electricity sectors. Finally, foreign direct investment profit remittances have increased, causing, among other things, inquiries from members of civil society and nongovernmental organizations regarding the net impact of foreign direct investment in capital flows over the medium term.[8] Still, foreign direct investment, which involves long-term commitment of investments, has remained resilient despite the Asian financial crisis and other problems. It is a fundamental source of financing for infrastructure and market penetration of services that are critical for growth and reaching the Millennium Development Goals (both directly through the impact of infrastructure on outcomes and indirectly through the impact of growth on outcomes).

Workers' remittances are monies sent by migrant workers to their home countries. Remittances have become the second largest capital flow behind foreign direct investment and ahead of official development assistance. Remittances, officially defined, are the sum of workers' remittances, compensation of employees, and migrant transfers. Thus defined, remittances received by developing countries rose from $31 billion in 1990 to $86 billion in 2001 and $167 billion in 2005 (World Bank 2006), representing more than twice the estimated amount of official development assistance. Accounting for unrecorded and informal flows, the actual amount of remittances could be twice the officially recorded amount. There are marked differences in remittance flows by region and country. In 2005 East Asia and the Pacific region received 26 percent of total worker's remittances; Latin American and the Caribbean, 25 percent; South Asia, 20 percent; the Middle East and North Africa, 21 percent; Europe and Central Asia, 20 percent; and Sub-Saharan Africa, 8 percent. The top five receiving countries in volume were India, China, Mexico, France, the Philippines, and Spain. On a per capita basis, the top five receiving countries were Jordan, Portugal, Barbados, Jamaica, and El Salvador. Data from a number of surveys indicate that the bulk of remittances are used for consumption, as well as human capital (health, education, and better nutrition).

Thus, official development assistance, especially technical assistance, should emphasize the need for appropriate policies and institutions to attract foreign direct investment to both middle- and low-income countries, if the Millennium Development Goals are to be reached. Similarly, the importance of remittances cannot be taken for granted, and both donors and recipients should strive for better ways to pool these resources to increase their impact on human development outcomes and growth. The emphasis on grant financing, although important, should not divert attention from these other, much larger, private sources of sustainable financing for development. Countries and companies should eventually be able to finance their needs from domestic and international capital markets. To achieve that goal, developing countries must make strong efforts to improve their international risk ratings. This requires, among other things, political stability, sound macroeconomic policies, sound institutions, and clear rules about complying with international contracts. Technical assistance should help countries meet the requirements to ensure a sustainable flow of resources beyond official assistance for development.

Trends in health aid

Development assistance for health has risen steadily since 1990 from about $2 billion to more than $10 billion in 2003.[9] Much of the post-2000 increase can be credited to an increasing number of global partnerships and a significant rise in private philanthropic funding—notably by the Bill and Melinda Gates Foundation. Partnerships and philanthropies have joined efforts to increase awareness and finance aimed at the eradication of major diseases. Global programs—such as the Global Fund to Fight AIDS, Tuberculosis and Malaria (GFATM); the Global Alliance for Vaccines and Immunization; Roll Back Malaria; the U.S. President's Emergency Plan for AIDS Relief (PEPFAR); and several others—represented roughly 15 percent of total health aid in 2002 and 20 percent in 2003 (Michaud 2003). Figure 4.3 reflects the increasing importance of global partnerships and private philanthropic funding in development assistance for health; such funding was considered negligible in 1990.

Estimates of the costs of reaching the Millennium Development Goals for health

Despite growth, health aid still falls far short of the estimated financing required to reach the health Millennium Development Goals. A World Bank study estimated that the additional health aid required to meet the health goals is about $25 billion a year, or almost three times the amount of development assistance for health in 2003. The Commission on Macroeconomics and Health of the World Health Organization estimated that an additional $40 billion to $52 billion would

FIGURE 4.3   Development assistance for health by source, 1997–2003

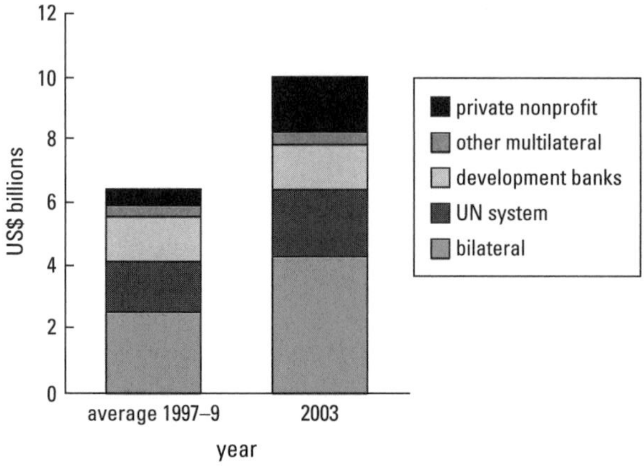

Source: Michaud 2005.
Note: The category of other multilateral includes the European Union and the Global Fund to Fight AIDS, Tuberculosis and Malaria.

be needed annually until 2015 to scale up the coverage for malaria, tuberculosis, HIV/AIDS, childhood mortality, and maternal mortality (Kumaranayake, Kurowski, and Conteh 2001). A third study estimated that between $25 billion and $70 billion of additional spending is needed to bring poorly performing countries up to the level of high performers (Preker and others 2003). A more recent estimate by the United Nations Millennium Project estimates that an additional $120 billion a year would be required by 2006 to reach all the Millennium Development Goals, and this amount would increase to $189 billion by 2015 (UN Millennium Project 2005). Of this amount, between $30 billion and $50 billion would be required for the health Millennium Development Goals.

Although the estimated cost of reaching the health goals ranges between $25 billion and $70 billion annually, all the studies acknowledge the need for additional investments, particularly for scaling up access to essential health services (Wagstaff and Claeson 2004). The increased financing available for health from donors does not match this need; that financing is mostly provided through disease- and intervention-specific programs that are off-budget, rather than as direct budget support to a country's health systems. Given the increased importance in health of these programs, they are examined here in more detail.

Disease- and intervention-specific health programs

The impact of disease- and intervention-specific programs on health care systems has recently become a major topic of debate. On the positive side, such programs are effective in increasing the awareness of major global concerns such as HIV/AIDS and immunizations. They have significantly increased the resources available in their areas of focus. They introduce new technologies to the countries in which they operate, and they seem to be more effective than general government programs in delivering services to the targeted populations. On the negative side, such disease- and intervention-specific programs potentially disrupt the country's health system. The expenditures they generate may not be sustainable within the recipient country's budget constraints. In addition, the global programs are not accountable to the recipient country. Thus, focusing solely on disease-specific initiatives can undermine the opportunity to integrate these initiatives with the country's overall health program, as well as fragment outreach, raise the demand for management skills that are already in short supply, and bleed the health system of financial and human resources in order to set up a parallel delivery operation—possibly delaying much needed institution building in the health sector (Lewis 2005).

Increased funding for HIV/AIDS. Resources available for HIV/AIDS have increased rapidly in recent years. Funding is heavily concentrated in a small number of countries. Donors are supporting activities in 140 countries, but approximately 72 percent of this funding is allocated to 25 countries, mostly in the highly affected countries in Africa and the Caribbean (OECD 2004). There has been steady growth in bilateral assistance for HIV/AIDS among members of the OECD's Development Assistance Committee (DAC). The upward trend in bilateral aid, however, is driven by the U.S. government's PEPFAR initiative. Excluding the United States, bilateral donor assistance for HIV/AIDS among DAC countries has been fairly stable since 2000.

Multilateral assistance for HIV/AIDS has also increased dramatically (figure 4.4). This has been due entirely to the establishment of GFATM. As of 2004 GFATM

FIGURE 4.4 Domestic and external financing for HIV/AIDS in developing countries by source, 2000–4

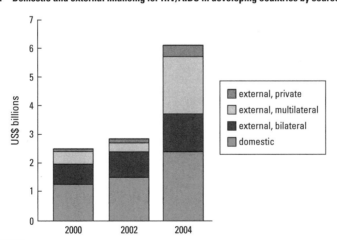

Source: Lewis 2005.

contributions among DAC countries other than the United States were roughly equal to these countries' bilateral HIV/AIDS assistance. However, there is a clear reversal in the trend in multilateral assistance outside of GFATM. The establishment of GFATM has not reduced bilateral assistance for HIV/AIDS but has had a negative impact on other multilateral assistance (box 4.1).

Impact on health systems. The increased prominence of GFATM has led to aid coordination challenges in many recipient countries. Lele, Ridker, and Upadhyay (forthcoming) examine several countries' experiences with GFATM related to donor aid coordination. They find that GFATM has led to

- duplication in institutional arrangements (for example, between national AIDS councils and country coordinating mechanisms);
- duplication in reporting requirements, increasing transaction costs;
- delay in implementation of other donor programs, particularly in small countries;
- concern among recipient governments over the uncertainty of future external resource flows;
- a focus on treatment that may be diverting attention from prevention.

Although some early conclusions can be drawn and anecdotal evidence is available, well-documented empirical analyses of GFATM's impact on health systems are lacking. PHR*plus* has organized a collaborative research effort to examine the impact of GFATM inflows on broader health systems functioning (PHR*plus* 2005). The early findings are summarized in box 4.1.

Mid-term sustainability. There is widespread concern that increased donor funding through disease and intervention-specific programs may lead to a reduction in domestic spending on HIV/AIDS. While donor funding for HIV/AIDS has only recently increased significantly, domestic spending has been growing at an aggregate level (see figure 4.4). However, such substitution may be taking place at the country level (Malawi, Mozambique, and Zambia, for example), as reflected in figure 4.5.

The sustainability of additional expenditures required for scaling up HIV/AIDS treatment is a particular concern in low-income countries. HIV/AIDS treatment will require hiring additional health workers and administrators, as well as importing almost all of the drugs to treat HIV/AIDS patients. If the resources or in-kind donations dry up, the government would need to take responsibility for funding antiretroviral therapy, because patients depend on continued therapy for survival. Interruptions in antiretroviral therapy because of funding gaps reduce the benefits of treatment and, more alarmingly, can lead to resistant strains of the virus, which compromise the efficacy of future treatment (Lewis 2005). To minimize the health and financial risks caused by the unpredictability of aid, donors

---

BOX 4.1 *Impact of the Global Fund to Fight AIDS, Tuberculosis and Malaria on health systems*

Policy processes

- The majority of proposals supported by GFATM appear to be in alignment with overall national health policies and plans; issues regarding incompatibility or divergence arise during the implementation phase.

- GFATM-related planning processes appear highly centralized, even in decentralized contexts; this has led to problems as countries begin to implement GFATM-supported activities, because of a lack of ownership at subnational levels.

Public-private mix

- In many countries, there has been rapid growth of nongovernmental organizations (NGOs), which appears to be at least partially attributable to partnership opportunities created by GFATM and other funding agencies. Country stakeholders expressed concerns about "briefcase" NGOs.

- GFATM support has contributed to innovations in public-private arrangements; many different types of partnerships were observed in different contexts.

Human resources

- None of the study countries had overarching national-level strategies or plans to address human resource constraints to scaling-up HIV/AIDS services. Plans that do exist relate to specific initiatives rather than the combined needs of all initiatives, and they do not typically take into account the potential implications of such scale-up on human resources for other programs within the health sector.

- In the face of staffing shortages and a lack of clear guidance or plans on how to motivate and retain key staff, countries and various stakeholders within countries are experimenting with alternative types of incentive packages (financial, nonfinancial, and in-kind). The effectiveness of such packages needs to be assessed.

Pharmaceuticals and commodities

- All participating countries experienced delays in procuring drugs and commodities, despite using different procurement models—working through government systems, through private parallel systems, and through multilateral agencies. Procurement through government systems appears to have led to the most substantial delays.

- Lack of consistency in the pricing of different commodities, pharmaceuticals, and services supported by different funding sources was observed to be problematic in many countries. Identical resources or commodities flowing through the same distribution systems were charged for and handled differently according to whether GFATM, other donors, or the government had paid for them.

Source: PHR*plus* 2005.

---

could commit to fund a cohort of AIDS patients for the duration of their lives instead of annually committing to fund an HIV/AIDS program. This course of action transfers risk from recipient countries to donors and makes donors accountable for their commitments. Taking on HIV/AIDS expenditures domestically is not a minor issue in many low-income countries. HIV/AIDS monies exceed total public health budgets in some countries. In 2003–4 Ethiopia's external flows targeted to HIV/AIDS were equal to the government's health budget, and in both Uganda and Zambia, AIDS funds exceeded all public health spending by almost 185 percent (Lewis 2005).

FIGURE 4.5 Domestic and external financing for HIV/AIDS in selected countries in Sub-Saharan Africa, 2000–4

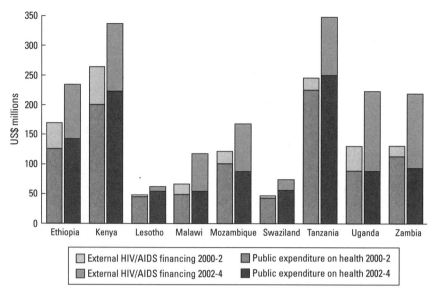

Source: Lewis 2005.

The effectiveness of aid

The large increases in official development assistance and additional commitments have led to renewed concerns about aid effectiveness. As discussed in the next chapter, donor funding seems to have had a limited impact on child and maternal mortality. These results can be explained by several factors, including fiscal sustainability, predictability, fungibility, and absorptive capacity.

Fiscal sustainability

Fiscal sustainability is often advocated, but rarely defined, for disease- and intervention-specific programs, sectors, and whole economies. Sustainability has generally been described in terms of self-sufficiency. In its broadest context, sustainability means that over a specific time period, the responsible managing entity will generate sufficient resources to fund the full costs of a particular program, sector, or economy, including the incremental service costs associated with new investments and repayment of external debt.

The exact definition of fiscal sustainability has also been the subject of recent debate (Bird 2003; Edwards 2002; Heller 2005). Traditionally, fiscal sustainability has been associated with the concept of debt sustainability. A common approach to assessing a country's fiscal sustainability has been its ability to meet a solvency and liquidity condition in terms of its debt. In practical terms, a country meets the solvency condition if it maintains a defined level of debt to GDP at a relatively constant rate from some defined period on (Edwards 2002).[10] Thus, if a country generates new debt, some time in the future it will be expected to make adjustments in taxes, spending, or both. A country meets the liquidity condition if its foreign resources allow it to meet its maturing obligations.

Defining the fiscal sustainability of a country's economy or its current fiscal situation is no easy matter. The IMF has been devoting increasing attention to these areas, particularly in light of the severe criticisms of IMF structural adjustment programs and fiscal ceilings (Tanzi and Zee 2000; Croce and Juan-Ramon 2003; Dunaway and N'Diaye 2004). Work is also under way to develop operational indicators of debt and fiscal sustainability (Dunaway and N'Diaye 2004). Although the practical definition of fiscal sustainability may change for programs supported by the IMF and IDA, it is extremely unlikely that such definitions will be divorced from a country's capacity to accommodate expenditures financed with aid within the domestic budget constraint in a reasonable period of time, while maintaining sustainable levels of debt to GDP and debt service to exports.

Certainly the discussions will hinge on what is meant by "reasonable period of time." The concept of a reasonable period of time must depend on the maturity and predictability of grants, which at this stage are short term and highly volatile. If a country receives reliable commitments of grants for a long period of time, say 20 years, these grants will be part of the revenue stream and sustainability would imply the capacity of a country to accommodate the expenditures initially financed with those grants within their own domestic envelope in the programmed 20 years.

Three features of this definition of fiscal sustainability are important:

- It strikes a compromise between the "resource constraint" definition of fiscal sustainability currently used by the IMF and the more "needs based" definition advocated by the UN Millennium Project and its director Jeffrey Sachs.
- It maintains internal (domestic) and external (debt management) prudence. Social expenditures are increased only to the extent of local capacity to overtake those expenditures within the domestic resource mobilization envelope, yet they are allowed to increase immediately based on donor grants.
- It generates the appropriate incentives for both donors and recipient countries.

To illustrate this last point, assume that donor grants are committed to a country in an unrestricted manner until 2020 and that the country does not have absorptive capacity constraints. The restraining factor to increased social expenditures would be the recipient country's commitment to expand domestic resources up to 2020 to progressively substitute for the donor funds. If it is estimated that the domestic envelope will allow such an expansion of health expenditures, the donors funds would be accepted, and the program of increased health expenditure with grant financing, later replaced by domestic resources, would be allowed. If, however, it is unlikely that the additional margin generated in the domestic envelope will accommodate such increases in health expenditures by 2020, or there is unwillingness in the recipient country to make such a commitment to health, expenditures would not be allowed to increase as much. If, however, donors can commit resources only until 2008, the total increase in health expenditures would be constrained by the capacity to increase domestic resources for health to the level of the additional grants by 2008. In that case, the shorter-term nature of the assistance reveals the absence of donor commitment to the effort.

There is nothing strikingly new about this discussion. Some low-income countries such as Uganda already use this type of analysis in their medium-term expenditure framework. The problem is that the adoption of such a definition or policy is unilateral by the recipient country and thus does not generate the appropriate incentives on either the donor or the recipient side. Because of the current short-term nature of donor commitments and the resultant lack of predictability of donor funding, the programmed increases in expenditures are limited to the possibilities of domestic funding in the next couple of years or the next medium-term expenditure framework cycle, at best. Thus increases in health expenditures are extremely constrained. If donor resources could be committed over a longer program period (say, 10–20 years) and be well invested, increases in health expenditures could be larger, and chances of making a difference in outcomes would improve.

Predictability

The core of the aid predictability problem is that low-income countries depend on vague indications of future aid commitments to fund long-term, recurring spending obligations. Though donors make substantial aid commitments, data show that commitments consistently exceed actual disbursements. Despite a poor record as predictors for disbursements, commitments continue to be used in budgetary exercises in aid-receiving countries (Foster 2005b). When coupled with the difficulty of reallocating budgets in the short term, this may have serious implications for the way governments use their domestic resources to fund their health priorities. Most notably, the unpredictability of donor aid creates fiscal sustainability problems in aid-receiving countries. Fluctuation in aid levels prevents countries from using donor aid to invest in projects that may generate recurrent costs because aid that may be available at the initiation of a project is not guaranteed to still be available over the long term.

For example, if revenues are secured for the long term, governments can pursue expenditure obligations that have future recurrent cost implications, such as taking on the cost of school fees and drug costs for the poor. If the money is available only for the next two years, however, countries will avoid making longer-term commitments, opting instead to make marginal improvements to existing services rather than aiming for bold expansions in coverage. The reason is obvious: when the money runs out, the cost of running the new facilities and paying the extra staff will stretch the available budget so far that the quality of existing as well as new services will suffer. Public expenditure plans are always subject to the risk of adjustment if resources are below expectation; the costs of making adjustments depends on the speed and predictability of changes in the availability of budget resources.

Figure 4.6 highlights the dramatic fluctuation in donor commitments that can occur over time. The variability reflects, among other things, exchange rate fluctuations, political and budgetary decisions by donors, administrative delays on the donor side, problems of absorptive capacity in recipient countries, and noncompliance with loan conditions. Commitments are reflected in U.S. dollars, and thus exchange rate fluctuations between the currency in which donors make their commitments and the U.S. dollar and between the U.S. dollar and the local currency strongly affected volatility. To illustrate, the franc in Burundi depreciated against the U.S. dollar an average of 27 percent per year between 1997 and 2000 for a cumulative depreciation of 104 percent. Moreover, the U.S. dollar depreciated against the euro, for instance, an average of 7 percent between 1997 and 2000 for a cumulative depreciation of 22 percent. Thus, in the case of Burundi, the increases in the ratio between commitments and actual health expenditures can partially reflect depreciation of the local currency in which expenditures are made against the dollar and the depreciation of the dollar against the currency in which the commitments are made, but it cannot fully explain the sharp decreases in the ratios.

Another major reason for the volatility in commitments has to do with political decisions in donor countries. Legislative constraints and the inability to compromise with successor governments inhibit donors from making long-term funding commitments. Commitments are never unconditional or irrevocable, and they require a high degree of trust by both partners. Donor preferences can change from one year to the next in response to changes in behavior in the recipient country or to political events in the donor country. The donor country's budget cycle can also be misaligned with the budget cycle of the recipient country, resulting in a serious mismatch between what is committed and what is actually disbursed.

Absorptive capacity at the country level is another reason donor commitments are often volatile and unpredictable. Absorptive capacity issues in more general terms are discussed later in this chapter; for the purpose of this discussion, absorptive capacity refers primarily to problems with spending resources made available by donors. Problems such as lack of administrative capacity or inefficiencies in public expenditure management (which inhibit already-disbursed resources from reaching projects or program executing units) may originate in the recipient country. Problems can also begin with donors, which may have burdensome procurement and reporting requirements.

FIGURE 4.6 **Donor commitments for health in seven African countries, 1997–2001**

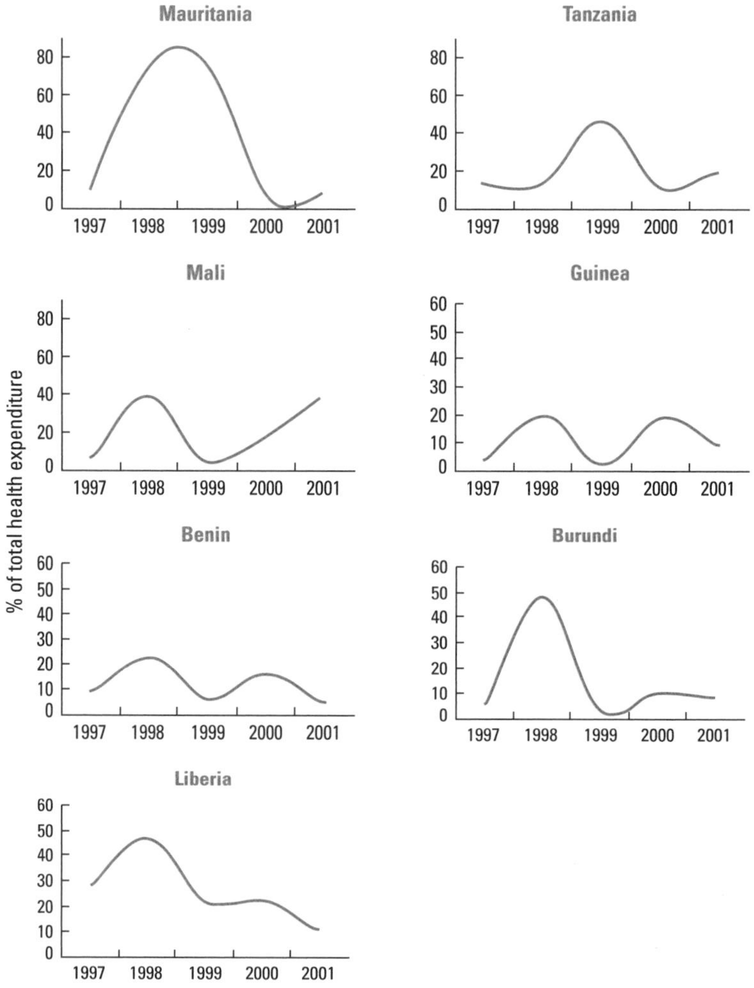

Source: WDI and OECD/DAC donor funding database and staff estimates.

Conditionality is another major reason why donor funding is unpredictable. The worst case scenario results when disbursements are stopped in all programs for noncompliance with conditions in one program or the macroeconomic framework. However, approaches to conditionality are evolving. Donor assessments of performance are being coordinated with the budget cycle and conditions applied with a lag, to avoid disrupting the current year's budget. Although new instruments, such as the poverty reduction support credit (see chapter 6) make the timing of disbursement no longer dependent on completion of a long list of actions, governments still need to agree on a forward-looking policy matrix and convince donors that they have made enough progress in implementation to merit further support. Current approaches leave governments vulnerable not only to donor assessments of their performance against existing conditions, but also to difficulty in negotiating future conditions.

Any solutions to the predictability problem must address each of the causes of volatility. Table 4.1 summarizes some of the main reasons for the discrepancies between donor aid commitments and disbursements and proposes some mitigating approaches.

TABLE 4.1 Reasons for aid volatility and possible mitigating alternatives

Reason for volatility	Possible mitigating alternative
Donor commitments are short term, but spending obligations are long term.	Longer donor commitment horizon if conditions are met
	Collective donor commitment to adjust for shortfalls by individual donors
Donor commitments are conditional and hard for governments to manage.	Partnership approach, joint review, and focus on implementation.
	Fewer, strategically negotiated conditions, within power and capacity of government to deliver consultation before sanction where there is "side tracking"; proportionate response to condition not being met
	Key spending programs for the poor maintained if program-specific conditions are met, even if other aspects (such as the macro economy) are temporarily off-track
	Conditions applied to future commitments not current budget, with time for government to adjust spending obligations if agreement cannot be reached
Pledges and commitments are not predictably linked to actual disbursements.	Transparent reporting system for significant commitments; discounting of donor figures based on past performance
	Continuous review of disbursement outlook
	Donor accountability through transparency on performance, peer review, and civil society pressure at global and country level
	Collective donor arrangements to ensure targets are met for donors as a whole; larger reserves to shield impact of shortfalls (such as the proposed aid stabilization facility of the UK Department for International Development); active use of foreign exchange reserves to manage fluctuations.
	Debt relief as predictable funding source.
Disbursements may be worth less than their nominal value.	Gaps in government poverty reduction strategies filled as first call on donor funds; collective government and donor group decision making on spending priorities; full disclosure of funding commitments and disbursements, transparency on funding intended to support public expenditure plans; harmonized government systems, strengthened as needed

Source: Foster 2005b.

Implementing these solutions will require major donor commitment and coordination efforts. Some of the solutions could generate additional problems, such as moral hazard or large transaction costs. Box 4.2 describes a proposed facility to be financed by donors, which may be helpful in diminishing short-term volatility of funding. It also is helpful in underscoring the issues of moral hazard and difficulties that the facility itself introduces.

Faster progress toward the Millennium Development Goals depends on governments' confidence that significantly higher aid flows will be maintained in the long term. The uncertainty surrounding future aid levels makes governments reluctant to commit to ambitious public expenditure plans that depend on continued and timely donor aid disbursements for their execution. Countries face significant risks if they establish health systems that cannot be maintained if donor preferences change.

BOX 4.2 *A solution to aid volatility? DFID's proposed aid stabilization facility*

At the High Level Forum 2004 in Abuja, Nigeria, the U.K. Department for International Development (DFID) proposed an aid stabilization facility to guarantee minimum overall funding levels for aid-dependent low-income countries. Additional detail was elaborated in a DFID study that recommended establishment of an aid stabilization facility (Foster 2005). This facility will guarantee countries that depend on aid to finance their public expenditure programs will not fall below certain defined limits and will not fall faster than a defined rate of decline. This recommendation provides the required assurances that aid will be broadly in line with commitments and will not be abruptly withdrawn. The aid stabilization facility is intended as a last resort, providing an insurance policy if donors fall short of their promises. The degree of security it is able to offer depends on the extent to which the donor community succeeds in taking other complementary measures to improve the medium- to long-term predictability of aid flows.

A specific mechanism for diminishing the difference between commitments and actual expenditures, although reasonable and desirable in principle, requires further analysis. Volatility in donor aid, defined as the difference between the commitment for a given year and actual expenditures in that year, is introduced by multiple factors. Some of these factors are the donors' responsibility (such as decreased commitments because of political and budgetary reasons or slow disbursement because of bureaucracy in the donor country); some are the recipient countries' responsibility (lack of capacity to disburse, public expenditure management difficulties, or noncompliance with conditionalities under the control of the recipient country); and some are due to exogenous factors outside the full control of either partner (such as deterioration of the terms of trade and natural disasters). The design of the fund will depend on what factors it intends to insure against. Moreover, the facility must be carefully designed to avoid moral hazard on the part of both donors and recipient countries. The consequences of a poorly designed facility could be more damaging than the problems it is trying to overcome. Finally, the facility as initially proposed does not lengthen the maturity of the funding provided by donors, which, in the case of the social sectors, is a major deterrent to increasing recurrent expenditures in a sustainable manner.

Fungibility

Development assistance has claimed many successes at the project level. However, at the macro level, many cross-sectional studies show little impact of donor aid on growth (Boone 1994; Burnside and Dollar 1997). Similarly, donor aid has had limited impact on child or maternal mortality (see chapter 5). What explains these apparent contradictions? The answer lies largely in the volatility of donor aid, as already discussed, and in its fungibility.

As discussed in chapter 5, the fungibility of donor aid is the diversion of funds to public expenditures other than those for which the aid is intended, including tax reduction or debt repayment. A vivid example comes from a statement in 1947 by Paul Rosentain-Rudin, then deputy director of the World Bank's Economics Department, who noted: "When the World Bank thinks it is financing an electric power station, it is really financing a brothel" (Devarajan, Rajkumar, and Swaroop 1999, p. 1). The reality is that in a resource-constrained environment, governments decrease their domestic funding of, for example, primary care, when they see that donors are funding such activities, so that donor funding may not generate additionality in spending, or at least not to the extent donors expected. Fungibility is likely to be larger when donor funding is provided off-budget and where there are a large number of donors in the country (Devarajan, Rajkumar, and Swaroop 1999). Chapter 5 discusses fungibility, including its impact on the effectiveness of donor funding and government expenditures on health outcomes, at length.

With dramatic increases in donor assistance for health, many stakeholders are wondering whether these resources actually reach the intended sectors or projects. Devarajan, Rajkumar, and Swaroop (1999) point out that this is an interesting question only if donor preferences are different from those of the recipient country. They also argue that it is not clear whether fungibility is good or bad: it all depends on what the government does with the resources that are released by the aid projects. However, the presence of fungibility, coupled with the difficulties that governments face in reallocating resources, may lead to a nonoptimal allocation of resources when donor funding is volatile.

For example, suppose that a donor gives aid to a country for primary care. Also suppose that the preferences of the donor and the recipient are not the same—the recipient does not want to increase primary care expenditures by as much as the donor does. The minister of finance is likely to argue that, because primary care is already funded from outside allocations, the government's budget will be directed only toward activities that are not receiving donor funding (secondary and tertiary care, for example). Ultimately, if donor aid is fully fungible, the final composition of expenditures (with both government and donor funding) may be exactly the same as if the government had received the resources as budget support and been allowed to make its own allocation decisions.

In this case, full fungibility may result in the optimal allocation of resources (several health subsectors are fully funded through a combination of donor aid and government funding) from the government's perspective, but not necessarily from the donor's perspective. Problems arise, however, even when donor aid is fungible, because donor resources are also volatile. When donors stop funding a project or even decrease funding levels, recipient countries find it difficult to transfer resources on short notice away from one subsector (such as higher-level care) to another (such as primary care). Budget reallocations can be asymmetrical: that is, it may be easy to increase expenditures to secondary and tertiary care (when resources have been released through aid funding of primary care expenditures), but cutting these expenditures may be difficult. This is particularly the case because higher-level care providers in the public sector have strong medical associations, are located mostly in urban centers where it is easier to get the government's attention through protests and other means, and tend to disproportionately benefit the voting middle class. Thus, recipient countries may end up, at least in the short run, with a nonoptimal allocation of resources—in this case overspending on higher-level care and underspending on primary care when the aid diminishes.

The fungibility and volatility of donor aid, combined with the inability of recipient governments to rapidly reallocate resources, can therefore lead to a result opposite from what either donor or recipient intended. In this example, the donor's objectives were for the country to expand expenditures in primary care, and the recipient country wanted to maintain primary care at its original level. However, after the donor pulled out, neither objective was achieved: primary care spending declined, and a nonoptimal allocation of resources resulted.

There is little analysis in the literature about the impact of fungibility on health-specific aid. Empirical studies that have estimated the degree of fungibility at the country level have examined how changes in total foreign aid affect total public expenditures, how categorical aid affects the targeted categories of expenditures, whether aid is fungible among public expenditure categories, and whether aid reduces a country's own revenue effort (Pack and Pack 1990, 1993, 1996; Feyziouglu, Swaroop, and Zhu 1997; Clements and others 2004). More recently, Devarajan, Rajkumar, and Swaroop (1999) found that governments in Africa do not spend all sectoral aid in the targeted sector, nor do they treat aid as merely budgetary support. They also found that the degree of fungibility could be partially explained by the importance of a particular donor and its aid level in a country. The larger the number of donors and the smaller the importance of aid in government expenditures, the more likely aid will be fungible.

Empirical analysis prepared for this study confirms that donor aid for health is fungible. The results indicate that the domestic resources diverted from the health sector as a result of the fungibility of aid would be significant. A 10 percent increase in off-budget donor funding generates a 0.87 percent reduction in domestically funded government health expenditures.[11] Taking the mean values of $19 per capita for domestically financed health expenditure and $1 per capita for off-budget donor funding for health, the regression results imply that a $1 dollar increase in off-budget donor funding leads to $1.65 dollar decrease in the allocation of government resources to health, holding everything else constant.[12]

A second important component necessary to explain the results of donor funding on child and maternal mortality is asymmetry in budgeting. To test the asymmetry hypothesis, the ratio of a change in hospital expenditures to changes in revenues was analyzed for a set of 61 countries (763 observations) over the period 1980–2001.[13] The hospital expenditures and revenues are all expressed in terms of percentages of GDP. These ratios are then divided into two groups, one with increasing revenue relative to the previous year (group 1) and the other with decreasing revenue relative to the previous year (group 2). A comparison of the mean values of these ratios by group shows evidence that revenue is significantly higher in group 1 (0.33) than in group 2 (0.04). Hospital expenditures respond in a more moderate way to a decreasing resource envelope than to an increasing resource envelop (figure 4.7).

Similar results are found at the country level. In Lesotho between 1984 and 1988, government health expenditures on hospitals maintained an increasing trend as a percentage of GDP, even though domestic revenues were decreasing (figure 4.8). To borrow a term from labor economics, hospital expenditure data reflects "downward stickiness"—resistance to decreasing beneath a certain level in response to declines in domestic revenues—during this time period. The same pattern was observed in Ethiopia, especially for the period from 1989 to 1992 (figure 4.9).

In addition to the effect of fungibility on the composition of spending, the specific form of aid (for example, grants as opposed to loans) can affect domestic revenue mobilization efforts. A recent study by Clements and others (2004) found

FIGURE 4.7   Model of government revenue and hospital expenditures over time

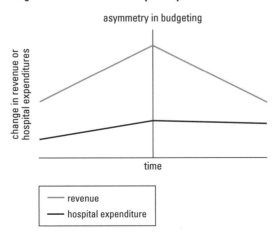

Source: Staff estimates from IMF and World Bank data.

FIGURE 4.8   Trends in domestic revenue and hospital expenditures in Lesotho, 1984–8

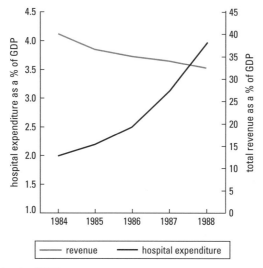

Source: Staff estimates based on IMF 2001.
Note: Domestic revenues are total revenues (net of grants) as a percentage of GDP.

FIGURE 4.9   Trends in domestic revenue and hospital expenditures in Ethiopia, 1981–92

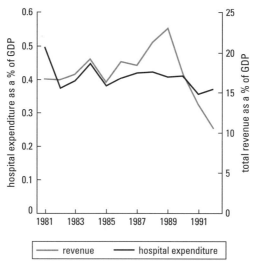

Source: Staff estimates based on IMF 2001.
Note: Domestic revenues are total revenues (net of grants) as a percentage of GDP.

that increases in grants to countries with weak policies and institutions resulted in a decline in total domestic revenue efforts. Thus, increases in grants to these countries do not necessarily imply net increases in resources available for expenditures. However, loans were not found to have a deleterious effect on domestic revenue mobilization. Thus, in addition to institutional arrangements, which have consistently been an important factor in aid effectiveness, and the effects of fungibility on expenditure composition, the form of aid could have important implications for domestic revenue efforts.

Absorptive capacity

Large (actual and promised) increases in health aid to low-income countries have raised the question of whether countries can use these new aid flows effectively. Absorptive capacity has macroeconomic, budgetary management, and service delivery dimensions (table 4.2).

Increased aid has important implications for macroeconomic management. There are potential impacts on exchange rates, inflation, import-export balances, overall competitiveness (Dutch disease), aid dependency, domestic revenue mobilization, and future recurrent cost generation. If aid flows are off budget, they can result in corruption and substitute donor priorities for country priorities. There may not be sufficient human resources, physical infrastructure, or managerial capacity in the country to use funds effectively, and resources that are both in short supply

TABLE 4.2   Constraints to absorbing more external resources

	Macro	Institutional	Physical and human	Social, cultural, and political
Macro/national government	• Debt sustainability • Competitiveness, Dutch disease	• Monetary and fiscal policy instruments • Exchange rate management	• Administrative, management, planning skills, trained technicians, sector specialists	• Stable national political institutions, power-sharing mechanisms, social stability
Fiscal instrumental/ allocative mechanisms			• Sector management skills • Connectivity and communications networks	• Cultural norms, weak institutions, power-sharing mechanisms
Service delivery/ local government			• Road accessibility, water control, geography • Local government skills and capacity	• Cultural norms; ethnic, caste, class relations • Local power structures

Source: World Bank 2004a.

and critical for effective service delivery may be diverted from other important activities or simply be overwhelmed, creating implementation bottlenecks. Additional burdens are imposed on countries through donors' cumbersome reporting and administrative requirements.

Supply and demand constraints in the health sector can also be obstacles for countries to effectively employ large increases in health resources. As shown in table 4.3, these constraints can occur at all levels of service delivery and governance (Hanson and others 2001). Additional funding alone is not sufficient for overcoming structural weaknesses.

A study for the High Level Forum 2004 held in Abuja, Nigeria (Foster 2005a) showed that for the 14 countries studied, concerns about absorptive capacity frequently reflected issues of governance and accountability, disbursement problems as a consequence of procedural requirements intended to address those concerns, and public financial management issues in general. In some cases, governance and expenditure management constraints are so pervasive that major reforms need to precede or accompany increased funding (Cambodia, Tajikistan). In other cases, government procedures are overly centralized and bureaucratic and need to be reformed to permit available funding to be spent (Benin, Burkina Faso).

Addressing public expenditure management and civil service reforms requires action not only by the health ministry, but by central authorities as well. Furthermore, coordinated action by government has to be mirrored by coordination within the donor agency to support both macro and sectoral reforms. Donors' procedures for project or pooled funding are usually part of the problem, because they not only cause low disbursement, but also divert capacity away from delivering services toward satisfying the donors' demand for meetings, field trips, reports, accounts, and audits. By absorbing the capacity of financial management staff, donors' procedures also get in the way of effective government action to address the systemic weaknesses that make parallel procedures necessary.

Recent efforts to revamp aid

Concerns regarding aid effectiveness have generated an intense global debate, as evidenced by the volume of literature on the subject (Burnside and Dollar 1997; Collier and Dollar 1999; Collier and Hoeffler 2002; Foster and others 2003; Clemens, Radelet, and Bhavnani 2004; Sagasti, Bezanson, and Prada 2005). These concerns have also led to some actions at the international level, such as the Paris Declaration on Aid Effectiveness, as well as efforts specific to the health sector, such as the strategy of sectorwide approaches.

The Paris Declaration on Aid Effectiveness

In March 2005, in the Paris Declaration on Aid Effectiveness, the ministers of developed and developing countries and the heads of multilateral and bilateral

TABLE 4.3   Constraints to improving access to health interventions

Level of constraint	Type of constraint	Likelihood of additional funds to help overcome constraints
Community and household level	Lack of demand for effective interventions	High
	Barriers to use of effective interventions (physical, financial, social)	High
Health services delivery level	Shortage and poor distribution of appropriately qualified staff	High
	Weak technical guidance, program management, and supervision	High
	Inadequate drugs and medical supplies	High
	Lack of equipment and infrastructure, including poor accessibility of health services	High
Health sector policy and strategic management level	Weak and overly centralized system for planning and management	Low
	Weak drug policies and supply system	Medium
	Inadequate regulation of pharmaceutical and private sectors and improper industry practices	Medium
	Lack of intersectoral action and partnership between government and civil society	Low
	Weak incentives to use inputs efficiently and respond to user needs and preferences	Low
	Reliance on donor funding that reduces flexibility and ownership	Low
	Donor practices that damage country policies	Low
Public policies cutting across sectors	Government bureaucracy (civil service rules and remuneration, centralized management system, civil service reforms)	Low
	Poor availability of communication and transport infrastructure	High
Contextual and environmental characteristics	Weak governance and overall policy framework	Low
	Corruption, weak government, weak rule of law and enforceability of contracts	Low
	Political instability and insecurity	Low
	Low priority attached to social sectors	Low
	Weak structures for public accountability	Low
	Lack of free press	Low
	Climatic and geographic predisposition to disease	Low
	Physical environment unfavorable to service delivery	Low

Source: Based on Hanson and others 2001.

development institutions agreed to emphasize the need for improvements in ownership, harmonization, alignment, results, and mutual accountability in aid effectiveness. Beyond the rhetoric, the most significant result of the High Level Forum on Aid Effectiveness was the establishment of specific goals and measurable targets regarding aid delivery. The indicators of progress to be measured in each country and monitored internationally are shown in table 4.4.

Establishing targets on ownership, harmonization, managing for results, and mutual accountability between donors and recipient countries is most important. The Paris Declaration on Aid Effectiveness is a good step in this direction. But more efforts are required to overcome problems of ownership and predictability of financing, which is necessary for the sustainability of health financing, fungibility of aid, and the effectiveness of aid and government expenditures in achieving the outcomes envisioned in the Millennium Development Goals. In particular, additional efforts and more ambitious targets need to be established for "aid flows [that] are aligned to national priorities" (goal 3), "more predictable aid" (goal 7), and the "use of common arrangements" (goal 9).

Coordinating donor funding through sectorwide approaches

To better coordinate donor funding to support a broad government program, many countries have adopted sectorwide approaches. This strategy seeks to address the limitations of project-based forms of donor assistance, to ensure that overall health reform goals are met, to reduce large transaction costs for countries, and to establish genuine partnerships among donors and recipients wherein both have rights and responsibilities. Sectorwide approaches also explicitly recognize the need to relate health sector changes to new aid instruments, macroeconomic and public sector management, poverty reduction, and achievement of the Millennium Development Goals (Cassels 1997). A key aspect of the sectorwide approach is to improve a country's overall policy-making processes and budget and public expenditure management by capturing all funding sources and expenditures and putting resource allocation decisions into a medium-term budget and expenditure framework based on national priorities.

The core elements of a sectorwide approach are as follows:

- The government is in the driver's seat.
- The partnership between development partners and government results in a shared vision and priorities for the sector.
- A comprehensive sector development strategy reflects all development activities to identify gaps, overlaps, and inconsistencies. The entire sector is considered when conducting sector analysis, appraisal, monitoring, and evaluation.
- An expenditure framework is developed to clarify sector priorities and guide all sector financing and investment.
- Partnering across development assistance agencies reduces transaction costs for government (McLaughlin 2003; 2004).

TABLE 4.4   Indicators of progress in the Paris Declaration on Aid Effectiveness

Goal	Indicator	Target for 2010[a]
	Ownership	
1	Partners have operational development strategies—number of countries with national development strategies (including poverty reduction strategies) that have clear strategic priorities linked to a medium-term expenditure framework and reflected in annual budgets.	**At least 75% of partner countries** have operational development strategies.
	Alignment	
2	Reliable country systems—number of partner countries that have procurement and public financial management systems.	**(a) Half of partner countries** move up at least one measure (i.e., 0.5 points) on the PFM/CPIA scale of performance. **(b) One-third of partner countries** move up at least one measure (i.e., from D to C, C to B, or B to A) on the four-point scale used to assess performance for this indicator.
3	Aid flows are aligned on national priorities—percentage of aid flows to the government sector that is reported on partners' national budgets.	**Halve the gap**—halve the proportion of aid flows to government sector not reported on government's budget(s) (with at least 85% reported on budget).
4	Strengthen capacity by coordinated support—percentage of donor capacity development support provided through coordinated programs consistent with partners' national development strategies.	**50% of technical cooperation flows** are implemented through coordinated programmes consistent with national development strategies.
5a	Use of country procurement systems—percentage of donors and of aid flows that use partner country procurement systems that either (a) adhere to broadly accepted good practices or (b) have a reform program in place to achieve these.	**Countries (a)** **All donors** use partner countries' procurement systems. **A two-thirds reduction** in the % of aid flows to public sector not using partner countries' procurement system. **Countries (b)** **90% of donors** use partner countries' procurement system. **A one-third reduction** in the % of aid flows to public sector not using partner countries' procurement system.

(continues)

TABLE 4.4 Indicators of progress in the Paris Declaration on Aid Effectiveness *(continued)*

Goal	Indicator	Target for 2010[a]
5b	Use of country public financial management systems—percentage of donors and of aid flows that use partner country public financial management systems that either (a) adhere to broadly accepted good practices or (b) have a reform program in place to achieve these.	**Countries (a) (PFM/CPIA of 5 or above)** **All donors** use partner countries' PFM systems. **A two-thirds reduction** in the % of aid flows to the public sector not using partner countries' PFM systems. **Countries (b) (PFM/CPIA of 3.5 to 4.5)** **90% of donors** use partner countries' PFM systems. **A one-third reduction** in the % of aid flows to the public sector not using partner countries' PFM systems.
6	Strengthen capacity by avoiding parallel implementation structures—number of parallel project implementation units per country.	**Reduce by two-thirds** the stock of parallel project implementation units (PIUs).
7	Aid is more predictable—percentage of aid disbursements released according to agreed schedules in annual or multiyear frameworks.	**Halve the gap**—halve the proportion of aid not disbursed within the fiscal year for which it was scheduled.
8	Aid is untied—percentage of bilateral aid that is untied.	**Continued progress over time.**
	Harmonization	
9	Use of common arrangements or procedures—percentage of aid provided as program-based approaches.	**66% of aid flows** are provided in the context of program-based approaches.
10	Encourage shared analysis—percentage of (a) field missions and/or (b) country analytic work, including diagnostic reviews that are joint.	(a) **40% of donor missions** to the field are joint. (b) **66% of country analytic work is joint.**
	Managing for results	
11	Results-oriented frameworks—number of countries with transparent and monitorable performance assessment frameworks to assess progress against (a) the national development strategies and (b) sector programs.	**Reduce the gap by one-third**—Reduce the proportion of countries without transparent and monitorable performance assessment frameworks by one-third.
	Mutual accountability	
12	Mutual accountability—number of partner countries that undertake mutual assessments of progress in implementing agreed commitments on aid effectiveness, including those in this Declaration.	**All partner countries** have mutual assessment reviews in place.

Source: Authors, based on Paris Declaration on Aid Effectiveness, September 2005, Table III (Indicators of Progress)

Note: PFM = public financial management; CPIA = country policy and institutional assessment.

a. Some of the targets require confirmation by OECD DAC member countries.

Sectorwide approaches are in various stages of development and implementation, and few fully conform to the basic specifications outlined above (Jefferys, Walford, and Pearson 2003). At this point in their evolution, sectorwide approaches are also heavily affected by new instruments, such as poverty reduction support credits, the IMF's Poverty Reduction Grant Facility, and medium-term expenditure frameworks. The following conclusions can be drawn from several recent evaluations of the effectiveness of sectorwide approaches in achieving the health Millennium Development Goals and other health system reforms (World Bank 2000; Foster and others 2000; Jeffreys, Walford, and Pearson 2003; Hill 2002):

- Sectorwide approaches are more relevant in low-income countries than in middle-income countries. Middle-income countries rely less on external agencies for financing; have more mature institutions and multiple agencies involved in financing, purchasing, and providing care; and in some cases have active reform programs affecting several types of institutions.
- There is often a lack of systematic analysis of implementation capacity. More could have been done to analyze and fix implementation weaknesses. The tendency for sector programs to be overly ambitious in relation to existing capacities, a corollary of their complexity, was noted.
- Indicators used to monitor and evaluate policy changes are often poorly identified or are not broken into annual indicators for assessing the rate of progress. Other programs have tended to include too many indicators, diluting the focus on key priorities.
- Sectorwide approaches are most effective when there is high-level commitment from the government and when the health sector strategy is linked to a credible medium-term budget process and civil service reform. Links to civil service and local government reforms and budget reform are still weak.
- An annual review that is focused on the important problems and the feasible solutions is important.
- Donors as a group need to focus on delivering coherent and consistent messages, thereby giving priority to essentials.
- Pressure for immediate results must be tempered by realism to avoid disappointment and damage to programs.
- Overloaded line ministries have to achieve and maintain high levels of momentum and productivity, especially when transaction costs have increased as a result of initial sectorwide negotiations. There is danger of burn out.

Results seem even less encouraging for linking the sectorwide approach to poverty reduction strategy papers and medium-term expenditure frameworks through the budget cycle and for including the approach in donor aid from disease- and intervention-specific programs. A review of experiences with sectorwide approaches in several low-income countries reveals key issues with which countries are grappling. The general view is that, although sectorwide approaches, poverty reduction strategy papers, and health plans may be aligned in terms of outcome indicators and overall objectives, there are large divergences in the resources required and the actual amounts reflected in medium-term expenditure frameworks, as in the cases of Cambodia and Uganda (Hill 2002). Chapter 6 discusses the links across different instruments in more detail.

In considering how to fit donor funds allocated to disease- and intervention-specific programs into sectorwide approaches in Uganda, it was reported that global initiatives have had a destabilizing impact, particularly in light of sectoral expenditure ceilings set by the Ministry of Finance. Inflows from the global initiatives are also substantial—likely to be more than $60 million next year—three-quarters of total projected donor spending on health ($80 million). The impact of introducing global initiatives part way through a sector program was also an issue for Bangladesh, Cambodia, Ghana, Mozambique, Senegal, and Tanzania (where only GFATM monies for malaria have been programmed into the medium-term expenditure framework) (Hill 2002).

In most of the countries examined, individual donors still undertake separate evaluations for bilateral projects and programs, even in countries that have had a sectorwide approach for more than five years. Over time this may be less of an issue, as fewer projects fall outside the sectorwide approach. In Tanzania and Zambia, evaluations are timed to coincide with the Joint Annual Reviews to reduce the burden. In Cambodia, which has yet to fully embark on the sectorwide approach, there are still multiple reporting, monitoring, accounting, and review systems for different donors.

Endnotes

1. Preliminary estimates show that official development assistance reached $78.6 billion in 2004. See World Bank 2005a.

2. The increase in official development assistance in 2003 is tightly linked to concerns of security and influenced by amounts earmarked to the start of reconstruction of Iraq and allocations to Pakistan, Colombia, and Afghanistan.

3. Spain, France, Italy, and Germany all had deficits of over 4 percent of their respective GDP in 2004 and, except for France, were all substantially below the 0.33 percent goal as of June 2004. The United State's deficit with respect to GDP was over 6 percent in 2004, and its ODA contribution was 0.12 percent of GNI that year. Japan's deficit for GDP was over 9 percent in 2004. The demographic transition in the European Union, increasing costs due to the rising costs of oil, and the accession into the European Union of new countries that have difficulties meeting increasing aid commitments also contribute to the uncertainty of ODA commitments.

4. For details on the IFF and on the proposed pilot IFF for Immunization (the IFFIm), see World Bank and IMF 2005.

5. These estimates by Nissanke (2003) assume that 80 percent of proceeds are used for development assistance and the rest are kept by rich countries. It is also assumed that volume of wholesale transactions is reduced by 5 percent to 15 percent as a result of the tax.

6. The other component is direct portfolio equity investments, which are a rather small part (about 5.4 percent of net equity flows) and unlikely to increase in the near future.

7. In 1990 East Asia accounted for 42 percent and Latin America for 32 percent of total net private capital flows (Sagasti, Bezanson, and Prada 2005). Between 1975 and 1995, 20 developing countries accounted for roughly 40 percent of total private capital flows, and this high level of concentration doubled to 80 percent in 1999, a level that has continued in recent years.

8. Protesters in Bolivia, Ecuador, and other countries claim that remittances of profit by multinationals are eventually larger than the resources invested by such companies.

9. These World Bank estimates are based on personal communication with Catherine M. Michaud at the Harvard Initiative for Global Health.

10. In technical terms a country meets the solvency condition if the present discounted value of the ratio of primary deficits to GDP is, at some defined future time, equal to the negative of the initial level of debt to GDP, that is, a government with debt outstanding must anticipate, sooner or later, to run primary budget surpluses in order for fiscal policy to be sustainable.

11. A fixed-effect generalized least squares model, similar to that of Pack and Pack (1990, 1993, 1996), was run. Model selection between random effect and fixed effects was based on the Hausmann test. Overall goodness of fit is 69.9 percent. Note that the regression does not include other control variables, such as literacy, under-five mortality rate, and maternal mortality ratio, which may lead to omitted variable bias. However, the omitted variable bias generated by the absence of these control variables is likely to bias the coefficient of donor funding off budget toward zero. This is because the coefficient on omitted under-five mortality is likely to be positive (the higher the under-five mortality rate, the more likely the government will increase spending on health), and the covariance between under-five mortality and donor off-budget health support is positive (donors will likely increase their support if the country has high under-five mortality rate).

12. Another related issue is whether there is fungibility within the health sector, independent of whether donor funding is fungible across sectors. In other words, is there a reallocation of domestic resources between primary care and higher-level care, for example, as a reaction to donor funding? The data used here do not permit analysis of this in any formal way. However, plotting time series data for some countries such as Ethiopia seems to indicate that this type of logical behavior by government is possible.

13. Revenues are domestic tax and nontax revenues net of grants as a proportion of GDP.

References

Bird, R. 2003. "Fiscal Flows, Fiscal Balance, and Fiscal Sustainability." Working Paper 03-021, International Studies Program, Andrew Young School of Public Studies, Georgia State University, Atlanta.

Boone, P. 1994. "The Impact of Foreign Aid on Savings and Growth." London School of Economics and Political Science, London.

Burnside, C., and D. Dollar. 1997. "Aid, Policies, and Growth." World Bank, Washington, D.C.

Cassels, A. 1997. "A Guide to Sector-Wide Approaches for Health Development: Concepts, Issues, and Working Arrangements." WHO/ARA/97.12, World Health Organization, Geneva; Danish International Development Assistance, Copenhagen; U.K. Department of International Development, London; European Commission, Brussels.

Clemens, M. A., S. Radelet, and R. Bhavnani. 2004. "Counting Chickens When They Hatch: The Short-Term Effect of Aid on Growth." Working Paper 44, Center for Global Development, Washington, D.C.

Clements, B., S. Gupta, A. Pivovarsky, and E. R. Tiongson. 2004. "Foreign Aid: Grants versus Loans." *Finance and Development* 41 (3): 46–9.

Collier, P., and D. Dollar. 1999. "Aid Allocation and Poverty Reduction." *European Economic Review* 46 (8): 1475–500.

Collier, P., and A. Hoeffler. 2002. "Aid, Policy, and Growth in Post-Conflict Societies." World Bank, Washington, D.C.

Croce, E., and V. H. Juan-Ramon. 2003. *Assessing Fiscal Sustainability: A Cross-Country Comparison.* Washington, D.C.: International Monetary Fund.

Devarajan, S., A. Rajkumar, and V. Swaroop. 1999. "What Does Aid to Africa Finance?" Policy Research Working Paper 2092, Africa Region, World Bank, Washington, D.C.

Dunaway, S., and P. N'Diaye. 2004. *An Approach to Long-Term Fiscal Policy Analysis.* Washington, D.C.: International Monetary Fund.

Edwards, S. 2002. *Debt Relief and Fiscal Sustainability.* NBER Working Paper 8939. Cambridge, Mass.: National Bureau of Economic Research.

Feyziouglu, T., V. Swaroop, and M. Zhu. 1997. "Foreign Aid Fungibility: A Panel Data Analysis." *World Bank Economic Review* 12 (1): 29–58.

Foster, M. 2005a. "MDG-Oriented Sector and Poverty Reduction Strategies: Lessons from Experience." Health, Nutrition, and Population Discussion Paper, World Bank, Washington, D.C.

———. 2005b. "Improving the Medium- and Long-Term Predictability of Aid." World Bank, Washington, D.C.

Foster, M., A. Brown, A. Norton, and F. Naschold. 2000. *The Status of Sector Wide Approaches.* London: Centre for Aid and Public Expenditure (CAPE), Overseas Development Institute.

Foster, M., A. Keith, H. Waddington, and A. Harding. 2003. *The Case for Increased Aid: Final Report to the Department for International Development.* Country Case Studies Vol 2. Essex, U.K.: Mick Foster Economics.

G-8 (Group of Eight). 2005. "Chairman's Summary." Statement presented at the G-8 Summit, Gleneagles, Scotland, July 6–8.

Hanson, K., M. K. Ranson, V. Oliveira-Cruz, A. Mills. 2001. "Approaches to Overcoming Health Systems Constraints at a Peripheral Level: A Review of the Evidence." CMH Working Paper Series WG5: 15, Commission on Macreconomics and Health, London.

Heller, P. 2005. "Understanding Fiscal Space." IMF Policy Discussion Paper PDP/05/4, International Monetary Fund, Washington, D.C.

High Level Forum. 2005. *Paris Declaration on Aid Effectiveness: Ownership, Harmonization, Alignment, Results, and Mutual Accountability.* Paris.

Hill, P. S. 2002. "The Rhetoric of Sector-Wide Approaches for Health Development." *Social Science and Medicine* 54 (11): 1725–37.

IMF (International Monetary Fund). 2001. *IMF Government Financial Statistics Manual 2001.* Washington, D.C.

Jeffreys, E., V. Walford, and M. Pearson. 2003. "Mapping of Sector-Wide Approaches in Health." Institute for Health Sector Development, Swedish International Development Cooperation Agency, London.

Kumaranayake, L., C. Kurowski, and L. Conteh. 2001. "Cost of Scaling Up Priority Health Interventions in Low-Income and Selected Middle-Income Countries: Methodology and Estimates." CMH Working Paper Series WG5: 18, Commission for Macroeconomics and Health, London.

Lele, U., R. Ridker, and J. Upadhyay. Forthcoming. "Health System Capacities in Developing Countries and Global Health Initiatives." Background paper prepared for the International Task Force on Global Public Goods, Washington, D.C.

Lewis, M. 2005. "Addressing the Challenges of HIV/AIDS: Macroeconomic, Fiscal, and Institutional Issues." Working Paper 58, Center for Global Development, Washington, D.C.

McLaughlin, J. 2003. "Accelerating Progress towards the Health MDGs: Important Lessons Learned from Development Assistance." World Bank, Washington, D.C.

———. 2004. "The Evolution of the Sector-Wide Approach (SWAp) and Explaining the Correlation between SWAps and Reform Initiatives." World Bank, Washington, D.C.

Michaud, C. M. 2003. "Development Assistance for Health (DAH): Recent Trends and Resource Allocation." Paper prepared for the Second Consultation of the Commission on Macroeconomics and Health, World Health Organization, Geneva, October 29–30.

Nissanke, M. 2003. "Revenue Potential of the Tobin Tax for Development Finance: A Critical Appraisal." School of Oriental and African Studies: University of London. Informal paper.

OECD (Organisation for Economic Co-operation and Development). 2004. *Analysis of Aid in Support of HIV/AIDS Control, 2000–2002.* Paris.

Pack, H., and J. R. Pack. 1990. "Is Foreign Aid Fungible?" *Economic Journal* 100 (399): 188–94.

———. 1993. "Foreign Aid and the Question of Fungibility." *Review of Economics and Statistics* 75 (2): 258–65.

———. 1996. "Foreign Aid and Fiscal Stress: The Case of Indonesia." University of Pennsylvania, Philadelphia.

PHR*plus* (Partners for Health Reform*plus*). 2005. "How the Global Fund Affects Health Systems." *PHRplus Highlights.* April: 5–6.

Preker, A., E. Suzuki, F. Bustero, A. Soucat, and J. Langenbrunner. 2003. "Costing the Millennium Development Goals: Expenditure Gaps and Development Traps." Health, Nutrition, and Population Discussion Paper, World Bank, Washington, D.C.

Sagasti, F., K. Bezanson, and F. Prada. 2005. *The Future of Development Financing: Challenges, Scenarios, and Strategic Choices.* Global Development Studies 1. Stockholm, Sweden: Palgrave Macmillan.

Tanzi, V., and H. H. Zee. 2000. "Tax Policy for Emerging Markets: Developing Countries." IMF Working Paper, International Monetary Fund, Washington, D.C.

UN Millennium Project. 2005. *Investing in Development: A Practical Plan to Achieve the Millennium Development Goals.* London: Earthscan.

Wagstaff, A., and M. Claeson. 2004. *The Millennium Development Goals for Health: Rising to the Challenges.* Washington, D.C.: World Bank.

World Bank. 2000. "Sector-Wide Approaches for Education and Health in Sub-Saharan Africa." Africa Region, Washington, D.C.

———. 2004a. "Aid Effectiveness and Innovative Financing Mechanisms." Paper prepared by the Development Committee for the 2004 Annual Meetings. Washington, D.C.

———. 2004b. *Global Development Finance 2004: Harnessing Cyclical Gains for Development.* Washington, D.C.

———. 2005a. "Aid Effectiveness and Aid Financing." Paper presented to the Development Committee, Document SecM2005-0435, September 25, Washington, D.C.

———. 2005b. *Global Monitoring Report.* Washington, D.C.

———. 2006. *Global Economic Prospects: Economic Implications of Remittances and Migration.* Washington, D.C.

World Bank and IMF (International Monetary Fund). 2005. "Moving Forward: Financing Modalities toward the Millennium Development Goals." Development Committee Paper DC2005-0008/add. 1, Washington, D.C.

5

Improving health outcomes

There is strong international support for increasing government expenditures and donor funding to accelerate progress toward the Millennium Development Goals. Additional government health expenditures and donor funding, although they may improve health outcomes, in particular maternal mortality and mortality of children under five, are not likely to be sufficient to reach the Millennium Development Goals for health by 2015. Reaching these goals requires broad economic growth and investment, significant change in the way donor funding is provided, and more efficient health spending.

With so many countries not on track to meet the health-related Millennium Development Goals, the international community is now reaching a consensus that current health expenditure levels in developing countries are too low and that more resources are needed (see chapter 7). These discussions take for granted, however, that the additional expenditures and resources will bring about the desired health outcomes. The discussions also often ignore the additional actions required to improve the ability of countries to absorb and mobilize additional resources to reach the Millennium Development Goals.

This chapter contains new findings on the impact of government health expenditures and donor funding on health outcomes. These findings indicate that government health expenditures do indeed affect under-five mortality and maternal mortality, contrary to results reported in much of the literature to date. The results also show that donor funding has a direct impact on under-five mortality, but not on maternal mortality. Nonetheless, donor funding indirectly affects maternal mortality by increasing the impact of governmental health expenditures on this outcome.

These effects of donor funding on health outcomes can be explained in part by the volatility and fungibility of donor funding, as well as by the difficulties that governments face in reallocating resources in the short term after a donor has decreased or discontinued funding. This chapter reviews these effects and their implications for reaching the Millennium Development Goals for child mortality and maternal mortality across different regions. The chapter concludes by addressing the fundamental issues for improving countries' chances of reaching the Millennium Development

Goals for health. These issues include stimulating economic growth and multisectoral investment, as well as changing the way donor funding is provided and government health expenditures are used, so that these critical resources produce better health outcomes. Three key lessons emerge from the discussion:

- Neither increased government health expenditures nor GDP growth alone are sufficient for reaching the health Millennium Development Goals. Although both expenditures and growth affect health outcomes, long-term investments in infrastructure, education, and water and sanitation are also needed. Furthermore, GDP growth is essential not only because it generates greater personal income, which directly boosts health outcomes, but also because it generates government revenues that can support a multisectoral approach to health investments.

- Recipient countries must improve their capacity to absorb and use additional health resources by strengthening policies and institutions for managing public expenditures. Resources, even if available, must be made accessible regularly and on time where health services are to be delivered; this effort requires efficient public expenditure management from central to local government and from local government to the service facility. It also implies appropriate accountability at all levels of government. (Such accountability is further reviewed in chapter 6.)

- Donors must carefully evaluate their role and desired impact in country-specific contexts to improve the consistency between donor and country objectives. Donor aid now has a limited direct impact on health outcomes, in part because of the fungibility, volatility, and asymmetry in budgeting (see chapter 4).[1] To improve outcomes, donors must

  ⬥ Exercise care in designing aid programs and evaluating the impact of their funds.

  ⬥ Give serious consideration to supporting government budgets directly through general budget support. Donors should agree with governments on a program, rather than directly finance projects that may crowd out the government's own resources.

  ⬥ Commit to predictable financing over long maturities to provide budget support to existing government programs. This action is especially important given the recurrent nature of many health expenditures, which make them unsuitable for financing through short-term grants.

  ⬥ Directly fund projects only in cases of major government failure, especially in public expenditure management.

  ⬥ Provide technical assistance as the first priority in cases of government failure to improve public expenditure management and government capacity.

Government health expenditures

The theoretical link between increases in government health expenditures and improved health outcomes is complex for several reasons. First, an increase in government health expenditures may result in a decrease in private health expenditures—a household may divert its funds to other uses once the government increases its basic health expenditures. Second, incremental government expenditures may be employed ineffectively (for instance, expenditures allocated to high-tech equipment or advanced hospitals may have little effect on public health if morbidity indicators show the need for increased resources for primary care). Third, even if extra funds are applied appropriately, they may yield little benefit if complementary services, both inside and outside the health sector, are lacking (for example, roads or transportation services to hospitals and clinics and easy access to water and sanitation) (Wagstaff 2002a).

The empirical literature has not shed much light on the link between public spending and health outcomes. Early studies (as summarized by Musgrove in 1996) find no evidence that total spending on health has any impact on child mortality. Filmer and Pritchett (1999) find that government health expenditures account for less than one-seventh of one percent of the variation in under-five mortality across countries, although the result was not statistically significant. They conclude that 95 percent of the variation in under-five mortality can be explained by factors such as the country's per capita income, female educational attainment, and choice of religion. Finally, using a model similar to that of Filmer and Pritchett, Wagstaff and Claeson (2004) showed more recently that good policies and institutions (as measured by the World Bank's Country Policy and Institutional Assessment or CPIA Index) are important determinants of the impact of government health expenditures on outcomes. In particular, as the quality of policies and institutions improves (as the CPIA Index rises), the impact of government health expenditures on maternal mortality, underweight children under age five, and tuberculosis mortality also increases and is statistically significant. However, the impact of government expenditures on under-five mortality remains not significantly different from zero.

New findings on the impact of government and donor funding

As discussed above, a large percentage of donor assistance for health is managed directly by the donor outside the recipient government's budgeting system—it is off-budget. A model developed for this report[2] attempts to capture both the direct and indirect impact of these off-budget resources on health outcomes. Donor funding levels and the volatility of donor funding are included in the model as explanatory variables.[3] In addition, the critical relationship and interaction between donor funding and public health spending is also taken into account to capture the impact of the fungibility of aid with respect to domestically financed public spending.[4]

The impact of government health expenditure is of key interest. In contrast to other results presented in the literature, this study found that a 10 percent increase in government health expenditures has a larger net impact[5] in reducing under-five mortality and maternal mortality than a 10 percent increase in education, roads, or sanitation. Government health expenditures also have as large an impact as income on under-five mortality but a smaller impact on maternal mortality.[6] In addition, for a 10 percent increase in government health expenditures, the decrease in maternal mortality is typically 1 percentage point more than the decrease in under-five mortality. In Albania, for example, a 10 percent increase in government health expenditures (from the current observed value of 92 Int$ per capita to 101.2 Int$) implies a 4.1 percent reduction in under-five mortality and a 5.5 percent reduction in maternal mortality.[7] In absolute terms, this would reduce under-five mortality from 26 per 1,000 to 24.8 per 1,000 and maternal mortality from 55 per 100,000 to 52 per 100,000.

Another important finding concerns the effect of donor funding on health-related outcomes. Donor funding can make an important dent in under-five mortality—but only when it is predictable and sustained. In contrast, neither the amount nor the volatility of donor funding has a direct impact on maternal mortality.[8] Donor funding does have an indirect impact on maternal mortality, however, through its impact on government expenditures. This likely arises from the fungibility of donor funding. If the recipient country takes these external and largely off-budget funds into consideration in the allocation of its own domestic resources and spends more of its own money on, say, secondary care such as hospitals, which typically are not funded by donors, the increased and sustained expenditure on secondary care may increase the effect of government expenditures on maternal mortality. Table 5.1 shows the regression results for under-five mortality and maternal mortality.[9]

Reaching the Millennium Development Goals for health

Will the Millennium Development Goals, at least for under-five mortality and maternal mortality, be reached? What are the implications for policy development? Several conclusions can be drawn from this model and other work in the literature.[10]

Continuing current levels of financing and growth and lack of coordination across sectors—"business as usual"—would mean that none of the developing regions of the world, according to the World Bank's regional classifications, will reach the Millennium Development Goal for under-five mortality (figure 5.1). Moreover, the slow progress from 1990 to 2000 implies that, to reach the under-five mortality goal in 2015, the annual rate of decline in mortality would have to be larger than the average 4.2 percent needed originally (as represented by the target

TABLE 5.1   Model regression results for under-five mortality
and maternal mortality

Variable	Under-five mortality	Maternal mortality
intercept	8.2591[++]	9.9084[++]
	(0.08477)	(1.4544)
lnE	0.0651	0.3082[++]
	(0.0427)	(0.0863)
lnR	−0.0868[++]	−0.1019[++]
	(0.0241)	(0.0415)
lnS	0.0493	0.1708
	(0.1115)	(0.1533)
lnVol	0.096[++]	0.0604
	(0.029)	(0.0408)
lnGDP	−0.3689[++]	−0.5320[+]
	(0.1348)	(0.2477)
lnGh	−0.3708[++]	−0.4286[+]
	(0.1082)	(0.2026)
lnDF	−0.0429[+]	−0.0348
	(0.0233)	(0.0367)
lnGh*DF	−0.0122	−0.0340[+]
	(0.01)	(0.0175)
R^2	0.8216	0.7414
Adjusted R^2	0.8079	0.7215

Source: World Bank staff estimates.

Note: Parameter standard errors are given in parenthesis. Estimates are based on the regression model presented in annex 5.1.

E = education, R = roads, S = sanitation, Vol = volatility of donor funding, GDP = gross domestic product per capita, Gh = government health expenditure, DF = donor funding.

[++] p-value = 0.01 or less; [+] p-value = 0.05 or less

bar on the figure).[11] For example, in East Asia and Pacific, under-five mortality would have to decline at a new rate of about 5 percent a year from 2001 to 2015 (black square on figure 5.1), almost double the current rate of 2.7 percent, as averaged over the period 1990–2000 and represented by the top shaded area. In the case of Sub-Saharan Africa, the rate of decline in under-five mortality has to accelerate from less than 0.5 percent a year between 1990 and 2000 to close to 8 percent a year between 2001 and 2015 to reach the Millennium Development Goal.

The outlook is more optimistic for maternal mortality (figure 5.2). Nonetheless, the business-as-usual trend will not be sufficient to reach the Millennium Development Goal, except in the Middle East and North Africa and East Asia and

FIGURE 5.1 **Progress toward reducing under-five mortality, by region**

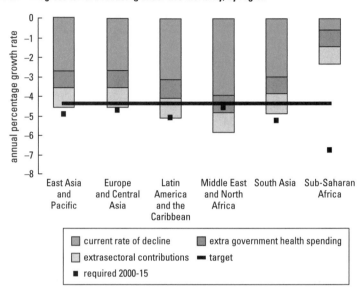

Source: World Bank staff estimates based on the model presented in annex 5.1.
Note: Extrasectoral contributions include contributions from the variables for income, education, roads, sanitation, and donor funding. Those contributions, as well as government health expenditure, are assumed to grow at 2.5 percent annually. Volatility of donor funding is assumed to be decreasing at 2.5 percent (by the end of 2015 donor funding will be one-third less volatile). Regional averages are population weighted.

Pacific regions. The annual rates of decline in maternal mortality will have to change in South Asia from about 3 percent in the 1990s to about 7 percent in 2000 to 2015 and in Europe and Central Asia from about 4 percent to 6 percent. The rate of decline in Sub-Saharan Africa and Latin America and the Caribbean would have to change from less than 2 percent a year to close to 8 percent. For Latin America and the Caribbean, this steep target may be partially due to the low baseline maternal mortality ratio in the region in 1990. The difficulty that the region is likely to have in reaching this target suggests that returns to delivery of appropriate services to reduce maternal mortality for the most marginalized women are diminishing. Efforts must be made to extend health services to remote areas and target the groups that are hardest to reach.

A multisectoral effort needed

Reaching the Millennium Development Goals requires a multisectoral effort plus growth in real GDP per capita. For most developing countries, anything short of this combined effort raises the likelihood that the goals will not be reached. For example, India has enjoyed an impressive real GDP per capita growth of 3.8 percent a year over the past four years. However, the model simulations show that

FIGURE 5.2   Progress toward reducing maternal mortality, by region

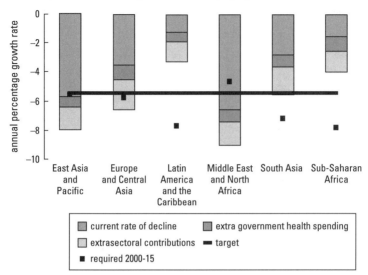

Source: World Bank staff estimates based on the model presented in annex 5.1.
Note: Extrasectoral contributions include contributions from the variables for income, education, roads, sanitation, and donor funding. Those contributions, as well as government health expenditure, are assumed to grow at 2.5 percent annually. Volatility of donor funding is assumed to be decreasing at 2.5 percent (by the end of 2015, donor funding will be one-third less volatile). Regional averages are population weighted.

even this impressive growth of income will fall short of the 15 percent increase in real GDP per capita needed over the period 2000 to 2015 if the Millennium Development Goals are to be reached through growth alone.

Similarly, resources devoted to health expenditures are insufficient by themselves to reach the goals. For instance, in Rwanda, per capita public expenditures would have to increase from $3.1 a year in 2004 to more than $56 in constant 2000 dollars by 2015. With no growth, the country would be spending more on health than the government collects in total revenues. A multisectoral approach with investments in infrastructure, education, and health is needed. Growth must occur, not only because of the direct impact of income on outcomes, but also because the financing of the multisectoral approach requires such growth and the revenues that it generates.

The combination of increasing health expenditures and growth would most likely help low-income countries come closer to reaching the Millennium Development Goals related to maternal and child mortality, but for a few countries even this formula would not work (figure 5.3). Kenya, Rwanda, and Sudan, for example, would not reach the under-five mortality goal even with ambitious increases in real per capita growth rates of 5 percent a year (above an average of –1.1 percent, 3.3 percent, and 3.9 percent, respectively, over the past four years)

FIGURE 5.3 **Under-five mortality targets and projected rates in Kenya, Rwanda, and Sudan**

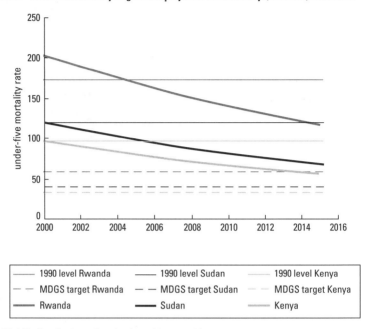

Source: World Bank staff estimates based on the model presented in annex 5.1.
Note: Projections for all three countries assume a positive 5 percent change per year in government health expenditures, education, infrastructure, water supply and sanitation, and donor funding. The solid line below the dotted line for Rwanda implies that under-five mortality in 1990 was below the 2000 estimate.

and increases of 5 percent a year in government health spending and the other explanatory variables of the model (education, roads, sanitation, and donor funding). According to the model, it would take very optimistic increases of 7 percent a year in real GDP per capita and government health expenditures, along with 5 percent annual increases in all the other variables, for these countries to reach the goal. To reach the Millennium Development Goal for maternal mortality by 2015, these countries would require similarly optimistic growth in GDP per capita and public expenditures.

Countries that strive to meet the Millennium Development Goals on health through a multisector and growth approach will have to emphasize not only increasing investments in sectors that directly promote improved health outcomes, but also pursue efforts that influence growth rates. Recent World Bank work in this area suggests that those efforts involve trade, infrastructure, and the policies and institutions required for attracting investment, such as mechanisms for the protection of property rights and reliable judicial systems (Leipziger and others 2003; Paternostro, Rajaram, and Tiongson 2004; Herrera and Pan 2005).

Donors and predictable resources

The model described in annex 5.1 shows that there is no direct impact of donor financing on maternal mortality ratios. Rather, the impact on maternal mortality occurs indirectly, by permitting an increase in the levels and sustainability of government health expenditures. Similarly, erratic donor financing does not have an impact on under-five mortality.

These results may be explained by the volatility and fungibility of donor funding, as well as by the difficulties governments have in reallocating resources from one priority to another. This implies that donors should not try to second guess recipient countries' priorities. Faster progress can be made by financing government programs, such as poverty reduction strategies, as the first priority. These programs must also be multisectoral, have appropriate growth strategies, and include efforts to improve policies and institutions. Donor funding must be predictable, stable, and sustained over a long period.

Improving policies and institutions

Wagstaff and Claeson (2004) have recently shown that policies and institutions are important for increases in spending to have a significant effect on health outcomes in achieving the Millennium Development Goals. The work shows that the impact of government health expenditures on outcomes is directly related to each country's policies and institutions, as reflected in the World Bank's measured assessment of country policies and institutions, the CPIA Index (see chapter 6). The authors conclude that increases in government health expenditures would not have an impact on any Millennium Development Goal outcome in countries with a CPIA below or at 3.25 (scale 1 through 5). Business as usual will not be sufficient in such countries. To reach the Millennium Development Goals, strong policy and institutional efforts are fundamental. These efforts include concentration on technical assistance to improve public expenditure management, administrative capacity, monitoring and evaluation, and mechanisms for ensuring accountability.

Annex 5.1 Government health expenditures, donor funding, and health outcomes: data and methods

The discussion in chapter 5 is based, in part, on the estimates of the following reduced form equation:

$$(1) \qquad \ln Y_m = \beta_{m1} + \beta_{m2} \ln E + \beta_{m3} \ln R + \beta_{m4} \ln S + \beta_{m5} \ln DF$$
$$+ \beta_{m6} \ln I + \beta_{m7} \ln Gh + \beta_{m8} DF \ln Gh + \beta_{m9} \ln V + v_m$$

where Y_m is either under-five mortality or maternal mortality.[12] The functional form is based on the assumption that these health outcomes are a function of government health expenditures (Gh), national income (I), education (E), roads (R) and sanitation (S) as well as the level of off-budget donor funding (DF) and volatility in donor funding (V). The percentage change in under-five mortality (or maternal mortality) due to a percentage change in government health expenditures (Gh), can be estimated from equation (1) as $\beta_{m7} + \beta_{m8} ln$DF. It should be noted that a small change in government health expenditures may be associated with a direct change in under-five mortality (or maternal mortality) as well as a change in other Millennium Development Goal health indicators such as proportion of 1-year-old children immunized against measles and proportion of population in malaria-risk areas using effective malaria prevention. Furthermore, any change in these latter indicators (which are not included in the right-hand side of the equation) would also cause a change in, for instance, under-five mortality. Thus our elasticity measure gives the net percentage change in indicator Y_m associated with a 1 percent change in Gh, holding I, E, R, S, DF, and V, but not the other Millennium Development Goals for Health indicators, constant. Finally, note that income and government health expenditures may both be correlated with the error term. We account for potential endogeneity of these variables through the use of instrumental variables within the generalized method of moments estimation techniques.

Data sources and description

Data on these variables were obtained from various sources and linked for 113 countries for the calender year 2000. The primary source was the World Bank's in-house online database, SIMA, which is a collection of variables from various data sources including *World Development Indicators*, Millennium Indicators Database, World Health Report, and *Human Development Report* by the United Nations Children's Fund.

Under-five mortality is measured as the under-five mortality rate per 1,000 live births and maternal mortality is measured as the maternal mortality ratio per 100,000 live births. The measure of national income is GDP per capita;[13] education is the percentage of the population age 15 or older who are illiterate; sanitation is the percentage of the population with access to improved sanitation facilities; and the measure for roads is paved roads (in kilometers) per unit area of country (in square kilometers). Data on government health expenditures are also in per capita terms and data for 2000 were obtained using the World Health Organization's *World Health Report 2004.*

Information on donor funding was obtained from the Creditor Reporting System table of the International Development Statistics online database. Funding commitments came from the Development Assistance Committee countries of the Organisation for Economic Co-operation and Development. These donations are bilateral and are usually used for specific off-budget health projects. Because bilateral donations are not counted as part of a country's government health budget, this variable was used as a measure of donor funding. However, this is the amount that the receiving countries were promised by donor countries in the given calendar year, not the actual amount received. The actual amount received is with a lag of a few years and may be different from the amount promised. For this reason the lagged value of the variable was used. For example, for the 2000 analysis the donor funding variable is per capita donor funding from Development Assistance Committee countries for health promised in 1998. For volatility, the standard deviation of the donor funding variable between 1994 and 1998 was used. Summary statistics of the log of these variables as used in the model are provided in table A5.1.

Endogeneity and instruments

Although many of the conditions of poverty—lack of clean water, sanitation, access to health services, and education—can lead to high levels of illness, micro theory suggests a reverse causality as well. Specifically, morbidity and ill health of the individuals in a family affects their ability to work and hence their income and can cause the household to fall into poverty. Similarly, it is possible that the government health expenditures variable may be correlated with the error term because governments may implicitly respond to poor health outcomes in prior years by adjusting health care spending in the current year. Here the source of endogeneity is not, per se, reverse causality—government budgets are set at the beginning of a year (with perhaps some deviations by the end of the year) while the health indicators are measured at the end of year—but rather due to omitted variables bias. Specifically, if current health outcomes are correlated with past health outcomes, and if the current government health expenditure is implicitly a function of prior health outcomes, equation (1) is misspecified to the extent that past health outcomes are not included in the equation.

To correct for potential endogeneity of income and government health expenditures, we estimate the models using instrumental variables techniques. The instrument that we use for national income is the consumption-investment ratio

TABLE A5.1   Variable names and summary statistics

Variable	Definition (N = 113)	Mean	Minimum[a]	Maximum	Standard deviation	Median
lnU5M	ln under-five mortality per 1,000 live births	3.9892	1.3863	5.656	1.0009	3.912
lnMM	ln maternal mortality per 100,000 live births	5.1603	0	7.6009	1.4905	5.0752
lnGDP	ln GDP per capita[b]	8.0187	6.1527	10.2681	0.9317	8.1634
lnGH	ln government health expenditures per capita[b]	4.2694	1.3863	7.688	1.2735	4.4188
lnE	ln education (percent of population age 15 or older illiterate)	2.4028	−2.3026	4.4313	1.5535	2.7535
lnS	ln sanitation (percent of population with access to improved sanitation)	4.1493	2.0794	4.6052	0.5381	4.3567
lnR	ln roads (paved roads per unit area)	1.3805	−8.8307	6.2198	2.3687	1.5023
lnDF	ln donor funding per capita for basic health in 1998[b]	−0.4775	−8.3192	4.1263	2.702	0.2836
lvol	ln standard deviation of donor commitment from 1994 to 1998	−0.0487	−9.1084	3.3009	2.251	0.4741
lnGH*DF	$(\text{lnGH} - \overline{\text{lnGH}}) \times (\text{DF} - \overline{\text{DF}})$	−1.1532	−34.0156	17.3859	5.2929	−0.6972

Source: Authors.

a. Log of zero was set equal to zero if the nonzero values were greater than one. However, if nonzero values were less than one, the log of zero was set equal to the log of the nonzero minimum value.

b. Converted to constant 2000 international dollars.

of the country because it is likely to be correlated with the GDP variable but not with under-five mortality or maternal mortality. Similarly, the instrument that we use for government health expenditures (and their interaction with donor funding) is military expenditures of neighboring countries (and their interaction with donor funding).

In addition to these variables, two other instruments were used. The World Bank staff annually assesses (and scores) the quality of polices and institutions in 4 broad areas with 20 criteria relevant to economic growth and poverty reduction of the countries borrowing from the International Bank for Reconstruction and Development and from the International Development Association.[14] Of these 20 criteria, 4 score the countries on a scale of 1–5 or 1–6 on the following issues relating to economic management: management of inflation and currency accounting, fiscal policy, management of external debt, and management and sustainability of developmental programs. The average score on these four criteria was used as an additional instrument for GDP per capita. Similarly, scores on three additional criteria partly assess the policies for social inclusion and equity: gender equity, equity of public resource use, and policies for building human resources. The average score on these three criteria was used as an additional instrument for government health expenditures.

Results

For each of the two indicators (under-five mortality and maternal mortality), equation (1) was estimated under a set of alternative assumptions about the error term: (a) no correlation between any of the right-hand side variables and the error terms (no endogeneity), (b) the government health expenditures variable and its interaction with the donor funding variable are correlated with the error term but the income variable is not correlated with the error term (only $lnGh$ and $lnGh \times DF$ are endogenous), and (c) the income variable is also correlated with the error term ($lnGh$, $lnGh \times DF$ and lnI are all endogenous variables). Furthermore, for each of the three assumptions above, the equations were estimated with and without accounting for the presence of an unknown form of heteroscedasticity. Thus under assumption (a) we estimated ordinary least squares (OLS) estimates with the usual standard errors as well as the heteroscedastic ordinary least squares (HOLS). Similarly, under assumptions (b) and (c), standard two-stage least squares (2SLS) estimates as well as the Davidson and Mackinnon's general method of moments heteroscedastic two-stage least squares (GMM-H2SLS) estimator was used to compute the estimates and the standard errors. Graphical methods indicate that mild heteroscedasticity is present. More formal White tests based on the interaction of all terms yield chi-square statistics that are significant in the p=.10 to p=.15 range. Results for the two indicators (under-five mortality and maternal mortality) are summarized in table A5.2. The six columns in the table correspond to estimates based on assumptions (a), (b), and (c) with and without heteroscedasticity.

Weak instruments, Hausman, and overidentification tests

The reliability of the instrumental variables estimates (2SLS and GMM-H2SLS) relies on the use of good instruments. To establish the empirical relevance of these instruments, the weak instruments test was performed. In all "first-stage" regressions, the joint F-test for the additional instruments alone was almost always above the rule-of-thumb recommended value of 10 (test statistics are given near the bottom of table A5.2).

Additionally, the validity of the instruments (under heteroscedasticity) was tested through the usual overidentification tests. Thus for specification (VI) for under-five mortality and maternal mortality, the maintained null that the instruments are valid could not be rejected at the usual levels (for under-five mortality, the Hansen's J-statistic was 0.331, with a p-value of 0.954, and for maternal mortality, the test statistic was 3.806, with a p-value of 0.283).

TABLE A5.2 Regression results

	GH exogenous and GDP exogenous		GH endogenous and GDP exogenous		GH endogenous and GDP endogenous	
	OLS (I)	H-OLS (II)	2SLS (III)	H2SLS (IV)	2SLS (V)	GMM-H2SLS (VI)
Dependent variable: log of under-five mortality						
Intercept	7.9642[++]	8.2199[++]	7.0014[++]	7.4697[++]	8.0852[++]	8.2591[++]
	(0.6425)	(0.5516)	(0.9122)	(0.7742)	(1.0634)	(0.08477)
lnE	0.1158[++]	0.1203[++]	0.0795[+]	0.1005[++]	0.0614	0.0651
	(0.034)	(0.0331)	(0.0406)	(0.038)	(0.0417)	(0.0427)
lnR	−0.1088[++]	−0.1015[++]	−0.0986[++]	−0.0773[++]	−0.089[++]	−0.0868[++]
	(0.0201)	(0.0196)	(0.0206)	(0.0233)	(0.0216)	(0.0241)
lnS	−0.0379	−0.1238	−0.0081	−0.0595	0.0562	0.0493
	(0.0935)	(0.081)	(0.0948)	(0.093)	(0.1031)	(0.1115)
lnV	0.0896[++]	0.1051[++]	0.1047[++]	0.1106[++]	0.0981[++]	0.096[++]
	(0.0267)	(0.0258)	(0.0282)	(0.029)	(0.0289)	(0.029)
lnGDP	−0.4036[++]	−0.3902[++]	−0.1666	−0.2422[+]	−0.3395	−0.3689[++]
	(0.1004)	(0.0764)	(0.1812)	(0.129)	(0.1966)	(0.1348)
lnGH	−0.1684[+]	−0.1726[‡]	−0.4003[‡]	−0.3405[‡]	−0.3886[++]	−0.3708[++]
	(0.0793)	(0.07)	(0.1574)	(0.1204)	(0.1495)	(0.1082)
lnDF	−0.0218	−0.0312	−0.0314	−0.0387	−0.0416[+]	−0.0429[+]
	(0.0224)	(0.0223)	(0.023)	(0.0241)	(0.0242)	(0.0233)
lnGH × DF[a]	−0.0027	−0.0063	−0.0016	−0.0081	−0.011	−0.0122
−	(0.0082)	(0.0061)	(0.0109)	(0.0081)	(0.0119)	(0.01)
R^2	0.8315	0.8286	0.8176	0.8208	0.8077	0.8079
Dependent variable: log of maternal mortality						
Intercept	8.5353[++]	8.2238[++]	7.0755[++]	6.8036[++]	9.8304[++]	9.9084[++]
	(1.1557)	(0.884)	(1.6184)	(1.3032)	(1.9175)	(1.4544)
lnE	0.3968[++]	0.4467[++]	0.3442[++]	0.394[++]	0.307[++]	0.3082[++]
	(0.0612)	(0.0593)	(0.072)	(0.0752)	(0.0751)	(0.0863)
lnR	−0.1273[++]	−0.1241[++]	−0.1157[++]	−0.1085[++]	−0.093[‡]	−0.1019[++]
	(0.0362)	(0.0354)	(0.0365)	(0.0414)	(0.039)	(0.0415)
lnS	−0.0615	−0.0545	−0.0201	0.0209	0.1284	0.1708
	(0.1682)	(0.1249)	(0.1682)	(0.1462)	(0.1859)	(0.1533)
lnV	0.0641	0.0508	0.0861	0.0907[‡]	0.0679	0.0604
	(0.048)	(0.0391)	(0.0501)	(0.0438)	(0.0521)	(0.0408)
lnGDP	−0.3664[‡]	−0.3944[++]	−0.0161	−0.0398	−0.4675	−0.532[‡]
	(0.1805)	(0.1312)	(0.3215)	(0.2533)	(0.3545)	(0.2477)

(Continues)

TABLE A5.2   Regression results *(Continued)*

	GH exogenous and GDP exogenous		GH endogenous and GDP exogenous		GH endogenous and GDP endogenous	
	OLS (I)	H-OLS (II)	2SLS (III)	H2SLS (IV)	2SLS (V)	GMM-H2SLS (VI)
Dependent variable: log of maternal mortality *(Continued)*						
lnGH	−0.2306	−0.1333	−0.5604[‡]	−0.5225[‡]	−0.498+	−0.4286[‡]
	(0.1426)	(0.1022)	(0.2792)	(0.2273)	(0.2696)	(0.2026)
lnDF	−0.0177	0.0108	−0.0312	−0.0283	−0.054	−0.0348
	(0.0403)	(0.0361)	(0.0409)	(0.0394)	(0.0436)	(0.0367)
lnGH × DF[a]	−0.017	−0.0155	−0.0103	−0.0106	−0.0352+	−0.034+
–	(0.0147)	(0.0112)	(0.0193)	(0.0161)	(0.0215)	(0.0175)
R^2	0.7541	0.7502	0.7411	0.742	0.718	0.7215

	First-stage statistics (for III and IV)		First-stage statistics (for V and VI)		
Dependent variable	lnGH	lnGH × DF[a]	lnGH	lnGH × DF[a]	lnGDP
R^2	0.691	0.7357	0.7166	0.7377	0.6837
Overall F-statistic	25.59	31.85	23.21	25.82	19.85
Weak instruments F-test	11.48	63.96	9.7	42.27	12.36

Source:

Note: Parameter standard errors are given in parenthesis.

a. The variable used in the regression was (lnGH − Ln$\overline{GH}$) * (DF − D$\overline{F}$), where x̄ stands for the mean value of the variable.

[++] p-value = 0.01 or less; [+] p-value = 0.05 or less; [‡] p-value = 0.1 or less

Finally, the Hausman statistic was employed to test for endogeneity of variables under assumptions (b) and (c) above. For 5 of 6 tests, the null hypothesis of no endogeneity was rejected.[15] The Hausman test statistics (under heteroscedasticity) are summarized in table A5.3. The conclusions of the Hausman test results were identical when homoscedastic errors were assumed. (These gave six additional test statistics that are not given in table A5.3.) On the basis of the remaining five tests, *Gh* (and its interaction with *DF*) as well as the income variable are treated as endogenous variables.

TABLE A5.3   Hausman X^2-statistics (with heteroscedastic error terms)

For under-five mortality equation		
II vs IV	5.1709	(Pr X^2 (2) ≥ 4.61) ≤ 0.1, hence can reject Null (at 10 percent)
II vs VI	9.0995	(Pr(X^2 (3) ≥ 7.81) ≤ 0.05, hence can reject Null
IV vs VI	16.05	(Pr (X^2 (1) ≥ 3.84) ≤ 0.05, hence can reject Null
For maternal mortality equation		
II vs IV	4.2918	(Pr X^2 (2) ≥ 4.61) ≥ 0.1, hence cannot reject Null
II vs VI	12.9342	(Pr(X^2 (3) ≥ 7.81) ≤ 0.05, hence can reject Null
IV vs VI	3.8282	(Pr(X^2(1) ≥ 2.71) ≤ 0.1, hence can reject Null (at 10 percent)

Elasticities

Given the results of the test statistics above, we use the coefficients in the last column of table A5.2 as the "correct" coefficients.

The coefficients on the education and roads variables have the correct sign, but for under-five mortality the coefficient for education in specification (VI) is no longer statistically significant. A 10 percent reduction in illiteracy reduces under-five mortality by 0.65 percent and maternal mortality by 3.1 percent. Similarly, a 10 percent increase in the network of paved roads per unit area of the country reduces under-five mortality by about 0.87 percent and maternal mortality by about 1 percent. Note that the OLS coefficients biased these results away from zero, thus exaggerating their impact on these two Millennium Development Goal outcomes. Nonetheless, these are large effects. By contrast, the sign on the sanitation variable is expected to be negative and significant for both the indicators. However the coefficient is not significant in any of the estimations. A similar result (of nonsignificance) was observed elsewhere as well. Although it is certainly possible that sanitation, as defined here, has no impact on the health outcomes, this result is suspect. It is more likely that this variable is measured with error and hence the lack of significance may be due to attenuation bias.

Elasticity for per capita income is −0.3689 for under-five mortality and −0.532 for maternal mortality, and both are statistically significant at the 5 percent level.

The coefficient on Gh is negative and significant for both under-five mortality and maternal mortality and increases in magnitude when the instrumental variable methods are used. The best point estimates of the coefficients on Gh are −0.37 for under-five mortality and −0.43 for maternal mortality. Due to the interaction with DF the elasticity estimates range from −0.33 (country with lowest donor funding) to −0.55 (country with highest donor funding) with a mean value of −0.37 for under-five mortality. For maternal mortality the elasticity ranges from −0.31 (country with lowest donor funding) to −0.93 (again country with highest donor funding) with a mean value of −0.43. Country-specific elasticities are give in table A5.4.

Elasticity for donor funding is negative and significant for under-five mortality but is not statistically significant for maternal mortality. This is likely because the off-budget bilateral funds are usually set aside for primary care, not secondary care projects.

Note that the elasticity of maternal mortality with respect to Gh is greater in magnitude than the elasticity of under-five mortality for countries that are above the mean value of donor funding. However, for countries that are at or below the mean value of donor funding the difference in the elasticity of maternal mortality and under-five mortality with respect to Gh is very small (in some cases the elasticity of under-five mortality is larger than the elasticity of maternal mortality). The fact that elasticity for Gh increases in magnitude with donor funding is because of the negative sign on the interaction term between Gh and DF, which in the case of maternal mortality is also significant at the 5 percent level.

TABLE A5.4 Elasticity of under-five mortality and maternal mortality for government health expenditures

	Under-five mortality	Standard error	t-value	p-value	Maternal mortality	Standard error	t-value	p-value
Albania	−0.414	0.1056	−3.9224	0.0002	−0.5494	0.1905	−2.8845	0.0048
Algeria	−0.3308	0.1204	−2.7483	0.0071	−0.3171	0.2286	−1.3869	0.1684
Argentina	−0.3305	0.1205	−2.7427	0.0072	−0.3162	0.2289	−1.3814	0.1701
Armenia	−0.3765	0.1071	−3.5142	0.0007	−0.4447	0.1999	−2.2247	0.0283
Azerbaijan	−0.3326	0.1196	−2.78	0.0065	−0.3221	0.2272	−1.4178	0.1592
Bangladesh	−0.3373	0.1178	−2.8617	0.0051	−0.3351	0.2236	−1.4986	0.137
Belarus	−0.3324	0.1197	−2.7763	0.0065	−0.3216	0.2274	−1.4142	0.1603
Belize	−0.33	0.1207	−2.734	0.0074	−0.3148	0.2293	−1.373	0.1727
Benin	−0.4387	0.1094	−4.0103	0.0001	−0.6182	0.1924	−3.2128	0.0018
Bolivia	−0.421	0.1063	−3.9623	0.0001	−0.569	0.1904	−2.9889	0.0035
Botswana	−0.3338	0.1192	−2.8017	0.0061	−0.3256	0.2262	−1.4391	0.1531
Brazil	−0.3302	0.1206	−2.7388	0.0073	−0.3156	0.2291	−1.3776	0.1713
Bulgaria	−0.3302	0.1206	−2.7387	0.0073	−0.3156	0.2291	−1.3776	0.1713
Burkina Faso	−0.3513	0.1131	−3.1073	0.0024	−0.3744	0.2137	−1.7518	0.0827
Burundi	−0.352	0.1129	−3.1189	0.0023	−0.3763	0.2133	−1.7642	0.0806
Cambodia	−0.382	0.1063	−3.5925	0.0005	−0.4601	0.1976	−2.3284	0.0218
Cameroon	−0.3537	0.1124	−3.1473	0.0022	−0.3809	0.2122	−1.7948	0.0756
Cape Verde	−0.389	0.1056	−3.6836	0.0004	−0.4796	0.1952	−2.4576	0.0156
Chad	−0.3805	0.1065	−3.5709	0.0005	−0.4558	0.1982	−2.2992	0.0235
Chile	−0.3302	0.1206	−2.7384	0.0073	−0.3155	0.2291	−1.3772	0.1714
China	−0.3306	0.1204	−2.7457	0.0071	−0.3167	0.2288	−1.3844	0.1692
Colombia	−0.3309	0.1203	−2.7494	0.007	−0.3173	0.2286	−1.3879	0.1681
Comoros	−0.4526	0.1131	−4.0009	0.0001	−0.6571	0.1963	−3.3464	0.0011
Congo, Dem. Rep.	−0.3388	0.1173	−2.8889	0.0047	−0.3395	0.2225	−1.5259	0.1301
Congo, Rep.	−0.3383	0.1175	−2.88	0.0048	−0.338	0.2229	−1.5169	0.1323
Costa Rica	−0.332	0.1199	−2.7693	0.0067	−0.3204	0.2277	−1.4073	0.1623
Côte d'Ivoire	−0.3773	0.107	−3.5261	0.0006	−0.447	0.1995	−2.2401	0.0272
Croatia	−0.3318	0.1199	−2.7665	0.0067	−0.32	0.2278	−1.4046	0.1631
Dominica	−0.4091	0.1052	−3.8872	0.0002	−0.5357	0.1909	−2.8065	0.006
Dominican Republic	−0.4485	0.1119	−4.0075	0.0001	−0.6456	0.195	−3.3109	0.0013
Ecuador	−0.3402	0.1168	−2.9133	0.0044	−0.3433	0.2214	−1.5504	0.1241
Egypt, Arab Rep.	−0.3361	0.1183	−2.841	0.0054	−0.3318	0.2245	−1.478	0.1424

(Continues)

TABLE A5.4 Elasticity of under-five mortality and maternal mortality for government health expenditures *(continued)*

	Under-five mortality	Standard error	t-value	p-value	Maternal mortality	Standard error	t-value	p-value
El Salvador	−0.3854	0.1059	−3.6379	0.0004	−0.4696	0.1964	−2.3914	0.0186
Equatorial Guinea	−1.0837	0.5729	−1.8915	0.0613	−2.4185	0.9728	−2.4861	0.0145
Eritrea	−0.3885	0.1057	−3.6769	0.0004	−0.4781	0.1953	−2.4477	0.0161
Estonia	−0.3361	0.1183	−2.8415	0.0054	−0.3319	0.2245	−1.4785	0.1423
Ethiopia	−0.3623	0.11	−3.2927	0.0014	−0.4051	0.207	−1.9567	0.0531
Gabon	−0.3877	0.1057	−3.6669	0.0004	−0.4759	0.1956	−2.4331	0.0167
Gambia, The	−0.3572	0.1114	−3.2072	0.0018	−0.3908	0.21	−1.8604	0.0657
Georgia	−0.3547	0.1121	−3.1648	0.002	−0.3838	0.2116	−1.8138	0.0726
Ghana	−0.425	0.1068	−3.9795	0.0001	−0.5801	0.1905	−3.0444	0.003
Grenada	−0.3591	0.1109	−3.2395	0.0016	−0.3961	0.2089	−1.8964	0.0607
Guatemala	−0.3961	0.1052	−3.7657	0.0003	−0.4993	0.1932	−2.5849	0.0111
Guinea	−0.3803	0.1066	−3.5688	0.0005	−0.4554	0.1983	−2.2964	0.0237
Guinea-Bissau	−0.5249	0.1462	−3.5905	0.0005	−0.8589	0.2436	−3.5263	0.0006
Guyana	−0.33	0.1207	−2.734	0.0074	−0.3148	0.2293	−1.373	0.1727
Haiti	−0.4115	0.1054	−3.9053	0.0002	−0.5425	0.1907	−2.8453	0.0053
Honduras	−0.3703	0.1083	−3.4206	0.0009	−0.4274	0.2028	−2.1076	0.0375
Hungary	−0.3329	0.1195	−2.7857	0.0063	−0.3231	0.227	−1.4234	0.1576
Iceland	−0.33	0.1207	−2.734	0.0074	−0.3148	0.2293	−1.373	0.1727
India	−0.3352	0.1186	−2.8262	0.0056	−0.3295	0.2252	−1.4633	0.1464
Indonesia	−0.3386	0.1174	−2.885	0.0048	−0.3388	0.2226	−1.5219	0.1311
Jamaica	−0.3317	0.12	−2.7636	0.0068	−0.3195	0.2279	−1.4018	0.1639
Jordan	−0.4269	0.1071	−3.9862	0.0001	−0.5853	0.1907	−3.0695	0.0027
Kazakhstan	−0.383	0.1062	−3.6058	0.0005	−0.4629	0.1972	−2.3466	0.0208
Kenya	−0.3684	0.1087	−3.3902	0.001	−0.422	0.2038	−2.0709	0.0408
Korea, Rep.	−0.33	0.1207	−2.734	0.0074	−0.3148	0.2293	−1.373	0.1727
Kyrgyz Republic	−0.4729	0.1203	−3.9295	0.0002	−0.7137	0.2054	−3.4739	0.0007
Lebanon	−0.3372	0.1179	−2.8602	0.0051	−0.3349	0.2237	−1.4971	0.1374
Lesotho	−0.33	0.1207	−2.734	0.0074	−0.3148	0.2293	−1.373	0.1727
Lithuania	−0.3308	0.1204	−2.7487	0.0071	−0.3172	0.2286	−1.3873	0.1683
Macedonia, FYR	−0.4836	0.1249	−3.8722	0.0002	−0.7435	0.2117	−3.5123	0.0007
Madagascar	−0.3574	0.1113	−3.2105	0.0018	−0.3913	0.2099	−1.864	0.0651
Malawi	−0.3748	0.1074	−3.4892	0.0007	−0.44	0.2006	−2.1928	0.0306

(Continues)

TABLE A5.4 Elasticity of under-five mortality and maternal mortality for government health expenditures *(continued)*

	Under-five mortality	Standard error	t-value	p-value	Maternal mortality	Standard error	t-value	p-value
Malaysia	−0.33	0.1207	−2.7343	0.0074	−0.3149	0.2293	−1.3732	0.1726
Mali	−0.3402	0.1168	−2.9137	0.0044	−0.3434	0.2214	−1.5507	0.124
Mauritania	−0.4167	0.1058	−3.9388	0.0001	−0.5568	0.1904	−2.9246	0.0042
Mauritius	−0.3331	0.1195	−2.7881	0.0063	−0.3234	0.2268	−1.4257	0.1569
Mexico	−0.3301	0.1206	−2.736	0.0073	−0.3151	0.2292	−1.3749	0.1721
Moldova	−0.3457	0.1149	−3.0096	0.0033	−0.3587	0.2175	−1.6489	0.1022
Mongolia	−0.3722	0.1079	−3.4497	0.0008	−0.4327	0.2019	−2.1434	0.0344
Morocco	−0.3354	0.1185	−2.8295	0.0056	−0.33	0.225	−1.4666	0.1455
Mozambique	−0.3914	0.1054	−3.7129	0.0003	−0.4864	0.1944	−2.5016	0.0139
Namibia	−0.5531	0.1632	−3.3882	0.001	−0.9376	0.2707	−3.464	0.0008
Nepal	−0.3384	0.1174	−2.8826	0.0048	−0.3385	0.2227	−1.5195	0.1317
Nicaragua	−0.3776	0.107	−3.5305	0.0006	−0.4478	0.1994	−2.2458	0.0268
Niger	−0.3569	0.1114	−3.2031	0.0018	−0.3901	0.2102	−1.8559	0.0663
Nigeria	−0.3306	0.1204	−2.7449	0.0071	−0.3165	0.2288	−1.3835	0.1695
Pakistan	−0.3325	0.1197	−2.7785	0.0065	−0.3219	0.2273	−1.4164	0.1597
Panama	−0.3322	0.1198	−2.7733	0.0066	−0.3211	0.2275	−1.4112	0.1612
Paraguay	−0.4544	0.1137	−3.9971	0.0001	−0.662	0.197	−3.3608	0.0011
Peru	−0.3701	0.1083	−3.418	0.0009	−0.4269	0.2029	−2.1044	0.0378
Philippines	−0.3519	0.1129	−3.118	0.0024	−0.3761	0.2133	−1.7632	0.0808
Romania	−0.3316	0.12	−2.7625	0.0068	−0.3194	0.228	−1.4008	0.1643
Russian Federation	−0.3354	0.1186	−2.8283	0.0056	−0.3298	0.2251	−1.4654	0.1458
Rwanda	−0.452	0.1129	−4.002	0.0001	−0.6555	0.1961	−3.3417	0.0012
Senegal	−0.4533	0.1133	−3.9995	0.0001	−0.659	0.1966	−3.3519	0.0011
Sierra Leone	−0.361	0.1104	−3.2706	0.0015	−0.4013	0.2078	−1.9315	0.0561
Singapore	−0.3301	0.1206	−2.7365	0.0073	−0.3152	0.2292	−1.3755	0.1719
South Africa	−0.3465	0.1146	−3.0229	0.0032	−0.3608	0.217	−1.6628	0.0994
Sri Lanka	−0.3341	0.1191	−2.8064	0.006	−0.3263	0.226	−1.4437	0.1518
St. Kitts and Nevis	−0.3521	0.1128	−3.1206	0.0023	−0.3766	0.2132	−1.766	0.0803
St. Lucia	−0.3616	0.1102	−3.2816	0.0014	−0.4032	0.2074	−1.944	0.0546
St. Vincent and the Grenadines	−0.3365	0.1181	−2.8479	0.0053	−0.3329	0.2242	−1.4848	0.1406
Sudan	−0.3461	0.1147	−3.0172	0.0032	−0.3599	0.2172	−1.6569	0.1006

(Continues)

TABLE A5.4 Elasticity of under-five mortality and maternal mortality for government health expenditures *(continued)*

	Under-five mortality	Standard error	t-value	p-value	Maternal mortality	Standard error	t-value	p-value
Swaziland	-0.33	0.1207	-2.7347	0.0073	-0.3149	0.2293	-1.3736	0.1725
Tajikistan	-0.3406	0.1166	-2.9206	0.0043	-0.3445	0.2211	-1.5577	0.1223
Tanzania	-0.3675	0.1088	-3.3771	0.001	-0.4197	0.2042	-2.0552	0.0424
Thailand	-0.3302	0.1206	-2.7375	0.0073	-0.3154	0.2291	-1.3764	0.1717
Togo	-0.3835	0.1062	-3.6123	0.0005	-0.4642	0.1971	-2.3556	0.0204
Trinidad and Tobago	-0.33	0.1207	-2.7347	0.0073	-0.3149	0.2293	-1.3737	0.1725
Tunisia	-0.3333	0.1194	-2.7919	0.0062	-0.324	0.2267	-1.4295	0.1558
Turkey	-0.3301	0.1206	-2.7364	0.0073	-0.3152	0.2292	-1.3753	0.172
Turkmenistan	-0.3412	0.1164	-2.9318	0.0041	-0.3463	0.2207	-1.5691	0.1197
Uganda	-0.4131	0.1055	-3.9163	0.0002	-0.5469	0.1905	-2.8702	0.005
Ukraine	-0.3438	0.1155	-2.9774	0.0036	-0.3535	0.2188	-1.6157	0.1092
Uruguay	-0.3319	0.1199	-2.7671	0.0067	-0.3201	0.2278	-1.4052	0.1629
Uzbekistan	-0.3438	0.1155	-2.9772	0.0036	-0.3535	0.2188	-1.6155	0.1092
Venezuela, RB	-0.3302	0.1206	-2.7386	0.0073	-0.3156	0.2291	-1.3775	0.1713
Vietnam	-0.3735	0.1077	-3.4692	0.0008	-0.4363	0.2013	-2.1676	0.0325
Yemen, Rep.	-0.3325	0.1197	-2.7776	0.0065	-0.3218	0.2273	-1.4155	0.1599
Zambia	-0.3506	0.1133	-3.0949	0.0025	-0.3724	0.2142	-1.7386	0.0851
Zimbabwe	-0.3979	0.1051	-3.7849	0.0003	-0.5044	0.1928	-2.6167	0.0102

That donor funding marginally increases the elasticity of maternal mortality with respect to government expenditures but not of under-five mortality is puzzling, especially because donor funding does not seem to have any direct impact on maternal mortality.

Endnotes

1. Asymmetry in budgeting refers to the difficulties that governments face in cutting expenditures when resources are declining.

2. A model developed for this book makes several adjustments to the Filmer-Pritchett and Wagstaff-Claeson models. Annex 5.1 provides a detailed technical explanation of the model. The model makes four econometric adjustments. First, both government health expenditures and income are treated as endogenous variables. This allows for a circular relationship between heath outcomes and income (heath outcomes may improve as income increases, but improved outcomes may also lead to increased income) and between government health expenditures and outcomes (for example, larger expenditures may lead

to improved outcomes, but the government may increase expenditures when outcomes are poor). Second, donor funding variables are lagged to account for the fact that commitments are disbursed at a later date but also solve endogeneity of donor funding. Third, endogeneity and choice of instruments were tested using Staiger and Stock (1997) weak instrument tests and Hausman (1978) tests. Fourth, the presence of heteroscedasticity was tested for and corrected (using a general method of moments heteroscedastic two-stage least squares estimator).

3. As in other studies (Filmer and Pritchett 1999; Wagstaff 2002b; Wagstaff and Claeson 2004), the model did not include private expenditures as part of the explanatory variables. Filmer and Pritchett (1999) explained that their main reason for not estimating health status as a function of private expenditures on health is that private expenditures are influenced rather than determined by policy. Economic agents spend out of pocket when a health event has taken place; thus, health expenditures and the dependent variables are endogenous and very hard to separate. In any event, the absence of private health expenditures as an explanatory variable could lead to omitted variable bias. Therefore, private expenditures were included in the model and shown not to be statistically significant. Their inclusion did not generate a significant change in other coefficients. Therefore, private expenditures were dropped from the model for comparative purposes with other models.

4. There are two related issues with the donor funding variable. First is the double counting of donor funding. Grants and loans provided by various donor agencies (such as the World Bank and the United Nations) are given directly to the government for health and other purposes, and hence are already counted in the government health expenditures variable. Information on donor funding that is actually available to various countries from all sources and that is reported "on budget" is not readily available. Information was used from the OECD/DAC for specific health projects that are off-budget. But this measure raises a second issue: the variable captures the amount of the donation receiving countries were promised by the DAC countries in the given calendar year, not the actual amount received in donations. The amount received can lag by a few years and even then may differ from the amount promised. For this reason, the lagged value of the variable was used. For example, for the analysis for 2000, the donor funding variable is per capita donor funding from DAC countries for health promised in 1998 (in 2000 Int$).

5. A small change in government health expenditures (Gh) will be associated with a direct effect and an indirect effect. The direct effect is the marginal impact that a change in government expenditures may have on under-five mortality or maternal mortality. However, governments may use their resources to influence other Millennium Development Goal indicators, such as nutrition, which may have an impact on under-five mortality; this is the indirect effect. Put another way, the coefficient on Gh represents the percentage change in the indicators under-five mortality or maternal mortality ratio associated with a 1 percent change in Gh, holding income (I), education (E), roads (R), sanitation (S), and donor funding (DF) constant but not the other Millennium Development Goal indicators. The coefficients in the table, therefore, provide the net impact of changes in the independent variables on the under-five mortality rate and maternal mortality ratio. For ease of exposition, this net impact of changes is called the net elasticity impact or just elasticity.

6. The under-five mortality rate is measured as deaths of children under the age of five years per 1,000 live births. The maternal mortality ratio is measured as a ratio of maternal deaths per 100,000 live births. The measure of income is GDP per capita in constant 2000

international dollars, education is the percentage of the population age 15 or older who are illiterate, sanitation is the percentage of the population with access to improved sanitation facilities, and roads are measured as paved roads (in kilometers) per unit area of country (in square kilometers). Donor funding refers to commitments made by donors with a two-year lag to finance health activities outside the government's budget. Volatility is the standard deviation of the per capita donor commitments from 1994 to 1998.

7. All currency measurements were converted to constant 2000 international dollars.

8. The results are robust to other measures of volatility of donor funding.

9. The coefficients in the table are not elasticities in the strict economic sense, but rather some sort of "net elasticities." It is not possible to separate the direct and indirect effects because the direct partial elasticity coefficients are not identified in the estimation model used. Thus, whenever the term "elasticity" of an outcome indicator with respect to a covariate is used, it refers to the net elasticity. Also, to estimate the elasticity of government health expenditures on under-five mortality and maternal mortality, the impact of donor funding on government health expenditures must also be taken into account (the interaction term). Thus, to estimate the impact of government health expenditures on under-five mortality or maternal mortality, some aggregation of coefficients is necessary. The interpretation of the government health expenditures coefficients in the table as elasticities is still correct for the average elasticity across countries (see annex 5.1 for details). Wagstaff and Claeson (2004) reported the elasticity for under-five mortality with respect to per capita income in the range of –0.3 percent to –0.5 percent, while Filmer and Pritchett (1999) had an estimate of –0.6 percent. Their studies treated Gh as endogenous but not GDP. The estimates across countries are presented in annex 5.1.

From an econometric perspective the S variable (sanitation) appears to be measured with error and hence the lack of significance may be due to attenuation bias rather than anything else. Two options for checking this hypothesis are to use a different measure of this variable (preferably from some other source) or to find some instruments for this variable. Currently, the data available fall short on both accounts, and so link between the lack of significance and attenuation bias was not tested.

10. The analysis and results are similar to Wagstaff and Claeson (2004) and figures 5.1 and 5.2 mirror their analysis. Differences arise largely as a result of the significant coefficient of the impact of government health expenditures on outcomes in the model here and the presence of donor funding.

11. The average rate of decline needed between 1990 and 2015 to reach the under-five mortality goal across all regions is 4.2 percent. However, given the slow progress from 1990 to 2000, the rate of decline needs to be larger from 2000 to 2015 and larger in some regions than in others.

12. This annex is based on the working paper "Government Health Expenditures, Donor Funding, and Health Outcomes" (2005) by Bokhari, Gottret, and Gai. For a copy of the working paper send an email to fbokhari@fsu.edu.

13. All currency measurements were converted to constant 2000 international dollars.

14. The four broad areas are economic management, structural policies, policies for social inclusion and equity, and public sector management.

15. There are three such tests for each indicator equation. Thus, the test statistics can be constructed by comparing: (1) coefficients under assumption (a) where no variable is exogenous to those under (b) where only government health expenditures (and their interaction)

are endogenous; (2) coefficients under assumption (a) where no variable is exogenous to those under (c) where income and government health expenditures (and their interaction) are endogenous; and (3) coefficients under assumption (b) where only government health expenditures (and their interaction) are endogenous to those under (c) where income and government health expenditures (and their interaction) are endogenous. Note that the third test statistic is an incremental test. It tests whether, given that government health expenditures (and their interaction with DF) are endogenous, income is endogenous.

References

Filmer, D., and L. Pritchett. 1999. "The Impact of Public Spending on Health: Does Money Matter?" *Social Science and Medicine* 49 (10): 1309–23.

Hausman, J. A. 1978. "Specification Tests in Econometrics." *Econometrica* 46 (6): 1251–71.

Herrera, S., and G. Pan. 2005. "Efficiency of Public Spending in Developing Countries: An Efficiency Frontier Approach." World Bank, Washington, D.C.

Leipziger, D., M. Fay, Q. Wodon, and T. Yepes. 2003. "Achieving the Millennium Development Goals: The Role of Infrastructure." World Bank, Washington, D.C.

Musgrove, P. 1996. "Public and Private Roles in Health." Technical Report 339, World Bank, Washington, D.C.

Paternostro, S., A. Rajaram, and E. Tiongson. 2004. "How Does the Composition of Public Spending Matter?" World Bank, Washington, D.C.

Wagstaff, A. 2002a. "Heath Spending and Aid as Escape Routes from the Vicious Circle of Poverty and Health." Paper prepared for British Association for the Advancement of Science Festival of Science, Leicester, U.K., September 12.

———. 2002b. "Intersectoral Synergies and the Health MDGs: Preliminary Cross-Country Findings, Corroboration, and Policy Simulations." Paper prepared for the Development Committee on Accelerating Progress toward the HNP MDGs, Washington, D.C., December 6.

Wagstaff, A., and M. Claeson. 2004. *The Millennium Development Goals for Health: Rising to the Challenges.* Washington, D.C.: World Bank.

6

Increasing the efficiency of government spending

Improving policies and institutions in developing countries is fundamental to reaching the Millennium Development Goals. Even if health care spending rises dramatically, the intended outcomes are not likely to be achieved without addressing weaknesses in government institutional capacity. To improve the effectiveness of government health spending, many of the instruments used to develop, implement, and assess policies, such as poverty reduction strategy papers, poverty reduction support credits, medium-term expenditure frameworks, and public expenditure reviews, need to be strengthened, and decentralization strategies need to be linked more closely to sector strategies. Country experiences using these instruments to address weaknesses in health sector performance have been mixed at best, and adjustments are needed to make the instruments more effective.

Consensus is emerging in the international community that current health expenditure levels in developing countries are too low. Often overlooked, however, are the other conditions that must be in place for countries to progress. Strong growth in national income, improvements in infrastructure quality and capacity, high literacy rates, and a host of other factors also drive health outcomes. Moreover, while much of the global debate focuses on the amount of additional resources required to meet the Millennium Development Goals, there is also a need to carefully examine the extent to which the policy environment and institutional capacity at the country level facilitate the efficient and equitable allocation of increased resources to the health sector.

This chapter first discusses the importance of the policy environment at the country level. Clearly, good public sector management and institutional capacity are important for government expenditures to be effective. The chapter then turns to the instruments and policy options available to governments to improve expenditure performance. These instruments include poverty reduction strategy papers (PRSPs), poverty reduction support credits (PRSCs), medium-term expenditure frameworks (MTEFs), public expenditure reviews (PERs), and public expenditure tracking surveys (PETS). Recommendations include:

- Ensure that the PRSP sets out clear priorities and criteria and that the priorities are reflected in the guidelines and ceilings sent to line ministries to guide budget preparation.
- Implement an iterative process for budget preparation in which proposals for sector plans and allocations are prepared by line ministries, scrutinized by central authorities, and adjusted in light of national priorities.
- Ensure that the MTEF reflects the annual budget for the first year and that the chart of accounts is structured in such a way that spending priorities for achieving the goals can be identified.
- Implement an annual review of sector-level progress and identify domestic and foreign finance requirements for the coming period, which should be timed to feed into the budget preparation cycle.
- Establish a system to ensure that carefully prepared budgets that are in line with nationally important goals receive favorable treatment in the final overall budget and the timely and full release of funds. This system would be maintained under the authority of the ministry of finance and the cabinet.
- Encourage line ministries to reallocate resources from lower-priority areas without fearing that their budgets will suffer as a result, by developing a system for the ministry of finance to provide credible medium-term assurances of sectoral budget levels or shares.

Decentralization of key functions is often advocated as a means of strengthening public sector management and improving overall health system performance. This chapter closes with an evaluation of country experiences with decentralization. Recommendations include:

- Before undertaking decentralization, ensure strong political backing at both the central and local levels, with stakeholder ownership of both the plan for decentralization and the process of organizational capacity building.
- Support political objectives with an appropriate legal and institutional framework, structure of responsibility for service delivery, and system of intergovernmental fiscal transfers.
- Delineate responsibilities among stakeholders and formally codify responsibilities in legislation, regulations, or other binding instruments.
- Although decentralization generally involves a diminished role for the central government in service delivery, certain functions are likely to be most efficiently undertaken at the central level—research and dissemination of research findings, national public goods, health information, standards, regulations, and accreditation. Decentralization still requires a strong central capacity for monitoring and enforcement of regulations and standards.

- Because local governments may have limited revenue-generating capacity and therefore are likely to remain reliant on transfers from the central government, determine intergovernmental transfers openly and objectively, ideally by a clear, simple, and verifiable formula.
- Link local financing and fiscal authority to service provision responsibilities and functions so that local politicians can deliver on their promises and bear the costs of their decisions.

Institutions and policies at the country level

One of the most significant constraints on the performance of health systems in developing countries is weak public sector management, particularly at the district or municipal level (Mills, Rasheed, and Tollman forthcoming). Within the health sector, weak public sector management manifests itself in poor planning, budgeting, and oversight at the central and district level, limited capacity for regulation, insufficient linkages with civil society, and excessive reliance on donor program management systems (Hanson and others 2003).

Mills, Rasheed, and Tollman (forthcoming) note that government institutional capacity constraints limit what the health sector can change on its own. The UN Millennium Project argues that reaching the Millennium Development Goals is primarily a financing problem, but it also recognizes the need to address institutional constraints and calls for a "governance plan" as a key element of country proposals for reaching the Millennium Development Goals (Foster 2005). The UN Millennium Project also suggests that this plan needs to address how increased spending will be carried out, as well as how to cover budget monitoring, audit, evaluation, oversight (with an explicit role for civil society), access to services for women and ethnic minorities, and plans to fight corruption and enhance the rule of law.

The World Bank's *Global Monitoring Report* also emphasizes the importance of improving governance—in particular, upgrading public sector management and controlling corruption—as an overarching agenda (World Bank 2005a). Although some aspects of governance are getting better in most countries, reforms need to be accelerated in others. Sub-Saharan Africa, for example, has seen encouraging progress on political representation, but less progress on public sector management and institutional effectiveness (World Bank 2005a). These management and institutional issues affect access to essential health interventions at all levels, from the local health center to community and national issues of public policy and environment.

Results of a study presented in *Rising to the Challenges* (Wagstaff and Claeson 2004) that measured the quality of policies and institutions in countries by the World Bank's Country Policy and Institutional Assessments (CPIA) Index, indicate the importance of institutions and governance in enabling effective health policy. The CPIA Index assesses how conducive the policy and institutional framework is to fostering poverty reduction, sustainable growth, and the effective use of development assistance. The index covers four broad categories: economic management, structural policies, policies for social inclusion and equity, and public sector management and institutions. Countries are rated on several performance criteria with scores ranging from 1 (poor performance) to 5 (as of 2004 the top of the range was expanded to 6).

Empirical analysis found that the elasticity of health outcomes to expenditure depended on a country's CPIA score. Spending had a larger impact on health outcomes at the margin in better-governed countries. For example, at a CPIA score of 4 (one standard deviation above the mean), a 10 percent increase in the share of GDP devoted to government health spending results in a 7.2 percent decline in the maternal mortality ratio. At CPIA levels below 3, the impact of increased spending is statistically insignificant (not different from zero). Clearly, policies matter.

Comparing CPIA scores across regions and through time indicates clearly that while some overall progress has been made—particularly in Africa—in strengthening policies and institutions in countries, public sector management remains the weakest component of the CPIA (figures 6.1 and 6.2). On average in every region, a country's capacities in rule-based governance, budgetary and financial management, revenue mobilization, public administration, transparency, accountability, and corruption in the public sector were all judged to be less conducive to growth

FIGURE 6.1   Country policy and institutional assessment scores by indicator and region, 2003

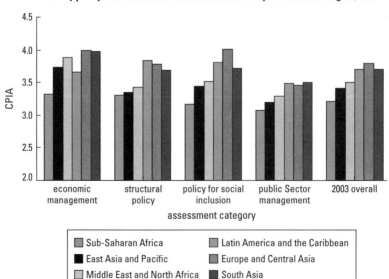

Source: World Bank data.

FIGURE 6.2 Country policy and institutional assessment scores by region over time, 1999–2003

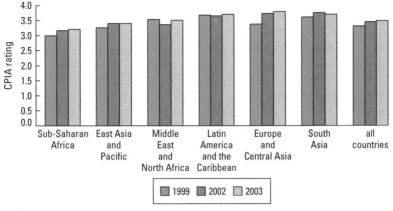

Source: World Bank data.

and poverty reduction than the country's policies and institutions for economic, structural, or social management.

Policy instruments to improve public sector management

The importance of policies and institutions is clear. But what instruments or policies are available to governments to improve public sector management? The remainder of this chapter discusses the role of instruments, such as PRSPs, PRSCs, MTEFs, PERs, and PETS in improving key public sector management functions. The roles of targeting mechanisms and decentralization are also discussed.

Poverty reduction strategy papers

Starting in the mid-1990s the World Bank and International Monetary Fund (IMF) began to radically change both the focus and the tools for providing development assistance to poor countries. In response to the high level of indebtedness in some of the poorest countries in the world, as well as criticism that previous development assistance efforts were ineffective, the World Bank and IMF focused on debt forgiveness, poverty reduction, and improved economic growth in the most heavily indebted poor countries. The quid pro quo for debt forgiveness required countries to reprogram the bulk of the savings from forgiven debt back into social programs such as health and education.

These efforts were formalized in 1999 when the World Bank and IMF stipulated that all concessionary assistance to some 81 eligible poor countries—through the World Bank's International Development Association (IDA) and the IMF's Poverty Reduction Grant Facility—would need to be based on a poverty reduction strategy as embodied in a PRSP. This new approach was intended to strengthen country ownership; enhance the poverty focus of country programs; provide a comprehensive and coordinated framework for the World Bank and the IMF, as well as other development partners; improve public governance and accountability; and strengthen priority setting. The principles underlying the PRSP process are country driven, involving broad-based participation, results-oriented and focused on outcomes that benefit the poor, comprehensive in recognizing the multidimensional nature of poverty, partnership-oriented, and based on a long-term perspective.

The PRSP process has made poverty reduction the top priority issue for development. Macroeconomic and sectoral strategies need to be formulated around the PRSP. Thus, health reform strategies for low-income countries must be embodied in PRSPs and focus on the poor. As of August 2005, 49 countries had developed PRSPs, which are serving as the basis for World Bank and IMF financing in these countries.

Extensive evaluations of PRSPs have painted a mixed picture (World Bank 2004a; IMF 2003; IMF and World Bank 2005). Evaluations suggest that

- PRSPs have the potential to encourage the development of country-owned, long-term strategies for poverty reduction and growth, but there are still tensions concerning ownership among countries and external partners. Many partners have not adapted the processes of their assistance programs in a coordinated manner around the PRSP processes. Better frameworks for accountability of both countries and partners are needed.
- Although broad-based participation in development efforts has improved, there is still room for much greater inclusiveness. Moreover, the PRSP has not strengthened domestic institutional policy-making processes or accountability.
- The PRSP process is an improvement over previous processes because it encourages a results-oriented approach to development, a focus on poverty reduction, and a long-term perspective.
- Although the PRS approach has initiated the intended fundamental change in the relationship between low-income countries and donors, it has fallen short as a strategic reform roadmap, especially in guiding structural reform, promoting economic growth, linking PRSPs with medium-term expenditure frameworks and budgets, integrating sectoral strategies into the macroeconomic framework, assessing the social impacts of macro strategies, understanding micro-macro linkages, and linking medium- and long-term operational targets.
- Capacity constraints have been serious impediments to effective implementation. There has been little focus on capacity building.
- Monitoring and evaluation is still a significant weakness.

Specific evaluations of the health components of PRSPs raise many of the same problems (WHO 2004). The treatment of health in new PRSPs has tended to be more extensive, but it is too soon to evaluate impact given the relative newness of the process and the learning curve for countries and partners. However, a recent study on the treatment of reproductive and adolescent health issues in PRSPs provides insight into some of the concerns related to health components of PRSPs (World Bank 2004b). The study found that

- Despite having to cover many topics, the PRSPs pay a reasonable level of attention to population and reproductive health issues. However, scope and quality vary enormously, and there is no exemplary PRSP as it relates to population and reproductive health issues.
- Participation by key population and reproductive health stakeholder groups in the PRSP process is uneven, and the process could better represent the interests of women, youth, and poor people. The participatory process can be strengthened and should give more voice to these groups and to civil society.
- Although PRSPs are not implementation documents, many basic implementation elements are missing from PRSP-related population and reproductive health policies. Only half of the recorded policies specify an institution responsible for implementing the policy, 44 percent of policies denote a basic timeline for implementation, and 17 percent of policies have a budget. Few policies (under 6 percent) include all three elements.
- The country assistance strategies reviewed address population and reproductive health issues, but in less detail than in the PRSPs.

Overall, PRSPs are still a work in progress. Although health and education strategies tend to be better developed than other sectors—due to the requirements for debt forgiveness in the heavily indebted poor countries, as well as the key roles that health and education play in poverty reduction and meeting the Millennium Development Goals—there has tended to be a focus on disease- and intervention-specific programs and less emphasis on systemic issues, such as human resources. The linkages to other sectors and to growth have been tenuous at best.

As more development partners join the process, and as increasing amounts of development assistance are funneled through PRSPs, the effectiveness of these development instruments and processes will depend on numerous factors, including countries' commitment and capacity and partners' flexibility and funding commitment.

Poverty reduction support credits

The World Bank introduced PRSCs in May 2001 as one of IDA's main vehicles to support low-income countries in implementing their poverty reduction strategies. The PRSC is a programmatic approach to development policy lending in low-income countries. It typically consists of three or four annual, single-tranche operations, phased to support the government's medium-term development

objectives. The overarching goal of the PRSC approach, and particularly of reinforcing the country ownership embedded in the initiative, was to be achieved
through several mutually reinforcing objectives (World Bank 2005b):

- *Flexible medium-term support.* To support a medium-term reform program
  that builds on and draws from the priorities and objectives of the government's
  PRSP through World Bank financing, policy dialogue, and analytic work.
- *Donor harmonization.* To support the medium-term reform program in coordination and harmonization with development partners, particularly with
  donors that provide budget support and with the IMF through its Poverty
  Reduction Growth Facility.
- *Resource predictability.* To improve resource predictability in well-performing
  countries through medium-term commitments that are disbursed in line with
  domestic planning, budgeting, and review processes.
- *Country ownership.* To reinforce country ownership by using policy-based and
  focused conditionality that reflects an understanding with governments on the
  priorities of their reform programs.

There are currently 18 countries with PRSCs, representing less than half of the
49 countries that have full PRSPs. The PRSC has emerged as a significant share of
new operations and commitments. In fiscal 2004, PRSCs composed 46 percent of
development policy lending to the poorest countries (those eligible for highly
concessional lending through the IDA arm of the World Bank). While the number
of PRSC programs has grown, the overall weight of World Bank investment lending has not changed significantly. Since PRSCs were introduced, the share of IDA
development policy lending has hovered at around 27 percent of total IDA lending, an increase from the 16 percent in fiscal 2000, but matching the average share
of development policy lending seen in the early 1990s.

A World Bank review of PRSCs and a review of country experiences with
PRSPs and PRSCs in the context of the health sector (World Bank 2005b; Foster
2005) draw several important conclusions related to PRSCs:

- In general, PRSCs are closely aligned with country PRSPs, with some variation
  depending on how well the PRSP prioritizes and operationalizes the government's medium-term development program. One drawback of this close link is
  that because PRSPs tend to be optimistic, using their targets in PRSCs tends to
  result in failure to meet the PRSC conditions for disbursement of credit.
- PRSCs have helped to improve coordination between central and line ministries and between central and local governments. Many cross-sectoral
  reforms, along with preparation and execution of the budget, have required
  close collaboration among various parts of the government.
- Since the launch of PRSCs, there has been a concerted effort to limit to a few
  priority actions the number of conditions related to the country's reform

agenda. Although the number of conditions has varied from a high of 44 in Vietnam to as low as 6 in Tanzania, the average number of PRSC conditions has decreased substantially from 30 in fiscal 2001 to approximately 12 in fiscal 2004.

- While the number of conditions has decreased, the length of the policy matrix has increased. Government officials often find the policy matrix to be over-loaded, particularly when it is driven by efforts to harmonize specific donor preferences. There are cases where the PRSC matrix seems to be overwhelmed by sector-specific detail. This is counterproductive to the intent of PRSC to concentrate on multisectoral issues or reforms that require multisector support.

- PRSC triggers or targets must be chosen appropriately. Governments do not control outcomes (mortality rates, literacy), just inputs (schools built, nurses trained). PRSCs should not hold governments responsible for something outside their control.

- Information on key PRSC results is often outdated because of countries' weak monitoring and evaluation capacity. PRSCs need to provide some support for governments to strengthen monitoring and evaluation systems, including linking the various ministries to the coordinating center.

- In almost all PRSC countries, but particularly in Africa, the PRSC has become a useful platform to facilitate donor coordination and harmonization within the common framework provided by countries' PRSPs. The aim is for governments to negotiate effectively one comprehensive reform program, with lower costs in terms of time, effort, preparation, reporting, and monitoring.

Medium-term expenditure frameworks

According to the World Bank's *Public Expenditure Management Handbook* (1998, p. 46), the MTEF "consists of a top-down resource envelope, a bottom-up estimation of the current and medium-term costs of existing policy and, ultimately, the matching of these costs with available resources . . . in the context of the annual budget process." The top-down resource envelope is fundamentally a macroeconomic model that indicates fiscal targets and estimates revenues and expenditures, including government financial obligations and high-cost governmentwide programs, such as civil service reform.

To complement the macroeconomic model, the sectors engage in bottom-up reviews that begin by scrutinizing sector policies and activities (similar to the zero-based budgeting approach), with an eye toward optimizing intrasectoral allocations. MTEFs are receiving renewed attention in the formulation of poverty reduction strategy papers as an appropriate instrument for incorporating PRSP strategies into public expenditure programs. The basic characteristics of MTEFs are described in table 6.1.

In practice, not all MTEFs have focused sufficiently on achieving a strategic shift in expenditures toward national priorities. The MTEFs in Cambodia and

TABLE 6.1   Stages of preparing a medium-term expenditure framework

Stage	Characteristics
Development of macroeconomic and fiscal framework	Macroeconomic model that projects revenues and expenditure in the medium term (multiyear)
Development of sectoral programs	Agreed sector objectives, outputs, and activities
	Review and development of programs and subprograms
	Estimated program cost
Development of sectoral expenditure framework	Analysis of inter- and intrasectoral trade-offs
	Consensus-building on strategic resource allocation
Definition of sector resource allocations	Medium-term sector budget ceilings (cabinet approval)
Preparation of sectoral budgets	Medium-term sectoral programs based on budget ceilings
Final political approval	Presentation of budget estimates to cabinet and parliament for approval

Source: World Bank 2002b.

Ghana and to some extent in Tanzania, for example, are based on detailed bottom-up activity costing, resulting in bulky documents that make it difficult or impossible to see how the changes in budget allocations relate to higher-level goals and targets. In addition, the effort devoted to preparing an MTEF can seem fruitless if the annual budget is not implemented, and the medium-term priorities are not respected. Cambodia, where health centers receive less than 10 percent of their budgets, is an extreme example.

Although there have been no evaluations of the MTEF experience specific to the health sector, it is useful to examine the general experience of governments with MTEFs. MTEFs have not been such a useful mechanism for detailed expenditure planning. Excessively detailed activity-based costing makes links to higher-level objectives difficult and obscures the main strategic choices that have to be made (Cambodia, Ghana, Malawi, Tanzania). A second constraint is that the program and activity basis on which the MTEF is prepared is often impossible to reconcile with the line-item basis by which the annual budget is reported and accounted (Benin, Ghana). This can make it difficult or impossible to know whether the budget priorities have been respected in budget execution and impossible to undertake disaggregated comparisons of the results achieved for the funds expended.

The technical problems of budget reporting can be solved as reforms to the chart of accounts and improvements in computer-based financial management systems. However, these improvements need to be accompanied by a simplified and standardized presentation wherein fewer activities are identified, thereby allowing easier aggregation for a more strategic analysis of shifting priorities.

An evaluation of MTEFs for the Africa region found no clear evidence that MTEFs have been successful in achieving the desired objectives (table 6.2). This evaluation suggests that in addition to the need to improve the quality of PRSPs and PRSCs, there is a need to improve the quality of MTEFs and to link them better to sector strategies. Although this example highlights the improvements needed, there are also examples of good practices, obtained from an analysis of 14 countries that have implemented PRSPs, PRSCs, and MTEFs (Foster 2005). This study found examples of good practices in countries where:

- The sectoral priorities of the PRSP and the allocations eventually agreed on in the budget are the outcome of an iterative process in which proposals for sector plans and allocations are prepared by line ministries, scrutinized by the central authorities, and adjusted in light of national priorities.
- The PRSP sets out clear priorities and criteria, and the priorities are reflected in the guidelines and ceilings sent to line ministries to guide budget preparation.
- The MTEF that is approved reflects the annual budget for the first year, and the chart of accounts is structured in such a way that spending priorities of particular importance for achieving the goals can be identified.
- There is an annual process for reviewing sector-level progress and the domestic and foreign finance requirements for the coming period, timed to feed in to the government budget preparation cycle.
- The ministry of finance provides credible medium-term assurances of sectoral budget levels or shares to encourage line ministries to reallocate resources from lower-priority areas without fear that their budget will suffer as a result. Credibility can be built through a medium-term track record of success, with year one of each year's budget preparation taking year two of the previous MTEF as the starting baseline. Agreements with external partners on the share of spending to be devoted to health are also widely used and helpful in reinforcing the confidence of line ministries in their likely future budget share.

TABLE 6.2 Preliminary impact assessment of medium-term expenditure framework reforms in Africa

Expected outcomes	Actual outcomes
Improved macroeconomic balance, especially fiscal discipline	No clear empirical evidence of improved macroeconomic balance
Better inter- and intrasectoral resource allocation	Some limited empirical evidence of reallocations to subsets of priority sectors
Greater budgetary predictability for line ministries	No empirical evidence of links to greater budgetary predictability
More efficient use of public monies	No evidence that MTEFs are developed enough to generate efficiency gains in sectoral spending

Source: World Bank 2002b.

Public expenditure reviews

Few developing countries take a comprehensive and systematic approach to their budget process. Public resource allocation decisions often do not reflect sound economic policy, and fiscally irresponsible subsidies often account for a significant part of the public budget. In such cases a PER can provide an important objective analysis of a country's public spending issues.

PERs typically analyze and project tax revenues, determine the level and composition of public spending, assess inter- and intrasectoral allocations (agriculture, education, health, roads), and review financial and nonfinancial public enterprises, the structure of governance, and the functioning of public institutions. Studies of public expenditure reviews over the past 10 years have suggested that the quality of analysis has been uneven, although their coverage has been comprehensive. General findings suggest that

• Most PERs do not examine the rationale for public intervention. Basic public economics concepts of market failure, public goods, and externalities are seldom used to analyze the efficiency of the public budget allocation.
• Most PERs do not integrate capital and recurrent expenditures and so sidestep the issue of the future recurrent cost implications of the capital budget. This introduces uncertainty regarding the sustainability of policies and projects. Such segmented analysis reinforces capital-led budgeting, which distorts public spending in favor of capital spending.
• Less than a quarter of recent PERs adequately focused on institutional issues, such as budget management or incentives in the public sector. Attention was restricted to incomplete (and often superficial) economic analysis of public expenditures.

Specific to the health sector, PERs provide important information on budget execution. For example, according to a PER in Latvia, late and uncertain budgets in the health sector undermine the health care institutions accountability to live within their annual revenue limits (World Bank 2002a). The response of health institutions to budget constraints in this environment is to defer expenditure in the hope of budget increases later in the fiscal year. When no increase is forthcoming, health care institutions are forced to finance overspending by accumulating debts to tax agencies and suppliers. Moreover, when budget cuts occur, they are perceived as arbitrary, made without explicit analysis of what outputs will be forgone or where efficiency gains will be made. Earmarked revenue for health is set on a basis that explicitly does not cover some elements of health care costs. In the absence of any decision about how these costs will be financed, or any accountability, costs are shifted to consumers in an ad hoc way or financed by arrears.

PERs also find that resources disbursed in the health sector do not always correspond to those budgeted through the MTEF. For example, in Nicaragua, total central government budget execution averaged 106 percent in 1997–8, but only 90 percent in the health sector. This low rate is attributable mainly to an inordinately low capital budget execution ratio of only 39 percent, which may reflect problems of absorptive capacity.

Uganda provides a second example of how PERs can show that resources disbursed in the health sector do not correspond to those budgeted through the MTEF. There, the budget performance for the health sector was 87 percent in 2003, compared with 90 percent the previous year. The underperformance was due to below-program (75 percent) wage releases to referral district hospitals, which, in turn, resulted from unfilled vacancies due to staff shortages. Nonwage recurrent releases to the health sector were at 94 percent, because of the late submission of accountability returns from local governments to the Ministry of Health (World Bank 2004c).

Public expenditure tracking surveys

Government resources for health care services often flow through several layers of bureaucracy down to the service facilities that are charged with responsibility for spending.[1] Information on public spending at the level of service delivery, however, is seldom available in developing countries. PETS follow the flow of government resources to determine how much of the originally allocated resources actually reach the service delivery point. They provide information on leakage of funds, corruption, and problems in the deployment of human and in-kind resources, such as staff, textbooks, and drugs.

PETS have uncovered considerable leakages in resource flows in the education and health sectors, and the surveys have led governments to improve institutional arrangements to address the leakages. A survey in Uganda in 1996 found that only 13 percent of the annual per student grant from the central government reached schools in 1991–5. Eighty-seven percent either disappeared for private gain or was captured by district officials for purposes unrelated to education. Almost three-quarters of schools received very little or nothing. About 20 percent of teacher salaries were paid to ghost teachers—teachers who never appeared in the classroom. In response to these findings the government required improved monitoring and reporting of the flow of funds. Although in 2001 schools were still not receiving the entire grant, leakage was reduced from an average of 80 percent in 1995 to 20 percent in 2001; the policy change accounted for two-thirds of this massive improvement.

A review of PETS carried out in African countries found leakage of nonwage funds on a massive scale in the health and education sectors. Salaries and allowances also suffer from leakage, but to a much lesser extent. Given that the availability of books and other instructional materials is key to improving the quality of schooling, the fact that between 87 percent (Uganda) and 60 percent (Zambia) of the funding for these inputs never reaches the schools makes leakage a major policy concern in the education sector. In designing interventions to reduce leakage, country experiences show that it may be more efficient to target reforms and interventions at specific problem spots within the public hierarchy instead of instituting more general public sector reforms. For example, the PETS pointed to the fact that nonwage expenditures are more prone to leakage than salary expenditures. The surveys also demonstrated that leakage occurred at specific tiers within the government. This knowledge can be exploited to design more efficient interventions.

A PETS was used in Honduras to evaluate civil servant behavior in the health and education sectors. The survey found that 2.4 percent of staff on the government payroll in the health sector were not working at all. Some 8.3 percent of general practitioners and specialists and 5.1 percent of staff were ghost workers. Absenteeism was also discovered to be a major concern; 39 percent of staff were absent without justifiable reason. This amounted to a productivity loss of 10 percent of total staff time.

Targeting health expenditures

Increasingly, governments are targeting resources in the health sector to specific priorities. The priorities may be based on geographic location, specific health care needs (immunization, antiretroviral therapy), household income levels, or demographic characteristics (Coady, Grosh, and Hoddinot 2004), among others. This section provides an overview of some of the key results from three types of targeting: geographic, levels of care, and bottlenecks. Issues related to targeting interventions with donor funding are covered in chapter 4.

Geographic targeting

In Mozambique, Zambezia receives seven times less government spending on health per capita than Maputo City. In Lesotho, the poorest district receives only 20 percent of the amount the capital city receives in per capita allocations of public expenditures on health. This inequity is not resolved by accounting for nongovernmental services. In Peru, per capita allocations through the regional budget (which excludes teaching hospital allocations) are 66 percent higher in the Lima region than in the very poor regions. In Bangladesh, more developed districts receive more per capita than less developed districts (Wagstaff and Claeson 2004).

As noted below in the section on decentralization, a well-designed, well-specified resource allocation formula can reduce such government spending disparities across regions. These formulas have an equity angle—they ensure that the poor also benefit from government spending. But they also have an efficiency angle—resources can be diverted from areas where the marginal benefit is fairly low (such as in high-tech hospitals in the capital city) to those where the marginal benefit is likely to be high (immunization programs in rural areas). Such formulas have narrowed regional gaps in developed countries and are beginning to be used in developing countries. They have been used, for example, as part of Bolivia's decentralization efforts since 1994, and in its allocation of newly available resources from debt forgiveness, Bolivia allocated funds to municipalities according to poverty indicators, with the mandate that municipalities spend such resources on specified health, education, and other social programs.

Changing the allocation of spending across levels of care

Developing countries allocate a surprisingly high share of health spending to secondary and tertiary infrastructure and personnel, despite low bed-occupancy rates. Armenian hospitals, for example, receive more than 50 percent of the government budget for health. Health clinics and ambulatory facilities—the preferred service providers for sick people in the poorest 20 percent of the population, according to household surveys—received just over 20 percent of expenditures. This pattern is also seen in low-income countries. In Tanzania, government spending in hospitals accounted for about 60 percent of the budget in 2000, compared with only 34 percent of spending on preventive and primary care facilities. Recent government efforts to change this brought the respective proportions to 43 percent and 48 percent in 2002.

Simply reallocating the budget toward primary care need not result in higher payoffs to government health spending in lowering child and maternal mortality and malnutrition. In many instances, service providers have failed to deliver quality care or to use resources efficiently. Thus, even though many key interventions for the Millennium Development Goals can be and are delivered at lower levels of the health care system, simply redirecting money toward these facilities will not necessarily yield higher returns. The trick is to couple expenditure reallocations with measures to improve the performance of primary care facilities and district hospitals and measures to ensure that households actually demand the relevant interventions.

Targeting spending to remove bottlenecks

Another approach is to assess—at the country level—the health sector impediments to faster progress, to identify ways to remove them, and to estimate both the costs of removing them and the likely impact of their removal on Millennium Development Goal outcomes. Work along these lines has begun in several African countries and in India. In Mali, for example, a number of key impediments to supporting home-based practices and delivering both periodic and continuous professional care were identified. These included low access to affordable health care supplies and the need for community-based support for home-based care, inadequate geographic coverage of preventive professional care (immunization, vitamin A supplementation, and antenatal care), shortages of qualified nurse-midwives, and an absence of effective third-party payment mechanisms for the poor for continuous professional care. Removal of these impediments would cost an estimated $12 per capita between 2002 and 2007 and might reduce under-five mortality by as much as 20–40 percent and maternal mortality by as much as 40–80 percent, depending on the poverty level of the region (Wagstaff and Claeson 2004).

If the estimates of these and other bottleneck costing exercises turn out to be right (validation will have to await the results of the program's implementation), the message is clear—higher returns to government health spending in terms of progress on the Millennium Development Goal indicators can be achieved by focusing marginal spending on the removal of carefully identified constraints.

Coady, Grosh, and Hoddinot (2004) provide a good summary of targeting programs in developing countries. As country incomes and inequality rise, so does the targeting performance of antipoverty interventions. Targeting seems to work better in higher-income countries because of their greater capacity to design and implement finer targeting methods. It also works better in countries having greater income inequality, perhaps because they recognize greater potential gains from targeting and have a greater ability to differentiate among households along different parts of the income distribution. Targeting is also better in countries where government accountability is better; this is consistent with the a higher level of accountability for the effectiveness of poverty reduction programs.

A review of targeting programs in developing countries (Coady, Grosh, and Hoddinot 2004) emphasized several lessons:

- Targeting can work. The best programs can concentrate a high level of resources on poor individuals and households. For example, a public works program in Argentina was able to transfer 80 percent of program benefits to the poorest 20 percent.

- Practice around the world is highly variable. Although median performance was good, targeting was regressive in approximately 25 percent of cases, so that a random allocation of resources would have provided a greater share of benefits to the poor.

- There is no clearly preferred method for all types of programs or all country contexts. More than 80 percent of the variability in targeting performance is due to differences within targeting methods, and only 20 percent to differences across methods.

- Interventions that use means testing, geographic targeting, and self-selection based on a work requirement are all associated with an increased share of benefits going to the bottom 40 percent, compared with targeting that uses self-selection based on consumption.

- Implementation matters tremendously to outcomes. Some, but by no means all, of the variability was explained by country context. Targeting performance improved with implementation capacity, the extent to which governments are held accountable for their actions, and the degree of inequality. Generally, using more targeting methods produced better targeting. Unobserved factors, however, explained much of the differences in targeting success.

Decentralizing health care

Decentralization of key functions is often viewed as a means of improving performance. The motivations behind decentralization are numerous. From a political standpoint, decentralization is seen as bringing decision making closer to the people, thereby increasing "democratization." From an efficiency standpoint, it is seen as a way of removing layers of bureaucracy or diseconomies of scale and of incorporating local information into decision-making processes. This section reviews the evidence on the impact of decentralization on the performance of health systems.

Generally, decentralization in the health care sector refers to the transfer of authority from central government to local government. Decentralization can take several forms (Bossert and Beauvais 2002):

- *Deconcentration* is the transfer of decision-making authority to regional, district, or subdistrict offices within the structure of the ministry of health.
- *Devolution* is the transfer of decision-making authority from the central to provincial or municipal governments.
- *Delegation* is the transfer of decision-making authority from central government to semiautonomous agencies.
- *Privatization* is the transfer of ownership from central, provincial, or municipal governments to private entities.

Each form of decentralization has different implications for the level of autonomy of the subnational authority. Moreover, in evaluating the impact of decentralization, it is important to track which functions are decentralized and which are not. Bossert and Beauvais (2002) identify these key health systems functions as finance (revenue generation, expenditure allocation), service organization (hospital autonomy, payment mechanism, contracts with private sector), human resources (salary setting, hiring and firing, terms of work), access rules (targeting), and governance rules (regulation, monitoring). Thus, in evaluating country experiences with decentralization in the health sector, it is important to consider the form of decentralization as well as the specific decision-making powers that are decentralized.

Proponents of decentralization argue that it improves health system performance through several channels (Bossert and Beauvais 2002; Khaleghian 2004; Hutchinson and LaFond 2004; Chernichovsky and Chernichovsky forthcoming). First, decentralization is thought to improve technical efficiency by making local governments more cost conscious and allowing more freedom in contracting with providers. Second, improved allocative efficiency can be realized by better aligning the mix of services and expenditures with the preferences of the local community. Third, decentralization is believed to improve equity, as local authorities are better able to target expenditures and services to vulnerable groups. Fourth, it also promotes service delivery innovations through experimentation and adaptation of service and financing models to unique settings. Finally, decentralization is thought to improve quality, transparency, accountability, and legitimacy as community involvement in decisions increases.

However, critics of decentralization point to the potential for diseconomies of scale and reduced investment in key public goods, such as research and development at the local level (Khaleghian 2004). Having separate administrative structures to manage health care provision and financing at the subnational level leads to duplication and inefficiency. With smaller populations covered by a particular health financing mechanism, risk pooling may become more difficult. Moreover, there is no clear evidence that local governments are better at targeting marginalized groups than central governments are. There is a potential for elites to "capture" decentralized authorities and prevent them from serving the interests of the needy.

The impact of decentralization

Of particular interest in examining evidence of the impact of decentralization on outcomes is the impact on efficiency and equity in two key areas of health systems: health service delivery and health financing. Several analysts note the paucity of sound evaluations of decentralization policies and the need for research in several areas.

Health service delivery. In general, the evidence base on the impact of decentralization on service delivery is weak, with few studies examining specific services. In general, experiences seem country specific, and it is difficult to draw general conclusions on the impact of decentralization on technical efficiency.

Khaleghian (2004) shows that decentralization (measured by the presence of subnational governments having certain powers, treated as a binary variable) increases the rate of immunization coverage in developing countries. On average, countries with decentralized governments have an 8.5 percent higher rate of immunization coverage. The results are based on cross-country time series data and rely heavily on cross-country variation. However, an analysis of the relationship does not hold for middle-income countries, and the author suggests several explanations. For example, local authorities in low-income countries may have more control over health care programs than local authorities in middle-income countries, even when both are decentralized. In addition, community members may play a more high-profile, pragmatic role in immunization campaigns in low-income countries than in middle-income countries.

Hutchinson and LaFond (2004) found that in Uganda, decentralization provided district governments the freedom to contract with nongovernmental organizations (NGOs) for service provision. The NGOs provided higher-quality care at lower cost in their facilities. They found similar results in Cambodia: NGOs proved more efficient at providing services—both in quality and quantity—than government facilities (box 6.1). In these cases, decentralization was associated with some improvement in technical efficiency in services. Other countries have

BOX 6.1 *Contracting nongovernmental organizations in Cambodia*

Cambodia has experimented with two models of contracting for health services. Districts were selected randomly and assigned to "contracting out" (two districts), "contracting in" (three districts), or "control" (four districts). In the contracting-out sample, NGOs were given full responsibility for the delivery of specified services in a district, including drug procurement and the hiring and firing of staff. In the contracting-in sample, NGOs worked within the existing system to strengthen district administrative structures. Control districts received only a small subsidy toward service delivery. Based on household and facility surveys 2.5 years after contracts started, contracted districts outperformed control districts in terms of predefined coverage indicators, such as immunization and attended deliveries.

The contracting-out model outperformed the contracting-in model. Much of the increase in health care utilization in contracted-out districts was attributed to increased use by households of low socioeconomic status. Because funding flows differed between the districts (contracted-out districts received larger per capita payments), some of the observed differences could have reflected differences in access to and levels of available resources.

Source: Mills, Rasheed, and Tollman forthcoming.

reported improvements in technical efficiency or quality through decentralization. In Tanzania, service use per facility was considerably higher in decentralized districts (Hutchinson and LaFond 2004).

According to Mills, Rasheed, and Tollman (forthcoming), the evidence related to the effect of decentralization on allocative efficiency is mixed. In some cases decentralization did not result in better alignment of health care service provision with the needs of the population. In the Philippines and Uganda, for example, expenditures were reallocated to curative care and away from primary care at the local level (Bossert and Beauvais 2002). Spending at higher levels of care is very visible and is seen as more politically rewarding for district governments, even though there were indications that primary care services are most needed in several of the developing countries examined.

There are also examples of decentralization leading to improved expenditure allocation across services. In Bolivia, for example, an analysis of expenditure patterns following decentralization showed that local government's better knowledge of local needs resulted in spending reallocations that improved access to health care services (Hutchinson and LaFond 2004). Decentralization improved equity in Chile and Columbia. In these countries, health care budgets were devolved to provincial or municipal governments on the basis of a per capita formula adjusted for various factors. The gap in health expenditures across income deciles decreased as a result of decentralization. Local government health expenditures on the wealthiest 10 percent decreased from 41 times that of the poorest 10 percent before decentralization to 12 times after decentralization.

One of the main reasons for the success in Chile and Colombia in improving equity is the acceptance and use of a clear formula for allocating resources to local governments that takes into account differences in health care needs. A second critical factor is adequate institutional capacity at the local level. In all positive experiences associated with decentralization, this was one of the key factors (Hutchinson and LaFond 2004). The evidence clearly indicates that having local health care managers who are highly skilled and have adequate support staff with access to high-quality information systems is a necessary condition for effective decentralization.

Capacity constraints have limited the effectiveness of many decentralization efforts. These constraints have included limitations in the absolute numbers of human resources and in their level of training and preparedness for their new functions. To successfully implement a decentralized system, the leadership capacity of new managers must be strengthened, as must the institutional capacity of new systems at the local level. It is clear that capacity building must occur both before and during decentralization.

Health financing—revenue generation and expenditure. Bossert and Beauvais (2002) examine the decentralization experiences, ranging from devolution to delegation, in Ghana, the Philippines, Uganda, and Zambia. They find that in all countries health expenditures increased at the local level and decreased at the central level as a result of the decentralization reforms. However, higher spending at the local level did not result from any significant increase in revenue generation at the level but rather from increased transfers from the central government.

With decentralization comes an increasing need to control costs at the local level. A logical cost center to target with cost control efforts is salaries for health care workers, which are a primary cost driver of health care spending. For example, salaries consume up to 80 percent of government health spending in developing countries (Joint Learning Initiative 2004). However, efforts at the local level to reduce the costs associated with health care workers' salaries are often restricted by unions, which exert political pressure not to change the terms of work or to hire and fire health care workers. In addition, evidence suggests that continued control from the central level over salary and personnel levels severely limits local fiscal autonomy and hinders cost control efforts (Bossert and Beauvais 2002).

Decentralization of revenue generation to district governments diminishes the ability of central authorities to reallocate expenditures. This has the potential to increase regional inequities in health care spending. For example, many Eastern European countries have devolved revenue generation to regional governments. The evidence indicates that in many of these countries the proportion of regional revenue that is collected and reallocated by the central authority has been inadequate, and regional inequality has increased significantly since decentralization (Langenbrunner forthcoming).

Main lessons of decentralization

A review of country experiences (Hutchinson and LaFond 2004) indicates that the main lessons related to decentralization in the health sector concern governance, service delivery, and financing:

Governance

- Decentralization requires strong political backing at both the central and local levels. Stakeholders should have ownership of both the plan for decentralization and the process of organizational capacity building.
- Political objectives must be supported by the legal and institutional framework, the structure of service delivery responsibilities, and the system of intergovernmental fiscal transfers.
- Changes in the roles and responsibilities of the different actors in the health sector, particularly local government health officials, should be accompanied by training and plans for building capacity.
- Decentralization should be accompanied by a clear delineation of responsibilities and mechanisms of accountability among the different stakeholders and should be formally codified in legislation, regulations, or other binding instruments.
- For decentralization to be successful, there must be willingness on the part of the central government to share power and on the part of local governments and communities to assume new responsibilities. In many countries, civil servants have objected to decentralization efforts for fear of status loss when these efforts involve a transfer of personnel from the central to subnational governments.
- Research institutions should monitor and evaluate practical aspects of the decentralization process.

Service delivery

- Although decentralization generally involves a diminished central government role in service delivery, certain activities such as research and dissemination of findings, provision of public goods, the development and enforcement of standards and regulations, and accreditation procedures are likely to be most efficiently undertaken at the central level.
- Communities must have the information on public sector performance that allows them to react and to hold officials and politicians accountable. For example, the costs of services provided at the community level, delivery options, and available resources must be transparent so that decision making can be informed and meaningful.
- There must be binding and credible mechanisms to allow communities to express preferences so that there are incentives for communities to participate.

- Decentralization has been motivated in many cases by theoretical considerations, rather than empirical evidence. The measurement of efficiency gains in decentralized service delivery remains open to empirical investigation, particularly in the developing world, where decentralization programs have been more ambitious and implemented more recently.

Financing

- Even under decentralization, local governments may have limited revenue-generating capacity and therefore are likely to remain reliant on intergovernmental transfers from the central government. Intergovernmental transfers should be determined openly and objectively, ideally by a clear, simple, and verifiable formula.
- Local financing and fiscal authority should be linked to service provision responsibilities and functions so that local politicians can deliver on their promises and be held accountable for their decisions.

Endnote

1. This section on public expenditure track surveys draws heavily from Dehn, Reinikka, and Svensson 2003.

References

Bossert, T., and J. Beauvais. 2002. "Decentralization of Health Systems in Ghana, Zambia, Uganda, and the Philippines: A Comparative Analysis of Decision Space." *Health Policy and Planning* 17 (1): 14–31.

Chernichovsky, D., and M. Chernichovsky. Forthcoming. *Decentralization in the Health Care System: A Framework for Design and Implementation.* Washington, D.C.: World Bank.

Coady, D., M. Grosh, and J. Hoddinot. 2004. *Targeting of Transfers in Developing Countries: Review of Lessons and Experience.* Washington, D.C.: World Bank.

Dehn, J., R. Reinikka, and J. Svensson. 2003. "Survey Tools for Assessing Performance in Service Delivery." In F. Bourguignon and L. Pereira da Silva, eds., *The Impact of Economic Policies on Poverty and Income Distribution: Evaluation Techniques and Tools.* Washington, D.C.: World Bank; New York: Oxford University Press.

Foster, M. 2005. "MDG-Oriented Sector and Poverty Reduction Strategies: Lessons from Experience." Health, Nutrition, and Population Discussion Paper, World Bank, Washington, D.C.

Hutchinson, P. L., and A. K. LaFond. 2004. *Monitoring and Evaluation of Decentralization Reforms in Developing Country Health Sectors.* Bethesda, Md.: PHR*plus.*

IMF (International Monetary Fund). 2003. *Evaluation of Poverty Reduction Strategy Papers and the Poverty Reduction and Growth Facility.* Washington, D.C.

IMF (International Monetary Fund) and World Bank. 2005. *2005 Review of the Poverty Reduction Strategy Approach: Balancing Accountabilities and Scaling Up Results.* Washington, D.C.

Joint Learning Initiative. 2004. *Human Resources for Health: Overcoming the Crisis.* Global Equity Initiative, Harvard University, Cambridge, Mass.

Khaleghian, P. 2004. "Decentralization and Public Services: The Case of Immunization." Policy Research Working Paper 2989, World Bank, Washington, D.C.

Langenbrunner, J. Forthcoming. *Health Care Financing and Purchasing in ECA: An Overview of Issues and Reforms.* Washington, D.C.: World Bank.

Mills, A., F. Rasheed, and S. Tollman. Forthcoming. "Improving the Performance of Health Systems." In D. Jamison, J. Berman, A. Meacham, G. Alleyne, M. Claeson, D. Evans, P. Jha, A. Mills, and P. Musgrove, eds., *Disease Control Priorities in Developing Countries,* 2nd ed., Washington, D.C.: World Bank; New York: Oxford University Press.

Wagstaff, A., and M. Claeson. 2004. *The Millennium Goals for Health: Rising to the Challenges.* Washington, D.C.: World Bank.

WHO (World Health Organization). 2004. *PRSPs: Their Significance for Health, Second Synthesis Report.* Geneva.

World Bank. 1998. *Public Expenditure Management Handbook.* Washington, D.C.

———. 2002a. "Republic of Latvia Public Expenditure Review." Poverty Reduction and Economic Management Unit, Europe and Central Asia Region, Washington, D.C.

———. 2002b. "Medium-Term Expenditure Frameworks: From Concept to Practice. Preliminary Lessons from Africa." Working Paper Series 28, Africa Region, Washington, D.C.

———. 2004a. *The Poverty Reduction Strategy Initiative: An Independent Evaluation of the World Bank's Support through 2003.* Washington, D.C.

———. 2004b. "A Review of Population, Reproductive Health, and Adolescent Health and Development in Poverty Reduction Strategies." Health, Nutrition, and Population Team, Washington, D.C.

———. 2004c. *The Republic of Uganda Country Integrated Fiduciary Assessment 2004, Volume II: Public Expenditure Review 2004.* Poverty Reduction and Economic Management, Washington, D.C.

———. 2005a. *Global Monitoring Report 2005: Millennium Development Goals, From Consensus to Momentum.* Washington, D.C.

———. 2005b. "A Stock Taking of Poverty Reduction Support Credits." Operations Policy and Country Services, Washington, D.C.

7

Financing health in low-income countries

Poverty magnifies the need for health care while shrinking the capacity to finance it. Low-income countries face 56 percent of the global disease burden but account for only 2 percent of global health spending (World Bank 2005; Mathers, Lopez, and Murray, forthcoming). With spending levels of some $30 per capita on average, over half of it out of pocket, low-income countries face severe challenges in providing their citizens with a basic package of essential services and a modicum of financial protection against the impoverishing effects of catastrophic illness. Most low-income countries, particularly those in Africa, are far off track for reaching the Millennium Development Goals for health. To improve the equity and efficiency of their health financing systems and to achieve the Millennium Development Goals, low-income countries will need to improve the efficiency and equity of their institutions, particularly public sector management; significantly increase their current government health spending levels through enhanced domestic resource mobilization, improvements in the efficiency of public spending, and large increases in grant-based and sustainable external assistance; improve financial protection to the extent feasible through appropriate risk pooling mechanisms adapted to country-specific circumstances; and improve the technical and allocative efficiency of government health-purchasing decisions. Low-income countries face difficult choices and trade-offs, and there are no one-size-fits-all solutions or magic bullets.

Every country wants a health care system that offers good health outcomes, affordable services, satisfied consumers and providers, and medical and financial equity. These objectives are hard to attain in low-income countries, where budget constraints are binding at low levels of overall expenditure, in particular in the public sector. As progress toward the Millennium Development Goals for health has faltered in the poorest countries, strong international pressure has been building to scale up efforts. Because health expenditures are largely out of pocket in low-income countries and there is limited capacity to increase domestic public expenditures, donors are expected to finance most of the scale-up. But even if donors make long-term commitments, health expenditures will eventually have to be absorbed within each country's domestic resource envelope. Moreover, donor assistance for health is most likely to focus on Sub-Saharan Africa, because of its large health needs and challenging economic circumstances, and on a few other low-income countries outside this region, leaving the remaining countries to find their own solutions.

This chapter reviews the enabling conditions for an expansion in health expenditures from efficiency, equity, and sustainability perspectives in the context of low-income countries (countries with a GNI of less that $766; World Bank 2005b). It examines mechanisms for increasing resources for health and the major restrictions on each method in low-income countries. Public and private financing arrangements for pooling health care revenues are also reviewed. Seven main lessons have emerged:

- Because economic growth is a precondition for reaching the Millennium Development Goals, low-income countries must not jeopardize overall growth and equity goals as they weigh decisions about additional taxation and resource allocation that could generate additional revenues for health. Although low-income countries should give priority to increasing their ability to tax in an effective and equitable manner, tax revenues cannot be expected to provide, in the short run, the large additional revenues needed for most countries to reach the Millennium Development Goals.

- Payroll-financed social insurance has many of the same limitations as general taxation in low-income countries, and it will be difficult for many countries to meet the enabling conditions that increase the probability of successful implementation of social health insurance schemes and guarantee their sustainability.

- In many highly indebted poor countries, debt relief is important for both growth and solvency. Debt relief does not, however, generate new resources for these countries, so they cannot count on debt relief alone to increase government expenditures in social sectors.

- To effectively increase recurrent health expenditures, donor funding should be in the form of predictable on-budget financing offered over extended periods (20 years or more in some countries). Without long-term commitments of assistance, low-income countries may not be able to handle the recurrent cost-related fiscal contingencies generated by such increases.

- Donors and governments alike must carefully consider the opportunity costs of their resource allocation decisions: what other uses might spur growth or generate increases in outputs and outcomes in other sectors, which could in turn improve health outcomes? The best way to approach overall expenditure allocation issues is through explicit country strategies, as described in poverty reduction strategy papers and medium-term expenditure frameworks. Countries must also carefully consider the distributional impact of their limited resources.

- Low-income countries are likely to have a larger and more equitable impact on health outcomes if they select a very basic universal package of mainly public goods, including some treatment services proven effective in moving toward the Millennium Development Goals. Other interventions should be considered in a targeted manner.

- The capacity of low-income countries to efficiently absorb additional resources may be a problem. To build capacity, donors need to work within governments' own programs and administrative mechanisms, rather than through independent initiatives. Low-income countries, in turn, need to improve public expenditure planning, management, and monitoring, particularly by upgrading financial management and procurement systems, improving accountability for results, and strengthening judicial systems. Decentralization, targeting, and contracting may all help improve the equity and efficiency of public expenditure management.

Health spending by region

As discussed in chapter 1, low-income countries in all regions spend much less on health care than higher-income countries and depend much more on private expenditures, mostly directly out of pocket. Severe institutional, fiscal, economic, and political constraints limit the use of all organized means of financing (which include tax revenue, social health insurance, community-based health insurance, and voluntary health insurance). The basic pattern of low health spending, heavy reliance on out-of-pocket financing, and limited domestic resource mobilization ability holds for low-income countries in all regions.

Asia

In low-income countries in South Asia, it is difficult to estimate total health expenditures, because households' out-of-pocket expenditures on health care, the largest source of financing, are not well quantified. According to World Health Organization (WHO) estimates, in 2002 total health expenditure (the sum of public and private health expenditure) was slightly above 6 percent of GDP in Afghanistan and India, about 5 percent in Nepal, 3.5 percent in Bhutan and Sri Lanka, and just above 3 percent in Bangladesh and Pakistan (figure 7.1).

On average across these countries, public sources of revenue for health accounted for less than 25 percent of total health expenditure, while most of the remaining 75 percent from private sources is in the form of out-of-pocket payments (chapter 1). There are three exceptions to this common pattern: Sri Lanka, Bhutan, and Bangladesh. In Sri Lanka public sources of financing for health services are significant, accounting for half of all spending. In Bangladesh, the share of total health expenditures from public sources is about 35 percent, because donor financing is more significant than in other low-income South Asian countries (about 13.5 percent).

By looking at the trends, one can also see that in low-income countries in South Asia, the proportion of total health expenditures paid out of pocket has been stable or increasing, while the share from government revenue sources has

FIGURE 7.1 Public and private health expenditures in South Asia, 1998–2001

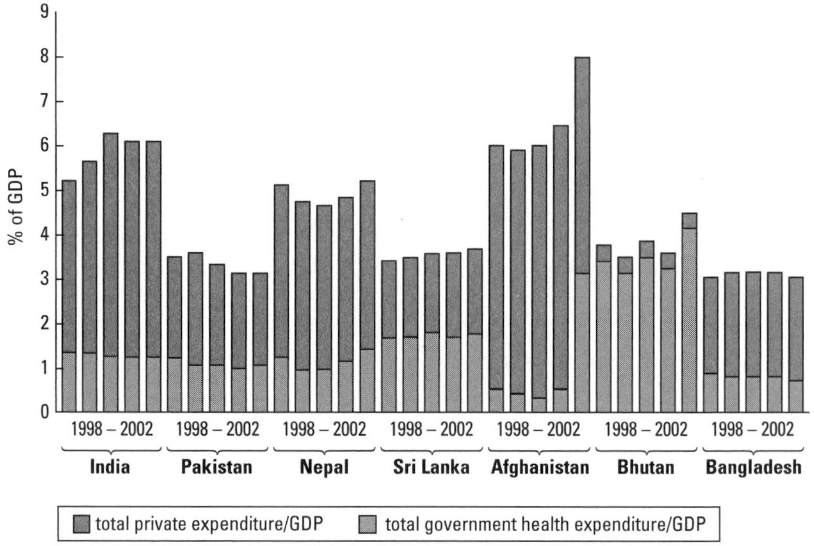

Source: WHO 2001.

been declining. For example, in India, the privately funded share of the total resources for health increased from 73.5 percent to 78.9 percent during 1998–2002 (Government of India Ministry of Statistics 1998, 2001). Almost all of it is directly paid by patients at the point of delivery. By contrast, over the same period, government expenditure on health and family welfare in India decreased from 9.2 percent to 7.3 percent of total government expenditure, and in 2002/3 it was equal to only $3.50 per capita. The share of government spending on health has also been decreasing in Nepal and Sri Lanka and has been stagnant in Pakistan. Governments in South Asia seem to be unable to respond to the expectations about increased levels of service, better quality standards, and greater diversification of care that is accompanying the steady increase in population, income, and education levels.[1]

The situation in low-income East Asian countries is very similar to that in South Asia; population-weighted average private expenditures represent 67 percent of total health expenditure, and these expenditures are mostly out of pocket (92 percent, on average). In low-income countries, such as Vietnam, where the private health spending share of GDP is 5 percent, and even more so in Cambodia— where the share is 6 percent—private health spending is almost entirely made up of out-of-pocket expenditures. WHO data also show a trend of increasing private expenditures in Vietnam, essentially stagnant levels in Lao People's Democratic Republic, and slight decreases in Cambodia during 1998–2002. Mongolia is a special case; private sources of revenue represent less than 30 percent of total health expenditure (and are tending to decrease even further). So is Papua Guinea, where private revenue sources are estimated to account for less than 15 percent of total health expenditure.

Africa

In Sub-Saharan Africa, government expenditures on health are also extremely low. However, because donor funding is an important source of revenue for health in these countries, on average, the sum of these two public sources of revenue is still substantial (chapter 1). Nonetheless, private spending exceeds public spending on health (see chapter 1 and figure 7.2). Furthermore, household out-of-pocket spending accounts for 80 percent of private spending and almost 50 percent of total health spending.

Nevertheless, with low per capita income, challenging growth prospects, limited domestic revenue mobilization potential, severe shortages of health manpower, and the highest disease burden in the world, Africa faces difficult health financing decisions. Africa accounts for 25 percent of the global disease burden and 60 percent of the people living with HIV/AIDS. But it accounts for less than 1 percent of global health spending and contains only 2 percent of the global health workforce (United Nations Population Division 1998; WHO 2004; WHO and UNAIDS 2004;

FIGURE 7.2   Private and public health expenditures in Sub-Saharan Africa, 2002

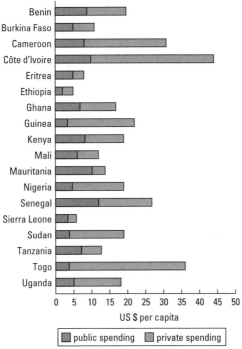

US $ per capita

☐ public spending   ☐ private spending

Source: Bitran forthcoming.

Joint Learning Initiative 2004). In this region, increasing the level of health expenditures and improving their efficiency is literally a life and death situation.

Other regions

Most low-income countries in Europe and Central Asia, Latin America and the Caribbean, and the Middle East and North Africa have public-private health expenditure patterns similar to those in Asian and African low-income countries. Health expenditures derived from private sources in Haiti and Tajikistan are above 60 percent, are mostly in the form of out-of-pocket spending, and show no recent declines. But the relative importance of private health expenditures is somewhat lower, at about 50 percent, in Latin American countries that have recently been classified as lower middle income (Bolivia, Honduras, and Nicaragua).

In the Kyrgyz Republic and Uzbekistan, two other low-income countries in the Europe and Central Asia region, the proportion of total health expenditures derived from private sources is lower, at about 50 percent, than in some countries in the region that are classified as lower middle income (such as Armenia, Azerbaijan, and Georgia), where the proportion is about 70 percent. These differences may reflect the different degrees of reductions in public health expenditures after the collapse of the Soviet Union. For example, Armenia and Georgia faced some of the largest declines in public health expenditures in the 1990s (Bonilla-Chacin, Murrugarra, and Temourov 2005).

The cost of the Millennium Development Goals

To integrate the Millennium Development Goals for health into national poverty reduction strategies, countries need to be able to estimate the costs. More attention must be paid to relative cost estimates than to absolute ones, to the short-term time horizon than to the long-term one, to domestic sources of funding than to foreign aid, and to national ownership than to donor-driven priorities (Vandemoortele and Roy 2004). This local and immediate orientation requires aligning health plans that have been developed with the Millennium Development Goals in mind with each country's medium-term expenditure framework and poverty reduction strategy. Moreover, it requires being cognizant of budget constraints and multisectoral priorities.

Estimating methods

The best methodology for estimating the costs of reaching the Millennium Development Goals remains a subject of debate. Some proposed methods are summarized in annex 7.1.

Table 7.1 provides a set of preliminary country-level estimates for removing bottlenecks to accelerate progress toward the health Millennium Development Goals (MBB method), what it will cost to achieve the health Millennium Development Goals (UN Millennium Project estimates), additional expenditure estimates

TABLE 7.1 Alternative estimates of the annual cost of meeting the Millennium Development Goals for health (U.S. 2000 dollars per capita)

Country	Model	Cost estimate for the year specified
Mali (one region)	MBB	$3.9 (2003)
	Elasticity	$6.8 (2003)
Madagascar (Toamasina)	MBB	$2.4 (2003)
	Elasticity	$6.7 (2003)
Ethiopia[a]	MBB/MP	$12.0 (2015)
	Elasticity	$11.0 (2015)
	MAMS	$15.0 (2015)
Bangladesh	MP	$20.6 (average, 2005–15)
	Elasticity	$16.9 (average, 2005–15)
Cambodia	MP	$22.5 (average, 2005–15)
	Elasticity	$37.4 (average, 2005–15)
Ghana	MP	$24.7 (average, 2005–15)
	Elasticity	$23.7 (average, 2005–15)
Uganda	MP	$32.1 (average, 2005–15)
	Elasticity	$40.6 (average, 2005–15)
Tanzania	MP	$34.7 (average, 2005–15)
	Elasticity	$66.9 (average, 2005–15)

Sources: MBB estimates from Soucat and others 2004 and country estimates using the MBB tool. MP estimates from UN Millennium Project 2004a. MAMS estimate from Bourguignon and others 2004. World Bank staff estimates.

MBB is marginal budgeting for bottlenecks; MP is Millennium Development Goal needs assessment; MAMS is maquette for multisectoral analysis.

Note: Elasticity estimates are expenditure per capita estimates by World Bank staff using the model in annex 5.1. Elasticity estimates in the table are based on assumptions of spending 1 percent per year increase in real GDP per capita, 5 percent increase in education, roads, water, and sanitation. For descriptions of models, see annex 7.1.

a. MBB estimate refers to the maximum access scenario with coverage up to 90 percent of the population for clinical care.

to reach the Millennium Development Goals in selected countries based on measured elasticities (elasticity estimates), and additional health expenditures per capita under an optimized allocation framework (MAMS). (See annex 7.1 for detailed information about these costing strategies.) The estimates illustrate orders of magnitude and should not be compared directly to each other or across countries; each methodology has a different estimating objective, and the numbers for each country are not comparable across methodologies.

The MP model estimates an average unit cost per capita and includes all Millennium Development Goals for health, including antiretroviral treatment and essential universal coverage of hospital care for childbirth. MBB estimates the costs of removing bottlenecks at different levels of care delivery: for Madagascar and Mali, the needed expansion of services is largely at the household and outreach levels of care, where the marginal impact on maternal and child mortality per dollar spent is expected to be large. When additional coverage of hospital care for mothers and treatment for HIV/AIDS is added to MBB costs per capita, per capita costs can reach $25–$35. Finally, the elasticity analysis measures expenditure per capita, under certain assumptions of growth in GDP, decline in illiteracy, and improved access to sanitation and roads. In the elasticity model, the expenditures per capita are especially high for countries for which under-five mortality increased between 1990 and 2000.[2]

Closing the health financing gap

Whatever estimation method is used, the conclusion of all the Millennium Development Goal cost estimate studies is the same: the financing gap between the costs of achieving the Millennium Development Goals and the potential for low-income countries to mobilize domestic resources is large. That gap can be closed only by external financing. Hence, all Millennium Development Goal cost estimate studies conclude that public expenditures on health must be increased and this additional spending must be financed largely by donor support, especially in the least-developed countries (CMH 2001; UN Millennium Project 2005).

To give a sense of this gap, actual and projected government health expenditures as a percentage of GDP are plotted for 10 low-income countries in Sub-Saharan Africa (figure 7.3). Projected expenditures per capita are derived for each country from the model presented in chapter 5 of this report under assumptions that GDP per capita would grow at 1 percent a year and that all other independent variables in that model (education, roads, water, sanitation, and donor funding) would grow at 5 percent a year.

For these countries, the ratio of government health expenditures to GDP would have to grow from an average of about 2.3 percent of GDP in 2000 (World Bank 2005a) to an average of 30 percent by 2015 to reach the goal for child mortality. For several of the countries, the level of public expenditures to GDP at the end of 2015 would have to be much larger than 20 percent, well above the ratio of total tax revenues to GDP (Kenya, Lesotho, Tanzania, and Zambia). All the other countries, except for Nigeria, are projected to need public spending on health well over 8 percent of GDP. This is obviously not realistic and suggests that the increases in spending would have to come mostly from donor grants and that these grants would have to be sustained for long periods. An independent study suggests that in the cases of Ethiopia and Tanzania, a doubling of aid as a percentage of GDP would require grant financing for 20 years before these grants can be substituted with additional tax revenue under reasonable assumptions of increased domestic revenues (Foster 2003).[3]

One way low-income countries might improve their health planning is to develop poverty reduction strategy papers under different scenarios of health sector assistance. For example, there is a strong push by certain advocates for governments to produce health plans and even broader poverty reduction strategies on a

FIGURE 7.3   Estimated government health expenditures required to meet the Millennium Development Goal on child mortality in 10 African countries, 1995–2015

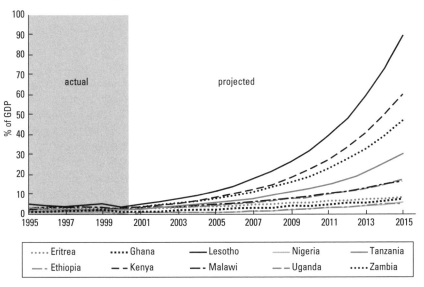

Source: World Bank staff estimates.

"needs basis," without consideration of budget constraints, under the assumption that any gap will be financed by donors after reasonable national efforts at resource mobilization (UN Millennium Project 2005). Others stress that to be a useful guide to action, the poverty reduction strategy paper needs to be linked to the national budget process, establishing clear priorities to guide public expenditure plans and budgets based on a realistic assessment of available resources.

Clearly, multiple scenarios of the poverty reduction strategy paper are useful for planning. By developing multiple scenarios based on alternative revenue and external assistance scenarios, as in the case of country assistance strategies, some countries have shown how the poverty reduction strategy paper can be used as a guide to the allocation of the resources they expect to have and as a bid for additional support—a "high-case" scenario is used to attract additional finance by showing what could be achieved with it, whereas realistic medium- or low-case scenarios set out how expenditure plans should be prioritized in the event that fewer resources are available. The World Bank and IMF have supported those countries wishing to adopt this approach. A strong case can be made for encouraging all countries to do so.

In any case, given the volatility and unpredictability of donor aid (chapter 4), the need for countries to eventually sustain their own increases in expenditure, and the need for realistic planning and prioritization, it is imperative to analyze the alternative financing mechanisms available to low-income countries and the major factors constraining their expansion.

Public sources of revenue for health

In principle, governments have various ways to increase health expenditure at a sustainable level—that is, to increase the fiscal space that can be available to health. Additional revenues can be raised by collecting new taxes or by strengthening tax administration. Lower-priority expenditures can be cut to make room for more desirable ones. Resources can be borrowed, from either domestic or external sources, or released through debt relief. Governments may benefit from the fiscal space arising from the receipt of grants from outside sources. Finally, governments can use their power of seignorage (having the central bank print money to lend to the government). The following sections review the constraints found in generating such fiscal space from the perspective of the health sector as well as the constraints faced by low-income countries in pooling and allocating resources.

Tax collection

One way of increasing fiscal space is to increase domestically available resources by raising tax revenues. However, raising revenues through tax reforms may be easier said than done. As shown in chapter 2, the low tax and nontax resource base and the slow growth rates of low-income countries imply that any increases in health expenditures derived from domestic financing will be slow to come, unless drastic changes take place in domestic revenue generation capacity. Yet, countries such as Benin, Ghana, and Zimbabwe have shown that such efforts are possible and can also support increases in expenditures in the health sector.

The evolution of tax and nontax revenue for 16 African countries during the 1990s shows that these countries had on average a low base of tax and nontax revenues, amounting to 16 percent of GDP in 1999. This average, however, conceals big differences across countries, four of which have shares above 25 percent (the Republic of Congo, Kenya, Lesotho, and Zimbabwe), seven between 15 and 20 percent (Benin, Burundi, Cameroon, Côte d'Ivoire, Ethiopia, Ghana, and Senegal), and five below 15 percent (Burkina Faso, the Republic of Congo, Guinea, Madagascar, Rwanda, and Sierra Leone). The evolution of tax and nontax revenues as a share of GDP also varies across countries. It decreased in five countries over the 1990s, grew at less than 2 percent a year in another four countries, and grew at faster rates (above the population growth rates) only in six countries (figures 7.4 and 7.5).

Low ratios of tax to GDP imply that developing countries have room to increase revenues from taxation to accommodate some increase in expenditures, including those for health. Developing countries may want to replace narrow, distorting tax bases that have widely differentiated rates and numerous loopholes

FIGURE 7.4   Annual percentage change of tax and nontax revenue in Sub-Saharan Africa in the 1990s

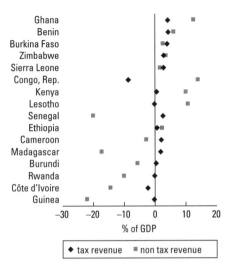

Sources: World Development Indicators (WDI) database and IMF Poverty Reduction and Growth Facility (PRGF).

FIGURE 7.5   Annual percentage change in total revenue in Sub-Saharan Africa in the 1990s

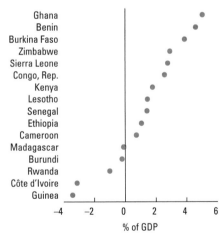

Sources: WDI database and IMF PRGF reports.

with broader tax bases that generate higher revenues at lower rates and that do not discriminate against the various sources and uses of income. Doing so would result in efficiency gains and greater administrative simplicity and horizontal equity.

However, the practical difficulties of implementing tax reforms must not be underestimated. Increasing revenues through tax reforms affects many interests and cannot be done effortlessly, especially when institutional changes in the tax authorities are required, rural and informal sectors are important, borders are large, and wealthy elites are politically powerful. Countries are unlikely to attempt tax reforms only to accommodate additional health expenditures within their budget constraints.

Budget reallocation

Governments may decide to reallocate resources from other lower-priority expenditures to generate fiscal space for health. This path, too, is difficult. From an economic point of view, the marginal social benefits derived from government expenditures should equal the marginal costs. Therefore, expenditures could theoretically be reallocated from unproductive public uses to more productive ones (or from uses that generate a lower marginal social benefit per dollar spent to those that produce more marginal social benefit per dollar spent). However, this rarely works in practice. In the first place, governments do not really have an optimizing function, so it is difficult to prove unproductive expenditures, beyond the obvious "white elephant investments," such as subsidies to the rich or excessive payrolls. Second, reallocation of expenditures implies cutting expenditures to a particular institution or program. Automatically, this raises a political or regional struggle. It is especially difficult when the reallocation of expenditures involves cutting payrolls.

Of course, inefficiencies are abundant and should still be addressed. For every rupee reaching the poor in a rice-subsidy program in India's Andhra Pradesh state in 1996, 3.6 rupees were lost in leakage to the nonpoor (Radhakrishna 1997). Although difficult, change is possible. In the late 1980s, only 30 percent of Bolivia's average government investments went to the social sectors; the remainder went primarily to public sector companies. But in 2000 the reverse was true: only 25 percent of government investments went to other sectors, while 75 percent was invested in the social sectors. This reversal, however, took almost 10 years and substantial structural reform, including the privatization of all major public companies (petroleum, energy, telecommunications, railroads, airline, and others). Therefore, although reallocation of resources is possible, it requires major political will and significant time for an important impact to take place.

Debt relief

Countries can increase their fiscal space through additional borrowing. However, a large number of low-income countries already have a large debt burden and do not have much room for additional borrowing. Moreover, scaling up health services requires increases in recurrent expenditures (such as salaries), which should not be financed with debt but rather with permanent sources of funding. The complement to additional borrowing is obtaining debt relief to release domestic resources that could be used for additional investment and recurrent spending in the country.

In principle, the Heavily Indebted Poor Countries Debt Initiative is a mechanism to increase the financing available for the social sectors in the target countries. It has important features to help address constraints to improve health, nutrition, and population outcomes. Debt relief is based on the delivery of measurable outcomes. Debt relief, and thus increased expenditures in the social sectors, are based on each country's poverty reduction strategy, taking into consideration the views of civil society and overall budget constraints. Poverty reduction strategy papers must look at overall constraints that affect absorptive capacity beyond the social sectors where expenditures are taking place.

Countries are eligible for the initiative if they receive concessional loans from the International Development Association (IDA) and would still have unsustainable levels of debt after full use of traditional debt relief mechanisms. Forty-two countries are now eligible, and another 38 are expected to qualify for debt relief. Countries reach the decision point, the first stage of debt relief, based on a three-year record of macroeconomic stability and preparation of an interim or full poverty reduction strategy paper. At that stage they begin to receive "interim" relief. Simultaneously, the criteria for the completion point are established. In addition to maintaining macroeconomic stability, finalizing a full poverty reduction strategy paper, and successfully implementing it for one year, countries must set performance benchmarks for structural and social reforms. Once a country reaches the completion point, the remaining debt relief is scheduled and is irrevocable. To date, 27 countries, including 23 in Africa, have reached the decision point and are receiving some interim debt relief. Nine African countries had reached the completion point (Benin, Burkina Faso, Ethiopia, Mali, Mauritania, Mozambique, Niger, Tanzania, and Uganda) as of May 2005.

The initiative provides eligible countries with substantial savings in debt service payments. The relief committed to the 27 countries that have reached their completion points or are in their interim period, together with other debt relief, represents a two-thirds reduction in the countries' overall debt stock (IMF/IDA 2004). But, from an expenditure perspective, what is relevant is whether the beneficiary countries had access to resources for additional expenditures as a result of debt relief. Debt service payments relative to fiscal revenue in these 27 countries have declined from an average of 24 percent in 1998–9 to 15 percent in 2003 and are expected to decline to less than half the 1998–9 average by 2006. Not surprisingly, there are large variations across countries. A recent study of 23 African countries shows that the ratios of debt service to government revenues in 2003 ranged from 6.1 percent in Rwanda to 30 percent in The Gambia and Malawi (Hinchliffe 2004).

An important question is whether the resources made available through debt relief were used to increase expenditures in the social sectors. Progress on this front is measured by IDA and the IMF as the share of poverty-reducing spending to GDP and to total spending. The definition of poverty-reducing spending is country specific and includes, for example, outlays on basic health, primary education, agriculture, infrastructure, housing, basic sanitation, and HIV/AIDS. The definition of such expenditure for each country is established in its poverty reduction strategy paper. According to the IMF and IDA 2004 Status of Implementation report, poverty-reducing expenditures in the 27 highly indebted poor countries have increased on average from 6.4 percent of GDP in 1999 to 7.9 percent of GDP in 2003 (Hinchliffe 2004).

As expected, the increase also varies across countries. According to Hinchliffe (2004), while poverty-reducing expenditures increased on average from 39 percent in 1999 to 48 percent in 2003 as a share of total revenues in 23 of the 27 highly industrial poor countries, it increased by as much as 76 percent in Mozambique and declined by 27 percent in Chad. Of 20 countries for which there was full information, 13 had significant increases in the share of total revenues directed toward poverty-reducing expenditures. Exceptions were Benin, Madagascar, and Niger, where the share remained roughly constant, and Chad, Ghana, São Tomé and Principe, and Zambia, where it fell.

Comparisons across countries make little sense, however, as the definition of poverty-reducing expenditures varies substantially from one country to another. The tendency has been for countries to widen the definition of "priority sectors." This wider definition can easily mask what is happening to expenditures in education and health, in particular. An analysis by Hinchliffe (2004) of the trend in health expenditures as a share of total government expenditures in 20 highly indebted poor countries between 1998 and 2002 (table 7.2) shows that the share increased on average from 6.2 percent to 8.1 percent. Of the 20 countries, 13 had increases. Exceptions are Guinea-Bissau, where data is not available for enough years to discern a trend; Malawi and Zambia, where the share remained essentially constant; and Burkina Faso, Ethiopia, Madagascar, and Mali, where the share declined.

Low-income countries have recognized the need for greater investments in health. In the 2001 Abuja Declaration on HIV/AIDS, Tuberculosis, and Other Related Infectious Diseases, African leaders pledged to increase health spending to 15 percent of government budgets. Achieving this larger proportion of expenditures in health is going to be a slow process, as the data in table 7.2 show. Debt relief for poor countries is important, but if the country did not have resources to repay the debt in the first place, it may have difficulty complying with the increases in poverty spending required by the program. Even though debt relief

TABLE 7.2   Share of health expenditures in total government expenditures in 20 highly indebted poor countries, 1998–2002

	1998	1999	2000	2001	2002
Benin	6.5	8.3	7.2	8.8	8.1
Burkina Faso	9.8	5.4	5.6	5.9	8.1
Cameroon	3.2	3.4	4.8	5.5	7.8
Ethiopia	5.8	4.3	3.4	4.8	4.4
Ghana	2.7	3.3	3.0	3.7	5.7
The Gambia	—	—	12.8	14.6	16.3
Guinea	4.4	4.4	4.2	7.5	6.5
Guinea-Bissau	—	—	4.3	3.5	—
Madagascar	3.6	2.8	2.7	4.4	2.7
Malawi	9.6	8.0	6.6	8.3	9.3
Mali	5.2	4.4	6.1	7.1	3.3
Mauritania	6.8	6.7	5.4	7.1	9.3
Mozambique	11.1	11.3	12.1	11.2	12.0
Niger	9.0	11.7	11.9	—	—
Rwanda	1.9	2.6	2.9	3.3	3.1
Senegal	4.9	5.2	5.8	8.7	11.7
Sierra Leone	—	4.7	5.4	6.8	8.1
Tanzania	—	8.5	7.3	9.1	10.1
Uganda	6.7	6.5	7.4	8.6	9.6
Zambia	6.9	5.5	4.7	4.7	6.9
Median	6.2	5.1	5.5	5.9	8.1

Source: Hinchliffe 2004.

— not available.

can generate significant savings in debt repayments, it does not automatically generate additional flows of resources to the recipient countries. Of the 20 countries in table 7.2, only 4 reported expenditures in health of 10 percent or more of total government expenditures in 2002. Reallocation of expenditures across sectors is a difficult political process, especially in a very constrained resource environment, as discussed later in this chapter.

Donor funding

As discussed in chapter 1, development assistance for health accounts for about 20 percent of country-weighted health expenditures in low-income countries. It plays an especially important role in Sub-Saharan Africa: all 12 countries in which external funding exceeded 30 percent of health expenditures in 2000 were in Africa (WHO 2001).

However, official development assistance in general and health aid in particular have serious problems (chapter 4). These include lack of predictability, increased focus on specific diseases or interventions, large numbers of new actors and donors, lack of responsiveness and flexibility to crises, and donors' lack of accountability for the absence of results and progress. Volatility is especially damaging, as is the fact that commitments are a bad predictor of disbursements. This hampers the ability of any government to plan appropriately. Commitments are made for short maturities (three years at best), but increased recurrent expenditures in health require long-term resources. Only a small share of aid (about 20 percent) is provided as budget support; the rest of financing is provided as either earmarked project support, off-budget support for disease- or intervention-specific programs, or even technical assistance that is not registered in the recipient country's balance of payments. Coordinating health plans is extremely difficult, if not impossible, under such circumstances.

Despite these problems, donor funding seems to be the only alternative in the short run for scaling up expenditures in health in many low-income countries, especially in Africa. Yet, to increase the effectiveness of such funding, additional efforts are necessary—to increase the maturity of resources, decrease volatility, and improve harmonization. It is particularly important for donors not to second guess recipient countries' preferences, but rather to fund gaps in country programs.

National health services

National health service systems have three main features (see box 3.1): funding comes primarily from general revenues, they provide (or at least aim to provide) coverage to the whole population, and they usually (though not necessarily) deliver health care through a network of public providers. Most low-income countries have a national health service run by the ministry of health. National health service systems finance a basic package of public health services for the entire population and some level of financial protection against catastrophic illness for at least some segments of the population. Financing also includes out-of-pocket payments and purchases of private services, limited social and private health insurance, and community risk pooling schemes.

The problems with national health service systems have been well documented (World Bank 2004b; Wagstaff and Claeson 2004). These include management, accountability, corruption, incentives, underfunding, and misallocation of expenditures. Poor countries with very limited resources have weaker institutions (chapter 6 and below) and limited resources to finance essential services and provide financial protection (chapter 1). The results are limited access and poor-quality health services as well as limited financial protection against catastrophic health expenditures, particularly for the poor in rural areas. More troublesome is that only one of the three basic financing functions (revenue collection), is fully under the control of the ministry of health.

Revenue collection. National health service systems receive their funding from general revenues. Thus, how much is collected and the proportion of the total amount collected that is allocated to health is largely outside the control of the ministry of health. Significant donor financing of health activities outside the government's budget may motivate ministries of finance to allocate domestic resources to uses other than health, thereby reducing the additionality of such funding and overall resources devoted to the ministry of health. In addition, the tax and revenue system is outside the control of the ministry of health, the ministry has little ability to affect the equity aspects of revenue raising.

Pooling. Given that collection of resources is outside the control of the ministry of health and the whole population is generally covered by the national health service, risk and equity subsidization will be determined by ministy of health decisions on resource allocation and purchasing functions and by service delivery functions. Risk pooling and prepayment functions are central to the creation of cross-subsidies between high-risk and low-risk individuals (risk subsidy) as well as between rich and poor (equity subsidy).

Resource allocation and purchasing. For a given budget, resource allocation and purchasing are the key endogenous functions of ministries of health. How a ministry of health allocates its resources will largely determine quality, efficiency, access, and equity of services. Ministries of health must determine, within their own political economy constraints, what to purchase, how to purchase, and for whom to purchase. But although these functions are fundamental to attaining access, equity, and efficiency in the health system, they are not solely under the control of the ministry of health.

National health service systems have usually been associated with the delivery of services by public providers. Problems such as capture by medical unions, misappropriation of public funds, lack of accountability, and interregional inequities in the distribution of facilities and personnel have been associated with public sector delivery. These problems may result in inequitable physical access to services for the poor, particularly in rural areas. Supply-side subsidies can further impoverish those who are already poor. For every dollar of services that is subsidized for the overall system, one less dollar is available to subsidize services for the poor, who often have access only to a very limited benefit package. As a result, the poor seek additional coverage from the private sector, becoming further impoverished. Although public sector delivery of services is not an inherent characteristic of all national health services, separation of financing from provision, as in Rwanda (box 7.2, later in the chapter), can generate the appropriate incentives to improve the services efficiency and equity.

Social health insurance

Social health insurance systems have been established in more than 60 countries all over the world (see chapter 3). Some low-income countries, especially in Africa, are considering introducing or implementing social health insurance. For instance, Tanzania implemented its National Health Insurance Fund in 2001, and Ghana passed a national health insurance law in 2003. Kenya introduced the National Hospital Insurance Fund in 1966 but is currently considering a major reform.

When low- and middle-income countries propose to adopt or reform social health insurance systems, the most common goals according to the ILO (2001) are to:

- mobilize funds for health care expenditures (introduce a new "tax"),
- improve insurance coverage (eliminate barriers to health care services and protect households against incurring large medical expenditures),
- improve equity (redistribute income and ensure equitable access to medical services), and
- build democratic and participatory institutions (promote solidarity and social cohesion, empower citizens, strengthen civil society organizations).

It is an open question whether these public policy goals can be reached through social health insurance, especially in low-income countries. The enabling conditions discussed in chapter 3 are especially difficult to meet in low-income countries.

First, while some countries have supportive economic conditions, with rapid growth and increasing formalization of the labor market, others are experiencing economic stagnation and have large informal sectors. Further constraints to developing social insurance schemes arise in economies that rely on exports of raw materials, agricultural products, or products with international market-set prices in which a competitive labor force is fundamental for the country to remain competitive. Moreover, policy makers should fully understand the equity implications of the slower growth that can result from implementation of a social health insurance system, as the population that might benefit from introducing such a system is not likely to be the same as the population affected by the slower growth or the population that benefits from government-contracted services.

Second, economies with large rural areas will face difficult challenges introducing social health insurance. Some countries in Latin America, such as Bolivia, Ecuador, and Peru, which have large rural populations and large informal sectors, have had difficulty increasing coverage beyond 25 percent of the labor force, despite having social insurance schemes in place for more than 60 years. Coverage has been expanded in some Latin American countries (Colombia, for instance) through demand-side subsidies from government for a predetermined population. Such subsidies must be analyzed from equity, efficiency, and sustainability perspectives.

Third, administrative capacity is an important constraint in low-income countries. Policy makers must consider the opportunity cost of using scarce administrative resources in the development and administration of a social health insurance system, which is likely to concentrate coverage among the formally employed and expand slowly to other, often more needy groups. More important, to function appropriately, a social health insurance system must be soundly governed. The supervisory structure and systems needed to attain the required quality of governance are difficult to find in low-income countries.

Private sources of revenue for health

Private spending plays a large role in health financing in low-income countries, where private spending invariably means out-of-pocket expenditures, not private insurance. The same is true of many lower-middle-income countries, such as China. The main consequence is that households have difficulty accessing health care services or are exposed to the risk of impoverishment because of catastrophic health expenses.

Evidence also suggests that exposure to the risk of catastrophic medical expenses as a result of highly limited insurance coverage causes rural households to hold more wealth and to keep it in liquid form (Wagstaff and Claeson 2004). This self-insurance is only partially successful at smoothing consumption when income shocks (due to a variety of factors including illness) occur. For example, in India, it has been estimated that nearly one-quarter of people admitted to hospitals were above the poverty line when they were admitted but were below the poverty line at the end of their stay because of the health expenditures they incurred. In Vietnam, health expenses are estimated to have pushed about 3.5 percent of the population into absolute poverty in both 1993 and 1998 (Wagstaff and van Doorslaer 2003). The risk of large-scale impoverishment is clearly greater the poorer the country.

Low-income countries' abilities to provide financial protection to their populations are limited by the scarce opportunities for risk pooling, as well as by very limited public and private resources to finance health expenditures.

Could enhanced pooling of private resources—whether through private health insurance or community-based health insurance—improve financial protection in low-income countries? Both of these kinds of voluntary insurance have some significant constraints on their potential, which require sustained efforts to overcome.

Voluntary health insurance

Voluntary health insurance can be a mechanism for harnessing and pooling private resources to finance health expenditures (see chapter 3). However, in low-income countries, private and community-based risk management and insurance schemes are in the initial stage of development. Voluntary health insurance represents less than 5 percent of health expenditures in low-income countries, and it plays more of a role in supplementing private care for middle- and upper-income groups. This section highlights some of the pros and cons often attributed to voluntary health insurance that were discussed in chapter 3. It is important to note, however, that these are largely untested in a low-income context.

Potential advantages. From the perspective of low-income countries, there are some good public policy reasons for exploring the development of both private and community-based voluntary health insurance systems:

- Mobilizing additional funding for the health care system
- Reducing the potential that catastrophic health costs could push the nearly poor into poverty
- Freeing public resources by inducing individuals, particularly those in the upper income groups, to opt out of the public sector in favor of the higher-quality private sector

If the poor had improved access to voluntary health insurance, they might obtain better access to health services. Nonetheless, this potential remains untested in low-income countries. Table 7.3 highlights the small percentage of private health expenditures originating from pooled funds within prepaid plans in several low-income countries.

Another possible advantage of voluntary health insurance is that it could encourage individuals to opt out of public sector health care in favor of the private sector, depending on the scope of coverage. Moreover, because private insurance is often concentrated among upper-income groups, expanded insurance coverage to

TABLE 7.3   Share of private health spending and prepaid insurance plans in private health expenditures in selected countries

Country	Private health expenditures (percent of total health expenditures)	Prepaid insurance plans (percent of private health expenditures)
Kenya	78.6	9.5
Nigeria	76.8	0.0
Ghana	40.4	0.0
India	82.1	—
Pakistan	75.6	0.0
Sri Lanka	51.1	1.1
Indonesia	74.9	8.2
Vietnam	71.5	4.2

Source: WHO 2004.

— not available.

TABLE 7.4   Barriers to expanding voluntary health insurance in India

Type of barrier	Key issue	Implications
Regulatory barrier	High capital requirement[a]	• High premium needed to compensate for investment, but volumes will be lower due to price sensitivities. • Need to grow very rapidly to break even.
Systemic barriers		
Customer attitude	No habit of prepayment	• High marketing cost to educate customers about insurance. • High transaction costs in terms of distribution (more than 72 percent of population lives in rural areas)
	High level of fraud	• Claims ratio will be higher for existing products.
Competitive scenario	Low premium	• Mediclaim[b] products priced at very low level for the level of benefits offered—has distorted standards and expectations.
Provider unpreparedness	Providers not standardized	• No standardization of treatment protocols and quality, through either registration or accreditation. • No way of controlling claims as prices vary (fee for service is the primary mode of provider payment system). • No information technology infrastructure. • Huge base of small practices limits rapid networking (average size of hospitals is about 22 beds). • Easier for providers to perpetrate fraud.
Payer unpreparedness	No socioeconomic health data	• Unable to design schemes that are profitable due to lack of comprehensive data on health requirements and usage patterns of different socioeconomic segments.

Source: McKinsey & Company 2002. *Healthcare in India—The Road Ahead.* New Delhi, India: Confederation of Indian Industry.

a. Minimum capital requirement to get an insurance company license to operate in the country is 1.0 billion rupees (Rs) (or about $23 million at the current exchange rate of US$1 = Rs 43.6).

b. Mediclaim is the most popular private health insurance product. It has more than 95 percent of the private health insurance market share. It is primarily a hospitalization and surgical insurance product. Mediclaim is used by major insurers to attract other profitable lines of insurance business, thus resulting in Mediclaim insurance being sold at less than the cost of risk being insured.

these groups might permit better targeting of public expenditures to the poor (Gertler and Sturm 1997). However, there is limited evidence of this occurring in OECD countries with widespread voluntary health insurance coverage, and the publicly financed system often continues to play a role for those with voluntary coverage (OECD 2004). Moreover, such opting out might result in reduced political support for the public system by those who no longer use it, to the detriment of those for whom it remains the only option.

Furthermore, the administrative and regulatory costs required to establish and maintain a voluntary health insurance market are not insubstantial. Regulatory, cultural, and systemic barriers also contribute to the low level of voluntary private health insurance penetration, some of which may not be easily tackled. Table 7.4 outlines some of the key barriers to the development of a voluntary health insurance market in India. One key barrier is a high capital requirement. Other low-income countries may face some or all of these barriers. It is therefore important to assess the potential for a voluntary health insurance market within the specific cultural, historic, and economic context of each country.

Community-based health insurance schemes

Community-based schemes have developed largely as a community response to the absence of alternative financial protection mechanisms (ILO 2002).[4] Most community-based health insurance schemes in Sub-Saharan Africa are based on voluntary participation of individuals and have fewer than 500 members (see chapter 3). The population covered by these schemes is still relatively small in most low-income countries.

There are exceptions, such as Rwanda, where the government and more than 90 community-based schemes have decided to subsidize premiums for the poor to encourage coverage of a defined package of services. As a result, coverage has risen to 4 percent of the total population. However, evidence shows that most community-based schemes do not reach the very poor. Another exception is the Yeshashvini scheme in the Indian state of Karnataka. The scheme concentrates on financial protection for surgical treatment and operates as a "cashless service" to the 2.1 million insured farmers in a network of 2 public hospitals and 73 private hospitals across the state. The scheme is managed by a third-party administrator, whose responsibilities include enrolling members, processing claims, and developing a network of providers.[5]

Realities of achieving significant risk pooling and financial protection

As discussed above, low-income countries are plagued by both low absolute levels of health spending and a high proportion of nonpooled out-of-pocket spending. The question remains: can low-income countries realistically finance universal coverage for a basic package of essential services and provide financial protection for their populations? Both the breadth and depth of coverage (the percentages of the population with public and private formal coverage and the percentage of out-of-pocket spending) need to be evaluated. In theory national health services cover everyone and may appear to provide universal coverage. In practice, that does not necessarily mean that services are available or accessible. Indeed, in most countries, services are rationed through supply- and demand-side constraints (unavailability of services in certain areas, waiting lists, need for under-the-table payments).

High-income countries have high absolute levels of health spending and a relatively small share of out-of-pocket spending—20 percent or 10 percent if country weighted (see chapters 1 and 9). Population health risks are pooled, and households have financial protection. In looking at the financial protection and depth-of-coverage issue in low-income countries, where out-of-pocket spending is around 60 percent of total health spending (40 percent if country weighted), one might initially[6] use the 20 percent out-of-pocket spending threshold of high-income countries as a measure of financial protection and coverage depth and pose the question: how many low-income countries meet this threshold? Examination of 2002 country-level spending information shows that of the 58 low-income countries for which data are available (WHO 2005) perhaps 7 would meet this criterion, almost all of them small Pacific islands.[7] In other words, almost no low-income countries, irrespective of their risk pooling mechanisms, have been able to provide their populations with high levels of financial protection.

This finding reinforces the need for low-income countries to use the most appropriate public and private mechanisms at hand, given their individual circumstances, to equitably, efficiently, and sustainably provide universal access to an essential package of public health and curative services and to provide financial protection to the extent feasible, particularly for the poor. There are no ideologically correct templates or one-size-fits-all solutions. The proposed scaling-up of aid and development assistance for health is likely to be a necessary condition to assist countries in providing universal access to essential services and financial protection, but in the absence of appropriate policies and targeting, that will not be sufficient. Given the extreme resource constraints in most poor countries, the entire armamentarium of available instruments including users fees, needs to be considered.

User charges

Few health policy issues are as controversial as user fees for health care.[8] Most countries in Sub-Saharan Africa impose user charges for health services. In China, user fees are widespread and account for a substantial share of total health financing. Cambodia has recently formally imposed user fees. In Eastern Europe and Central Asia, informal user fees have proliferated to make up for major shortfalls in public financing brought about by economic transition.

In the 1980s, the pervasive lack of public financing for basic health services, particularly for primary health care and drugs, led to calls for the expansion of user fees. User fees were considered an appropriate financing mechanism to make resources available at public facilities to improve the quality of services and health outcomes. The adopting countries, other proponents of user fees, and the literature at the time recognized that the introduction of user fees could limit access to services by the poor, as well as limit overall utilization of preventive and primary health care. Therefore, policy papers recommended that fees be accompanied by appropriate systems of waivers for the poor and exemptions for preventive and some primary health services.

Given the current focus on countries achieving the Millennium Development Goals, the recognition that demand-side constraints may be one of the impediments to achieving the goals, the poor progress (especially in Africa) in reducing poverty, and the large actual and proposed increases in donor aid for health, there has been a strong push by several global development partners to eliminate user fees. Unfortunately, much of the debate has been clouded by rhetoric, selective interpretation of the global evidence, and a lack of clarity about context and definitions, including confusion between goals and instruments, as well as a lack of understanding of how user fees for publicly covered services are a small part of consumers' overall out-of-pocket payments.

Distinguishing goals and instruments. The goal of most proponents of the elimination of user fees (Save the Children 2005) is improved access, especially by the poor, to essential health services in low-income countries. Nonetheless, user fees are merely one of many instruments (others include domestic resource mobilization, external assistance, and improved technical and allocative efficiency of spending) used to provide the revenues needed to achieve this goal. The political discussion surrounding the abolition of user fees often does not deal with this broader overall revenue question. In other words, raising sufficient revenues to ensure access to essential services and financial protection for a country's population in an equitable, efficient, and sustainable manner must be addressed in terms of a holistic assessment of all public and private financing instruments.

Distinguishing user fees for public services and overall out-of-pocket health spending. There is a lack of clarity in the precise definition of user fees, as well as a lack of distinction between user fees and out-of-pocket payments for costs incurred in the use of health services. In the classic public finance definition, user fees are charges for publicly provided services. Others define user fees as payments for publicly and privately provided services. Whatever the definition, there are other direct and indirect "costs" and payments incurred by families in their use of health services. These include the opportunity costs of the individual's and family's time in lost wages, work at home, studying, and so on; transportation costs to and from the health care provider; and costs that the patient and accompanying relatives or friends incur for food and lodging while seeking and obtaining care (box 7.1).

BOX 7.1 *Payments for health care*

The health care system imposes many payments on individuals and households. They are shown as ovals in the figure below. Some payments are indirect, not connected with the act of obtained health care, whereas others, known as user payments, are directly linked with health care seeking. There are many user payments. Removing user fees from government health facilities may partly reduce user payments. But, it does not eliminate other user payments such as transport, food, and lodging. And the removal of such user fees, if not appropriately compensated by other public funding for the provider, may actually increase the financial burden to patients, by forcing them to incur additional private user payments to purchase needed medical supplies or other health care elsewhere.

Indirect payments

Some of the payments are made irrespective of people's actual use of health services (the gray ovals). They include the taxes that individuals and households pay, a part of which eventually are used by government to finance its health care system. They also include the contributions people make to mandatory or voluntary health insurance and other prepayment schemes. Finally, they also include payments or contributions to local health cooperatives. Because these payments are not directly linked to individuals' consumption of health services, they are called indirect payments for health care.

Direct payments

These payments, shown as white ovals, are also known as *user payments,* because they occur in connection with using services. A first kind of user payment, which does not involve

an actual disbursement of money, is known as the *opportunity cost of time.* It represents the income and other economic costs that the individual and family incur because they have to spend time seeking and obtaining care instead of spending that time on their usual activities, such as work, study, and home duties. A second user payment is that made for transportation to and from the health care provider. A third user payment consists of the costs that the patient and his or her accompanying relatives or friends incur on food purchases while seeking and obtaining care. A fourth user payment includes disbursements made on lodging while away from home for medical care. A fifth kind are the purchases of drugs and other medical supplies made in connection with the medical problem for which health care was sought. The sixth and seventh kinds are the user fees charged by the provider. User fees can be of two kinds. There are fees that the provider must forward to the country's treasury and that are not retained by the provider and are therefore not available to improve the quality of care or to finance other costs of provision. These fees tend to exist only with government providers, not with private providers. The other kind of user fee is the payment made by the patient to the provider, which remains with the provider and which can be used by it to improve health care quality (to buy medicines, to update the facility, to pay bonuses to the medical staff). This user fee can be charged by both public and private providers.

In summary, individuals and households must make a variety of payments to finance the health care system. Some payments are indirect and are not connected with obtaining health care. Others, known as user payments,

(Continues)

Moreover, the debate never takes into account that a large portion of the user payments made at the facility level are informal or under the table, such as in China and India, and will not disappear merely with the approval of legislation (Lewis 2000).

Arguments for and against user fees. Most of the debate has focused on required direct payments by households to providers for publicly provided health services.

BOX 7.1 *Payments for health care (Continued)*

are directly linked with health-care-seeking behavior. Removing user fees from government health facilities may reduce direct user payments. But, it does not eliminate other indirect user payments related to accessing health care (such as transport, food, and lodging costs).

In addition, the removal of such user fees, if not compensated for by other public funding, may increase the financial burden to patients by forcing them to incur additional private user payments to purchase needed medical supplies or more health care elsewhere.

Payments for health care

Source: Bitran forthcoming.

Such payments include charges for the use of publicly covered or provided services (the abolition of these public charges is at the center of the current debate) and charges to consumers made by private providers for direct purchase of their services, including drugs, physician care, and diagnostic tests. While public and private providers may charge user fees, regulatory mandates (law, presidential decree, or other) can eliminate only the user charges for publicly covered services.

Charges for privately financed nonpublic services remain. It is extremely rare for a country to restrict its citizens' ability to purchase privately provided health services on a purely commercial private basis.[9] Abolition of user fees at public facilities may not lead to a substantial reduction in the total out-of-pocket payments because the user fee charged by public programs is likely to be small relative to all the other payments (direct and indirect) incurred by the user. Moreover, if the quality of service declines as a result in public facilities (which previously retained the fees), then consumers may go to private facilities and pay higher fees, resulting in an increase instead of a decrease, in out-of-pocket payments. Table 7.5 summarizes some of the arguments for and against user fees.

Evidence of the impact of user fees on access to quality health services by the poor is mixed (Bitran forthcoming; World Bank 2004b; Pearson 2004; Wilkinson and others 2001). This evidence shows that where user fees have been removed, demand by the poor has increased in some places and decreased in others. It also shows that demand can be both price inelastic and price elastic. This diverse and seemingly contradictory body of evidence may result from varying circumstances where the studies have been undertaken and from the use of different research methods.

A key variable is what is done with user fee revenue, specifically whether it is used to finance improvements in health care quality at the local level. Evidence shows that where the revenue has been kept locally and spent on drugs or salary improvements, quality of care has improved, leading to increased demand and improved welfare for both poor and nonpoor patients (Niger and Cameroon are

TABLE 7.5   Arguments for and against user fees

Arguments for user fees	Arguments against user fees
• Generate additional revenue with which to improve health care quality	• Are rarely used to achieve significant improvements in quality of care, either because their revenue-generating potential is marginal or because fee revenue is not used to finance quality improvements
• Increase demand for services owing to improvement in quality	
• May reduce out-of-pocket and other costs, even for the poor, by substituting public services sold at relatively modest fees for higher-priced and less-accessible private services	• Do not curtail spurious demand because in poor countries there is a lack, not an excess, of demand
• Promote more efficient consumption patterns, by reducing spurious demand and encouraging use of cost-effective health services	• Fail to promote cost-effective demand patterns because the government health system fails to make cost-effective services available to users
• Encourage patients to exert their right to obtain good-quality services and make health workers more accountable to patients	• Hurt access by the poor, and thus harm equity, because appropriate waivers and exemption systems are seldom implemented; where they are, the poor receive lower-quality treatment
• When combined with a system of waivers and exemptions, serve as an instrument to target public subsidies to the poor and to reduce the leakage of subsidies to the nonpoor	

examples). There seems to be growing evidence that the demand for health care is more price responsive among the poor (Indonesia, Peru), and therefore the need to find well-functioning waiver systems for better targeting public subsidies to the poor remains a priority. Evidence from Africa, Asia, and Latin America is showing that the adoption of effective waiver systems by poor countries is possible, albeit difficult. Evidence has also shown that implementation of user fees can lead to quality improvements, but that such a link is not automatic and requires careful design and implementation.

The recent decision by the government of Uganda to remove user fees has helped fuel the debate, because of the reported impact of the removal on the poor's use of services in public sector facilities. Indeed, the more rigorous studies show that the benefit incidence in public facilities after abolition has improved (for example, utilization by the poor has increased relative to the nonpoor) (Xu and others forthcoming). Unexpectedly, however, the incidence of catastrophic health expenditures among the poor did not fall. Xu and others (forthcoming) claim that the most likely explanation is that the frequent unavailability of drugs at government facilities after 2001 forced patients to purchase from private pharmacies. Informal payments to health workers may also have increased to offset the lost revenue from fees. This occurred in spite of Uganda's track record of improving public expenditure management, increasing government health expenditures, and other restructuring in the health sector before the abolition of user fees.

As low-income countries emerge from poverty over the coming decades, they are likely to move toward greater public financing of health care and universal coverage, either through the establishment of national health service systems or through social health insurance. But while they transition to those systems from their current situation of underfinancing and user fees, countries will require help from their development partners to lessen any detrimental impact of fees on the poor. During this transition, blanket abolition of user fees may appear to be an attractive policy option. In reality, however, the abolition of user fees may result in the exclusion of many basic services, or worse, a reduction in quality and even access for the poor, the population the policy is intended to help. There are a range of policy options that could mitigate negative effects caused by user fees, each of which should be adapted with consideration for the individual country context. Some governments may decide that user fees should remain a policy option, even when new health financing systems are adopted.

Donors should focus on helping countries promote demand for preventive, primary, and other health services that can make the greatest contributions to achieving the Millennium Development Goals. They should also help countries find mechanisms for increasing poor people's access to needed medical care without jeopardizing their consumption of other basic goods and services. In addition, support should be given to local and national initiatives aimed at raising additional revenue for health care (such as local taxes and local health insurance) and ensuring that part of that revenue is targeted to the poor (with waivers or other targeting systems) and to underprovided, cost-effective health services.

The importance of country-specific factors and the resulting multitude of organizational and health financing arrangements suggest that no single solution can be formulated for all. The overall operational sustainability of health systems may depend on user fees for some time to come. Although small as a source of health financing at the aggregate health system level, user fees may constitute an important resource for the payment of variable costs, especially for primary care at the individual facility level. This flexible (not earmarked) income for primary care facilities will be difficult to replace with other funding sources until a number of conditions are met, most notably improvements in governments' ability and readiness to mobilize funding for health care through alternative sources and to make those resources reliably available at the facility level. The international community must assist low-income countries to obtain equitable, efficient, and sustainable financing to provide their citizens with an essential package of basic services and financial protection against the impoverishing effects of catastrophic medical expenses.

Equity and efficiency of health spending in low-income countries

Although government health expenditures are likely to increase in low-income countries attempting to reach the Millennium Development Goals for health, budget constraints will surely remain, and low-income countries will continue to face allocation decisions that have important implications for equity and efficiency.

The use of currently available resources may not be directed toward interventions that have the greatest marginal impact on health outcomes. Tradition, corruption, political pressures, and other factors generate incentives to use increased health resources as additional subsidies to university hospitals, sophisticated equipment, specialized diagnostic laboratories, or elite cardiovascular or cancer institutes (World Bank 2002).[10] The mix of recurrent inputs in the health sector is unique, demanding a large scope and scale of labor skills, as well as the continued availability of a large variety of drugs and supplies. To make adequate use of additional funding, each country will require individual support to understand clearly the production function and to maximize the impact of services on improved outcomes for the Millennium Development Goals.

However, progress toward the Millennium Development Goal targets could be achieved through a pattern that benefits primarily the better-off, while largely bypassing the poor (Gwatkin and others 2000). As mentioned above, there is an incentive to use increased available resources in tertiary hospitals, where utilization trends tend to favor the rich (Castro-Leal and others 1999). Moreover, a study in 2000 of the benefit incidence of public spending on health in Africa showed that among seven countries only Kenya and Tanzania exhibited a pro-poor pattern of utilization of primary care services (Sahn and Younger 2000). In the remaining five countries (Côte d'Ivoire, Ghana, Guinea, Madagascar, and South Africa), the richest 20 percent of the population accessed primary care, as well as higher-level care facilities, more than the poorest. This implies that shifting resources to primary services alone will not necessarily increase their use by the poor. Other efforts will be required.

To overcome the allocative and technical efficiency problems and increase the probability that the additional resources will have the desired effect on health outcomes, countries will need to strictly monitor and adjust their poverty reduction strategies. And they will need technical assistance to improve their capacity to absorb and make efficient use of any additional resources derived from debt relief and other initiatives. Given budget constraints, countries must carefully answer some fundamental questions through the health plans imbedded in their poverty reduction strategy (Preker and Langenbrunner 2005):

- What services should the government purchase?
- How should it purchase those services?
- From whom should it purchase services?
- For whom should it purchase services?

What services should the government purchase?

The answer to this difficult question is determined by economic, social, and political factors. In low-income countries, budget constraints impose restrictions or become binding at relatively low levels of expenditure per capita. This implies that states must make their financing choices with careful consideration of whether they are merited. A small but important collection of health-related activities must be financed by the state if they are to be provided at all or provided at the socially optimum level of consumption. These interventions appear to account for much of the impact of health spending on health improvements (Musgrove 1996). These public health activities are especially important at low income levels, for both epidemiological and economic reasons, so that public financing may be particularly crucial for health in poor countries. However, as Musgrove (1996) points out, numerous other criteria influence government decisions to finance and directly provide health services.

From the perspective of reaching the Millennium Development Goals, effective health interventions exist for all health targets. There is an impressive array of interventions to fight child malnutrition, child mortality, maternal mortality, and communicable disease mortality (Wagstaff and Claeson 2004, pp. 47–54). Many of these interventions should be financed by the public sector, because they provide public goods or generate externalities. Many of these interventions are underused, especially by the poor. Public financing of the portion of these interventions that are private goods can also be justified from an equity perspective for a targeted population.

In 1993 the World Bank recommended a basic package of health services that costs about $12 per capita (World Bank 1993). More recently, more inclusive packages with costs of $30–$40 per capita have been recommended (CMH 2001). These packages include treatment of AIDS with antiretroviral therapy, which is very costly. In Ethiopia, a package of services that is designed to reach the maternal and child health Millennium Development Goals and includes prevention and treatment of other communicable diseases (except for HIV/AIDS) was estimated at $16 per capita. Treatment for HIV/AIDS would essentially double the cost per capita. Moreover, with increases in life expectancies afforded by antiretroviral therapy, HIV/AIDS can, in some cases, become a chronic as well as an infectious disease, imposing the challenge of maintaining treatment levels over an extended period (Lewis 2005). From this perspective, the inclusion of antiretroviral therapy in publicly financed interventions needs to be weighed against the high opportunity cost of other investments not undertaken and the implications of this decision for economic growth, education, and other health interventions.

Determining which health services the government should purchase or cover is a difficult decision that low-income countries must face. This decision is usually made on social and political grounds rather than economic reasoning alone. Yet the decision has important implications for the opportunity cost of the resources used and the impact on outcomes and growth. Moreover, it can generate far-reaching fiscal contingencies, even if financed in the short and medium terms with donor funding. Governments are encouraged not to promise what they cannot deliver. It would seem to be best for these governments to first finance a universal, small package of services, essentially encompassing public goods, goods with externalities, and other interventions with proven impact on the health Millennium Development Goals or other goals set by each country and reflected in its poverty reduction strategy.[11] Any other clinical care and catastrophic expenditures would then be financed for the poor through some targeting mechanism.

How and from whom should the government purchase services?

Public funds may be used to pay for the provision of services by public providers (budget allocation), to purchase services from private or public providers, or to contract managed care institutions, which in turn do the purchasing and/or provision.[12] Once resources are available to a low-income country, restrictions on how to use them are determined by the country's absorptive capacity. Although absorptive capacity constraints are usually discussed in relation to international aid, they also relate to any increase of expenditures (independent of the source of funding), especially at the sector or regional level. For instance, the ministry of health may have difficulty spending additional resources allocated in a given year or a municipal government may have difficulty executing a budget.

From the perspective discussed above, absorptive capacity includes the ability of the public sector to design, disburse, coordinate, control, and monitor public spending. This coordination is both vertical (between central and local governments) and horizontal (between line ministries at any given level). The question is whether governments or even institutions such as health ministries have the capacity to manage a large increase in real expenditures beyond a usual trend. These issues have to do with public expenditure management but also with more general administrative systems, such as registries for contracts and property, systems for arbitrating contractual conflicts, and transparent judicial systems.

As discussed in chapter 6, the World Bank's Country Policy and Institutional Assessment (CPIA) Index rates countries on a composite scale of 1 (low) to 6 (high). The Africa region, where further efforts are required with respect to Millennium Development Goals, had the lowest CPIA score of all regions in 2004. Only five countries in the region scored 4 or higher. On another indicator of institutions, Transparency International's Corruption Perceptions Index, more than a third of the countries in the Sub-Saharan region scored below 3 (on a scale from 1 to 10, with 1 being most corrupt) in 2001. The perception of corruption, payment delays and difficulty adhering to contractual agreements, and the overall lack of absorptive capacity in African governments negatively affect prices and terms offered to African countries for pharmaceuticals and medical supplies as well as for other services and result in delays or cancellation of donor financing to the health sector. They may lead ministries of finance to conclude that health financing is excessive, thereby inhibiting further budgetary increases to the health sector.

Thus, programs to improve public expenditure management are an important priority and may even constitute a necessary precondition for scaling up programs in health or other social sectors. Well-designed health plans need to be part of a multisectoral strategy, reflected and costed as part of poverty reduction strategies. Moreover, poverty reduction strategies need to be reflected in medium-term expenditure programs, disbursed and monitored according to compliance with objectives measured in outputs.

Good practices in these areas were discussed in chapter 6. Box 7.2 illustrates the case of Rwanda, where the government costed a health strategy that was part of a poverty reduction strategy. The costs of the poverty reduction strategy—in particular, the cost of the health plan—were negotiated with the Ministry of Finance and included in the medium-term expenditure framework, with important increases in the health budget. What is to be accomplished, in terms of outputs, is clearly established in the strategy and is part of the medium-term expenditure framework. The Ministry of Finance is clear about what it will provide from the increased budget and may cut future allocations in cases of nonperformance, thus generating a clear mechanism of accountability. The World Bank supports the program through a poverty reduction support credit.

BOX 7.2 *Rwanda: aligning a health strategy with the poverty reduction strategy and medium-term expenditure framework*

Rwanda is like other postconflict countries that suffered massive loss of lives in that its overall health status has deteriorated. Mortality rates for infants, children under five years old, and mothers are some of the highest in the world, even though the major causes of mortality and morbidity, such as malaria, acute respiratory infections, intestinal parasites, and diarrheal ailments are largely avoidable. Although there have been important improvements in health indicators in recent years, the continuing high mortality rates primarily reflect inadequate access to high-impact health services, especially by the poorest segments of the population, as well as the increasing incidence of HIV/AIDS.

The government is seriously committed to improving the health of its population and meeting the Millennium Development Goals. Over the past three years the government, with the assistance of development partners, has improved the quality of its health centers and the availability of drugs and has created incentives among health staff to increase the availability of human resources in rural areas. To finance these efforts, the government budget allocation to health has increased substantially: an almost twofold nominal increase (185 percent) occurred between 2002 and 2004. Yet the budget allocation to the health sector remains relatively low, amounting to only about 1.6 percent of GDP, equivalent to about $3.2 per capita in 2004.

To ensure there are enough resources to meet the Millennium Development Goals by 2015, the Ministry of Health involved the Ministry of Finance upfront in health strategy development. As part of the process, the health strategy was costed using the marginal-budgeting-for-bottlenecks model, and performance targets were linked to expenditures to justify funding increases.

The main objective of the program is, through budget support, to reduce under-five mortality rates and maternal mortality ratios and improve other health indicators through increased utilization of a set of evidence-based interventions, increased access to these interventions by the poor, improved accountability and efficiency in the health system, and fiscal sustainability of the budget support effort.

Increased utilization of evidence-based interventions
The set of interventions to be delivered through the health system has been selected on the basis of the most recent research regarding the impact of such interventions for the particular causes of illness and death in Rwanda.

(Continues)

For whom should the government purchase services?

A major problem with allocations of resources is that increased expenditures often may benefit the better-off more than the poor. Studies have repeatedly shown that the poor benefit much less than the nonpoor from government health expenditures in many countries. Supply-side subsidies (such as the financing of public hospitals) and gratuities (under-the-table payments to physicians) are common in Eastern Europe, and together they imply a subsidy to the rich, who take advantage of a public facility by paying an amount that does not cover the full cost while receiving a privileged service because of their ability to pay the gratuity to the doctor. Similarly, supply-side subsidies to deficit-ridden social insurance institutions in Latin America (for example, Argentina) imply a subsidy to the nonpoor, since such institutions cover mostly formally employed urban workers.

BOX 7.2 *(continued)*

**Increased access for
the poor population**
Access for the poor would be obtained through a universal (available to the whole population) package of basic services to be delivered at the household, community, and health center levels and financed through the budget. Increased access to referral clinical care for the poor population would be obtained through the payment by government of the premium for a package of such services in Mutuelles de Sante. Targeting will be carried out by the administrative districts.

**Improved accountability and efficiency
of the health system**
To improve the accountability and efficiency of the health system the government will introduce conditional transfers from the budget to administrative districts and provinces for the purchase of specific packages of services for targeted populations. The government will also purchase a limited set of clinical services for the poor from district and national hospitals, using performance-based contracts. The block grants from the central budget will be transferred to the administrative districts or the provinces conditional on compliance with certain actions as established in specific contracts to be underwritten by the Ministry of Health and the corresponding local authorities. Similarly, the

Ministry of Health will purchase from the hospitals a set of specific interventions for the poor population on the basis of specific contracts. Only on verification of compliance of contract clauses will the Ministry of Health request the transfer of resources by the Ministry of Finance to the administrative district or the province or make the payment to the hospital.

Fiscal sustainability
The health sector contribution to fiscal sustainability will be accomplished through close coordination of additional budget requirements with the Ministry of Finance to ensure that such requirements fall within the envelope of the medium-term expenditure framework and longer-term government fiscal program.

Planning and negotiation with the Ministry of Finance led to an increase in the budget allocation directed to health. The initial medium-term expenditure framework ceiling allocated to health for the medium-term expenditure framework period of 2004–7 implied a constant expenditure per capita of $3.2. The negotiations resulted in an increased budget allocation to health—6.2 percent of the government budget in 2004 to 10.4 percent in 2007—implying an increased expenditure per capita from $3.2 in 2004 to $5.6 in 2007.

Source: Authors.

How can governments improve the allocation of resources so that they favor the poor? There is no conclusive evidence that either of the collective resource generation mechanisms for health services—social insurance (Bismarck model) or general taxation (Beveridge model)—works better for the poor. To favor the poor, both require some level of cross-subsidy—through either differential premiums or progressive taxes (World Bank 2004b). However, in a low-income country, given the limits of the formal economy, as well as the binding constraints faced by government at low levels of per capita expenditures, the options for reaching the poor are even less clear. Beyond a basic universal package, special targeting mechanisms are needed to ensure financing of needed services for the poor population. These were discussed in chapter 6. The enabling conditions for decentralization were also discussed in chapter 6. Box 7.3 on Vietnam shows how growth and even

BOX 7.3   *Vietnam: leaving the poor behind?*

In the 1980s Vietnam was one of the poorest countries in the world. A rough estimate of its GNP per capita in 1984—$117—made it the second poorest country in the world, barely ahead of Ethiopia and just behind Bangladesh (as reported in World Bank 1986). By 1999 Vietnam's GNP per capita had increased to $370, so that Vietnam ranked 167 of 206 countries. This rapid improvement began in 1986, when the first Doi Moi ("renovation") economic policies started to transform Vietnam from a planned to a market-oriented economy. In particular, the government disbanded state farms and divided agricultural land equally among rural households, removed price controls, legalized buying and selling of almost all products by private individuals, stabilized the rate of inflation, and opened up the economy to foreign trade and investment. In the 1990s Vietnam was one of the 10 fastest-growing economies in the world, with an average real GDP growth of 8.4 percent a year from 1992 to 1998. This rapid economic growth led to a dramatic decline in the rate of poverty, from 58 percent in 1993 to 37 percent in 1998.

Health outcomes—good progress
By international standards, especially given its relatively low per capita income, Vietnam has achieved substantial reductions in mortality among infants and children under five. By the mid-1980s, its rates were among the lowest in the developing world. The Vietnamese government's own goal was to reduce the infant mortality rate to 30 per 1,000 live births by 2000.

The infant and under-five mortality rates appear to have continued to fall under Doi Moi. The infant mortality rate was below the 2000 target of 30 per 1,000. Indeed, the evidence suggests that this target was probably reached in the mid-1990s, and the figure now may well be around 25 per 1,000 or even lower. There have also been large decreases in the rate of stunting among Vietnamese children and improvements in other health outcomes.

**Growth can potentially
leave the poor behind**
Nevertheless, inequalities in child survival between poor and less poor children now exist in Vietnam, and these inequalities appear to be a recent phenomenon. Reductions in child mortality appear not to have been spread evenly and are heavily concentrated among the better-off. Poorer Vietnamese children do not appear to have seen any appreciable improvement in their survival prospects in recent years.

(Continues)

improved health outcomes may leave the poor lagging behind and thus the need to give special consideration to the targeting mechanism.

Conditional cash transfers: seeking results from targeting

A recent social safety net innovation from Latin America and the Caribbean, which constitutes a de facto "negative" user fee, is the conditional cash transfer (Rawlings 2004). Conditional cash transfers provide direct cash payments to poor households contingent on certain behavior, such as completing a full set of prenatal visits or attending health education classes. In some pilot programs, cash grants were based on an estimate of the economic cost of travel and waiting time for the beneficiary and so represent a negative user fee. The focus of conditional cash transfers is both on short-term income support and on longer-term human capital accumulation and not necessarily on strict financial protection against illness shocks. Nonetheless, the cash grants can be fairly large, up to 25 percent of household income, and

---

BOX 7.3 *(continued)*

What explains this inequality and what policy options are available for accelerating the pace of decline of child mortality among Vietnam's poor?

Extensive analysis of data from several sources points to two important factors: declining education levels among poor mothers and declining use of skilled birth attendants and medical facilities among the poor. In 1993, mothers in the bottom income quartile averaged 5.8 years of schooling. In 1998, this figure had fallen to 5.4 years. In 1993, 62.7 percent of births in the poorest quartile were attended by a medically trained person, and 43.1 percent of births took place in a medical facility. In 1998, these figures had fallen to 57.3 percent and 33.3 percent, respectively. Reversing the decline in maternal schooling and in deliveries in medical facilities and attended by medical personnel would reduce the under-five mortality rate by an estimated 11 percent.

Success factors

Econometric analysis shows that growth in household incomes accounted for only a small proportion of the improvement of

child and maternal health in Vietnam from 1993 to 1998. Looking to 2015, even under quite optimistic assumptions about annual income growth, the projected levels of child mortality are likely to be higher than the targets. In other words, economic growth is not enough. Ensuring that it is not just the better-off who benefit from improvements that increase the impact of health determinants on child survival is central to achieving the Millennium Development Goals.

What policies can promote this objective? Better targeting is essential. In improvements in health services, drinking water, and sanitation, where the poorest quartile of children lag far behind the best-off are also necessary. Closing these gaps—by bringing the poor up to the levels enjoyed by the better-off—is likely to have a sizable effect on child mortality. The largest impact would come from raising health service coverage among the poorest quartile to the level of coverage enjoyed by the best-off three quartiles.

Source: World Bank 2004a; WHO [www.who.int].

---

so potentially constitute a buffer against financial shocks due to illness (in addition to having a direct effect on incentives to use mandated health care interventions) (Gertler 2000). Evaluation of the programs has been rigorous, usually involving random assignment designs. The results are generally positive; the programs have demonstrated gains in human capital outcomes, including health.

The applicability of such programs to health care financing in low-income countries is still unresolved. The evidence suggests that well-designed conditional cash transfers have the potential to improve human capital and health outcomes and to reduce poverty, with relatively modest administrative costs. However, testing of the programs has been confined almost exclusively to middle-income countries, many in Central and South America, where the programs constitute social sector spending on top of existing health spending. Further research is needed to determine whether conditional cash transfer programs can be an effective means of improving health outcomes and cushioning households from illness shocks and whether they can be effectively implemented in low-income country settings.

Annex 7.1 Four models to estimate the cost of the Millennium Development Goals for health at the country level[13]

Millennium Development Goal needs assessment (MP) model developed by the UN Millennium Project (UN Millennium Project 2004a)—The MP model yields total cost estimates for full coverage of the needs of a defined population with a comprehensive set of health interventions in a given year.[14] It uses the unit cost of covering one person multiplied by the total population in need in a given year to yield the direct health cost. Resource requirements are added (on the basis of assumptions rather than actual inputs) for improving the health system; increasing salaries for human resources, administration, and management; and promoting community demand and research and development (UN Millennium Project 2003).

Marginal budgeting for bottlenecks (MBB) model developed by the United Nations Children's Fund (UNICEF), the World Bank, and WHO (Soucat and others 2004)—The MBB model determines the additional resources required for removing a set of health system bottlenecks, which are thought to hinder the delivery of essential health services, through family/community, outreach, and clinical delivery modes. The MBB method also estimates the impact on outcomes (for instance, child and maternal mortality) of increased coverage and use of health services. First, a set of high-impact services are selected on the basis of a country's epidemiological needs. Second, health system bottlenecks hindering delivery of these services are identified. Then strategies for removing the bottlenecks are discussed and the inputs for improving coverage (for example, in a village) are identified. Cost estimates are based on these inputs by scaling up the cost to cover the district, province, or nation (Soucat and others 2004).

Elasticity estimates through econometric modeling developed by World Bank staff—A few studies use econometric techniques to analyze the impact on Millennium Development Goal outcomes of certain cross-sector determinants (such as economic growth, water and sanitation, education, road infrastructure), as well as government expenditures on health (Filmer and Pritchett 1997; Wagstaff and Claeson 2004; Bokhari, Gottret, and Gai forthcoming). Econometric analysis has been used mostly to analyze the impact of changes in government health expenditures on outcomes, using cross-sectional or panel data at a global scale. But in one study in India, the methodology was used to estimate the marginal costs of averting a child's death at the state level. The estimates could vary from as low as $2.4 per child death in a low-income state to $160 in a middle-income state.

Maquette for multisectoral analysis (MAMS) of Millennium Development Goals under development by the World Bank—the basis for this new approach is that development aid is a key ingredient of the development process of a country, but its effectiveness has to be assessed at the country level within each country's local implementation and macroeconomic constraints. The objective of the model is to calculate the financial needs to attain a targeted path to 2015 and determine an optimal allocation of additional funding directed to different social sectors for the Millennium Development Goals. The model captures some aspects of absorptive capacity (such as the impact of increased demand for skilled labor on public sector overall wages); spillovers across sectors and across Millennium Development Goals; implications of additional financing, such as grants, on the macroeconomy (for instance, on the exchange rate); and interactions between growth and the Millennium Development Goals (Bourguignon and others 2004).

Endnotes

1. Sri Lanka is the only low-income country in South Asia where public sources of financing for health services are significant, accounting for half of the spending.

2. An alternative methodology establishes a "production" frontier using the health expenditure level (total and public) for the 20 percent of countries in a sample of 135 that performed best on health indicators such as under-five mortality, maternal mortality, and HIV prevalence (Preker and others 2003). The gap in expenditures between each country and the production frontier is calculated, adjusting for population and controlling for level of income (measured by GDP per capita). The methodology was used to estimate a global expenditure gap to reach the Millennium Development Goals—estimated to be between $25 billion and $70 billion—by aggregating individual country expenditure gaps.

3. Obviously, a more ambitious assumption of real GDP growth per capita would reduce health expenditures as a percentage of GDP. However, the percentages are likely to be high unless very ambitious GDP per capita growth rates are assumed. If GDP per capita grows at an average of 3 percent a year in real terms, the average expenditure per GDP in the countries in figure 7.3 would have to increase from 2.3 percent in 2000 to 16 percent in 2005. Ghana, Kenya, Tanzania, and Zambia would still be spending on health more than they tax.

4. For a detailed discussion of organizational, institutional, and management constraints of community-based health insurance schemes see Dror and Preker (2002).

5. The scheme basically leverages an existing institutional mechanism in order to minimize adverse selection and moral hazard issues by restricting coverage to members of the cooperative and insuring a huge number of members (2.21 million lives were insured as of March 2005); reduce the transaction costs in providing insurance coverage for people in rural areas, which are thinly populated; and ease administration, as an existing administrative set-up is used to administer the scheme.

6. Leaving aside the low levels of absolute spending, which clearly make it more difficult to provide large amounts of financial protection against catastrophic illness costs.

7. The seven countries meeting the threshold are Timor-Leste, Solomon Islands, Papua New Guinea, Bhutan, São Tomé and Principe, Mozambique, and Lesotho. The information for Mozambique is clearly suspect and not consistent with data from other sources.

8. This section of the report relies heavily on Bitran (forthcoming).

9. A recent decision by the Supreme Court of Canada has called into question the validity of some Canadian provinces' restrictions on people's ability to buy private health insurance to cover privately provided health services. In this case, the court ruled that the Quebec government cannot prevent people from paying for private insurance for health care services obtained from private providers outside the publicly reimbursed system (*Chaoulli v. Quebec,* June 9, 2005).

10. In 2000, Mauritania allocated most of the additional HIPC resources for its tertiary hospital. Senegal allocated HIPC funds to building a secondary hospital, although the Ministry of Health had proposed allocating the funds to recurrent cost requirements of existing primary-level infrastructure.

11. Included in the package for instance would be preventive and treatment interventions for child and maternal mortality as established in Wagstaff and Claeson (2004, figure 3.2). If resources were not available to guarantee universal coverage of such services, limits would be based on morbidity and mortality indicators. If additional resources were available, still other interventions would be undertaken and targeted to the poor though alternative mechanisms.

12. For a detailed analysis of purchasing, see Preker and Langenbrunner (forthcoming).

13. Claeson and others forthcoming.

14. These methodologies have different objectives and produce different estimates, which cannot be compared with each other. Each methodology has strengths and weaknesses, the discussion of which is beyond the scope of this report. It is, however, fundamental to have a clear objective of what is to be measured in order to select the appropriate tool.

References

Bitran, R. Forthcoming. *User Fees for Health Care in Developing Countries: A Review of Current Issues and Experiences.* Santiago: Bitrans & Asociados.

Bokhari, F., P. Gottret, and Y. Gai. Forthcoming. *Government Health Expenditures, Donor Funding, and Health Outcomes.* Washington, D.C.: World Bank.

Bonilla-Chacin, M. E., E. Murrugarra, and M. Temourov. 2005. "Health Care during Transition and Health Systems Reform: Evidence from the Poorest CIS Countries." *Social Policy and Administration* 39 (4): 281–408.

Bourguignon, F., M. Bussolo, H. Lofgren, H. Timmer, and D. van der Mensbrugghe. 2004. "Toward Achieving the Millennium Development Goals in Ethiopia: An Economywide Analysis of Alternative Scenarios." World Bank, Washington, D.C.

Castro-Leal, F., J. Dayton, L. Demery, and K. Mehra. 1999. "Public Spending on Health Care in Africa: Do the Poor Benefit?" *World Bank Research Observer* 14 (1): 49–72.

Claeson, M., A. Wagstaff, P. Gottret, Q. Fang, R. Hecht. Forthcoming. "Millennium Development Goals: What Will It Take to Accelerate Progress?" In D. Jamison, J. Berman, A. Meacham, G. Alleyne, M. Claeson, D. Evans, P. Jha, A. Mills, and P. Musgrove, eds., *Disease Control Priorities in Developing Countries,* 2nd ed., Washington, D.C.: World Bank; New York: Oxford University Press.

CMH (Commission on Macroeconomics and Health). 2001. "Macroeconomics and Health: Investing in Health for Economic Development." Report presented by Jeffrey Sachs to the World Health Organization, Geneva, December 20.

Dror, D., and A. Preker. 2002. "Social Re-Insurance: A New Approach to Sustainable Community Financing." World Bank, Washington, D.C. and International Labour Organization, Geneva.

Filmer, D., and L. Pritchett. 1999. "The Impact of Public Spending on Health: Does Money Matter?" *Social Science and Medicine* 49 (10): 1309–23.

Foster, M. 2003. "The Case for Increased Aid." Final report to the Department for International Development, London.

Gertler, P. 2000. *Final Report: The Impact of PROGRESA on Health.* Washington, D.C.: International Food Policy Research Institute.

Gertler, P., and R. Sturm. 1997. "Private Health Insurance and Public Expenditures in Jamaica." *Journal of Econometrics* 77 (1): 237–57.

Government of India Ministry of Statistics. 1998. *National Sample Survey 1998.* New Delhi.

————. 2001. *National Sample Survey 2001*. New Delhi.

Gwatkin, D. R., S. Rustein, K. Johnson, R. P. Pnade, and A. Wagstaff. 2000. "Socio-Economic Differences in Health, Nutrition, and Population." Health, Nutrition, and Population Discussion Paper, World Bank, Washington, D.C.

Hinchliffe, K. 2004. "The Impact of the HIPC Initiative on Public Expenditures in Education and Health in African Countries." Human Development Department, Africa Region, World Bank, Washington, D.C.

ILO (International Labour Organization). 2001. *Social Security: A New Consensus*. Geneva.

————. 2002. *Extending Social Protection in Health through Community Based Organizations*. Social Security Policy and Development Branch. STEP Unit, Universitas Programme, Geneva.

IMF (International Monetary Fund). 2005. *Poverty Reduction and Growth Facility Reports*. Washington, D.C.

IMF/IDA (International Monetary Fund/International Development Association). 2004. "Heavily Indebted Poor Countries (HIPC) Initiative: Status of Implementation." Prepared by the staffs of the World Bank and the IMF. Washington, D.C.

Joint Learning Initiative. 2004. *Human Resources for Health: Overcoming the Crisis*. Cambridge, Mass.: Harvard University Press.

Lewis, M. 2000. "Who Is Paying for Health Care in Eastern Europe and Central Asia?" Human Development Sector Unit, Europe and Central Asia Region, World Bank, Washington, D.C.

————. 2005. "Addressing the Challenge of HIV/AIDS: Macroeconomic, Fiscal, and Institutional Issues." Working Paper, Center for Global Development, Washington, D.C.

Mathers, C. D., Lopez, A. D., Murray, C. J. L. Forthcoming. "The Burden of Disease and Mortality by Condition: Data, Methods, and Results for 2001." In: Lopez, A. D., Mathers, C. D., Ezzati, M., Murray, C. J. L., Jamison, D. T., editors. *Global burden of disease and risk factors*. Washington, D.C.: World Bank; New York: Oxford University Press.

Musgrove, P. 1996. "Public and Private Roles in Health." Technical Report 339, World Bank, Washington, D.C.

OECD (Organisation for Economic Co-operation and Development). 2004. "Private Health Insurance in OECD Countries." Health Project, Paris.

Pearson, M. 2004. "Issues Paper: The Case for Abolition of User Fees for Primary Health Services." Health Systems Resource Centre, U.K. Department for International Development, London.

Preker, A., and J. Langenbrunner, eds. 2005. "Spending Wisely: Buying Health Services for the Poor." World Bank, Washington, D.C.

————. Forthcoming. The World Bank/ILO/WHO Resource Allocation and Purchasing (RAP) Project. World Bank, Washington, D.C.

Preker, A., E. Suzuki, F. Bustreo, A. Soucat, and J. Langenbrunner. 2003. "Costing the Millennium Development Goals: Expenditure Gaps and Expenditure Traps." Health, Nutrition, and Population Discussion Paper, World Bank, Washington, D.C.

Radhakrishna, R. 1997. "India's Public Distribution System: A National and International Perspective." Discussion Paper, World Bank, Washington, D.C.

Rawlings, L. B. 2004. "A New Approach to Social Assistance: Latin America's Experience with Conditional Cash Transfer Programs." Social Protection Discussion Paper Series 0416, World Bank, Washington, D.C.

Save the Children. 2005. "An Unnecessary Evil: User Fees for Health Care in Developing Countries." London.

Soucat, A., W. Van Lerberghe, F. Diop, S. N. Nguyen, and R. Knippenberg. 2004. "Marginal Budgeting for Bottlenecks: A New Costing and Resource Allocation Practice to Buy Health Results—Using Health Sector's Budget Expansion to Progress toward the Millennium Development Goals in Sub-Saharan Africa." Unpublished paper, World Bank, Washington, D.C.

Sahn, D., and S. Younger. 2000. "Expenditure Incidence in Africa: Microeconomic Evidence." *Fiscal Studies* 21 (3): 329–47.

UN Millennium Project. 2003. "Millennium Development Goal Country Case Studies: Methodology and Preliminary Results." New York.

———. 2004a. "Millennium Development Goals Needs Assessments: Country Case Studies of Bangladesh, Cambodia, Ghana, Tanzania, and Uganda." Unpublished working paper for the Millennium Project, New York.

———. 2005. *Investing in Development: A Practical Plan to Achieve the Millennium Development Goals.* London: Earthscan.

United Nations Population Division. 1998. *Briefing Packet, 1998 Revision of World Population Prospects.* New York.

Vandemoortele, J., and R. Roy. 2004. "Making Sense of Millennium Development Goal Costing." UNDP Poverty Group, New York.

Wagstaff A., and M. Claeson. 2004. *The Millennium Development Goals for Health: Rising to the Challenges.* Appendix A, pp. 169–74. Washington, D.C.: World Bank.

Wagstaff, A., and E. van Doorslaer. 2003. "Paying for Health Care: Quantifying Fairness, Catastrophe, and Impoverishment with Applications to Vietnam, 1993–98." *Health Economics* 12 (11): 921–33.

WHO (World Health Organization). 2001. *National Health Accounts.* Geneva.

———. 2004. *World Health Report: Changing History.* Geneva.

———. 2005. *World Health Report: Make Every Mother and Child Count.* Geneva.

WHO and UNAIDS. 2004. *AIDS Epidemic Update, 2004.* Geneva.

Wilkinson, D., E. Gouws, M. Sach, and S. Karim. 2001. "Effect of Removing User Fees on Attendance for Curative and Preventive Primary Health Care Services in Rural South Africa." *Bulletin of the World Health Organization* 79 (7): 665–71.

World Bank. 1986. *World Development Report.* Washington, D.C.

———. 1993. *World Development Report: Investing in Health.* Washington, D.C.

———. 2004a. "Economic Growth, Poverty, and Household Welfare in Vietnam." Washington, D.C.

———. 2004b. *World Development Report: Making Services Work for People.* Washington, D.C.

———. 2005a. "Improving HNP Outcomes in SSA." Washington, D.C.

———. 2005b. *World Development Report: A Better Investment Climate for Everyone.* Washington, D.C.

Xu, K., D. Evans, P. Kadama, J. Nabyonga, P. Ogwang, and P. Nabukhonzo. Forthcoming. "Understanding the Impact of Eliminating User Fees: Utilization and Catastrophic Health Expenditures in Uganda." *Social Journal of Science and Medicine.*

8

Financing health in middle-income countries

While low-income countries are still struggling to raise sufficient resources to fund essential health care, countries in the middle-income group are focusing on a somewhat different set of priorities. With the ability to deliver basic health services, most middle-income countries are increasingly turning their attention to the issues of universal health coverage, financial protection, and health system efficiency. These objectives require an overhaul of the current financing structures—a prospect that raises technical, institutional, and political challenges. This chapter summarizes common issues confronting middle-income countries and offers viable alternatives for health financing reforms. It first reviews the background of health financing systems in middle-income countries and their financing priorities. Secondly, it describes issues specific to each of the three financing functions: collecting revenue, pooling risk, and purchasing services. Finally, it discusses the need for governance and regulations to support financing functions.

This overview of health financing challenges yields these policy recommendations for middle-income countries:

- Efficient revenue mobilization should be a top priority for health, because funding must be sustainable and must match long-term needs.
- Domestic revenues and funding sources will need to supply the bulk of financing.
- Tax-raising ability should increase and resources should be mobilized equitably and efficiently for health, possibly through better payroll collection, tax reform, or other structural reforms.
- Increased risk pooling is needed to improve allocative efficiency, equity, and financial protection. This would entail increasing the pooling of out-of-pocket health spending—estimated to compose about 40 percent of total health spending —as well as integrating informal sector workers into coverage schemes.
- Risk pools should be consolidated to provide maximum financial protection and universal coverage. The associated benefits are greater purchasing power and efficiency through lower transaction costs.

- An appropriate package of benefits should be designed for covered populations, because the level of benefits affects the efficiency of risk pooling and resource allocation as well as the degree of financial protection. Standard or minimum benefit packages should have the right mix of coverage breadth and depth, so that trade-offs among the goals of universal coverage, financial protection, health outcomes, and cost containment are well balanced.

- Health spending should be parsimonious so that coverage can be expanded to more people. Overall efficiency in the health system can be increased by reforming procedures for purchasing services and by instituting incentive-based payment mechanisms. Furthermore, payment policies should be in line with overall cost containment and cost-effectiveness objectives.

- The specific form of health insurance scheme, whether based on a national health service system, social health insurance, or a private health insurance model (or some combination of the three), is less important than ensuring that the scheme focuses on improving revenue collection, risk pooling, and service purchasing. Depending on the context, a combination of insurance schemes may be necessary to accomplish the dual goals of universal coverage and financial protection.

- Lessons and best practices from the health-financing reform experiences of middle-income countries, especially those that address ways to overcome institutional impediments, are valuable for low-income countries as their economies grow. Development partners should document such experiences to expand global knowledge.

- The international community should not overlook the disparities in the health status of different populations within middle-income countries, a situation that also prevails in low-income countries and some high-income countries.

Commonality and variations in health systems

Middle-income countries, as defined by the *World Bank Atlas* method, are countries with 2003 gross national income (GNI) per capita of $766–$9,385 ($3,035 is the dividing line between lower-middle-income and upper-middle-income economies) (World Bank 2005). In general, middle-income countries are diversified and well integrated within the world economy. Compared with low-income countries, they tend to have a greater institutional and administrative capacity for economic growth and for the introduction, implementation, and management of social programs. Many have achieved measurable results in reducing poverty and providing basic health services.

Nonetheless, poverty and income inequality are still common (Linn 2001). For example, approximately 28 percent of Thailand's population, 18 percent of Turkey and Mexico's, and 17 percent of Brazil's still live on less than $2 a day. In the education, employment, and social security sectors, many middle-income countries are lagging behind. In Latin America, only 60 percent of the population is enrolled in secondary education, and 10 percent of adults are illiterate. High unemployment rates and social exclusions are widespread throughout middle-income countries (Linn 2001). These social challenges provide the context for any discussion of these countries' desire to achieve equity in health.

Because of their economic situation, middle-income countries have the capability to provide essential public health services and deliver basic primary care, usually through a combination of public and private delivery systems. Their current health expenditures average some 6 percent of GDP. In addition, with the exception of some countries in Eastern Europe, middle-income countries rely on high levels of out-of-pocket expenditures to fund their health systems. Out-of-pocket payments are estimated to account for some 50 percent of total health expenditures in lower-middle-income countries and about 35 percent in upper-middle-income countries (see chapter 1).

Health financing arrangements in middle-income countries vary widely by geographic region and cultural context. A variety of health reform efforts—with varying approaches—are under way in this cluster of countries as well. But at present, the predominant features of the countries' health financing systems are influenced by the historical dynamics of institutional development in each region. The distinctions are worth noting because the evolution of current frameworks and institutions strongly depend on their historical, cultural, and political genesis. In turn, this backdrop continues to frame (at least to some degree) the challenges faced by and the policy solutions considered in each country.

The modern health care systems of the middle-income countries of Eastern Europe and Central Asia largely began with a preexisting Semashko model system (a centrally planned national health services entity similar to that found in the former Soviet Union) (Langenbrunner and Adeyi 2004). The financing structures within such systems were grossly inefficient, because of misalignment between the budget and the demand for services (Langenbrunner 2005). Although such systems achieved good results for communicable diseases, they were less successful for noncommunicable diseases. After the fall of Communism in the early 1990s, middle-income countries in the region, such as Estonia, Hungary, Poland, Romania, and the Russian Federation, immediately moved to revamp their health financing structures. Today, most countries in Eastern Europe and Central Asia have organizational and financing structures that can be traced to Bismarck's social insurance model. However, their health funding has in many cases been adversely affected by economic downturns, and the transition to more market-based systems has been slow (Langenbrunner 2005).

In the Latin America and the Caribbean region, middle-income countries have developed a mix of arrangements to finance health care—social health insurance, private health insurance, and national health service systems. The current structures evolved from the corporatist relations between workers and the state that developed as Latin American political elites consolidated their power at the end of the nineteenth century (Savedoff 2005). Workers in the public and formal sectors were first incorporated into Bismarck-style social health insurance entities. Later, between 1940 and the 1960s, other groups, including the poor and the uninsured, were covered through national health services (Baeza and Packard forthcoming). These different financing arrangements coexist to varying degrees in Latin America and the Caribbean, ranging from an even split between the national health service system and social health insurance coverage in Mexico to a predominantly social health insurance model in Argentina (Baeza and Packard forthcoming).

Most countries in the Middle East and North African region are middle-income countries, and their financing systems are built on a combination of the national health service system and social health insurance models (Schieber 2004). Some countries, such as Bahrain, Lebanon, Morocco, Saudi Arabia, and Tunisia, have a rapidly expanding private health insurance sector, and more countries seem to be following this trend (Sekhri and Savedoff 2005). However, a few places are involved in conflict situations, in particular, Iraq and the West Bank and Gaza. Given the political instability in the region, reforming health financing is not currently a principal concern for many of these countries (Raad 2005).

Middle-income countries in the East Asia and Pacific region are politically and socially diverse. Traditionally, social health insurance has not been as developed in this region as in Eastern Europe or Latin America (Saadah 2005). Despite their diversity, however, many of these countries share the common trait of having achieved the so-called economic miracle within the past 25 years. They have used the additional resources to make major investments in their health systems. Many systems are in transition, and a few economies (such as the Republic of Korea and Taiwan, China) have already achieved universal coverage.

Common health financing challenges

Despite their regional differences, middle-income countries have similar health financing priorities and goals: universal coverage, financial protection, and efficiency. These priorities spring from pressures facing health systems in the form of cost increases due to demographic, epidemiological, and technological change; large out-of-pocket payments; inequitable and ineffective health financing systems; and inefficiencies in the health care systems.

Demographic and epidemiological transitions

Currently, the overall health outcomes in middle-income countries are fair, and life expectancies are catching up with those in high-income economies. But like high-income countries, middle-income countries are experiencing aging demographics and an increasing burden of noncommunicable diseases (WHO 2003). Additionally, the demand for expensive technologies and pharmaceuticals is projected to rise with income levels. In the face of demographic, epidemiological, and techno-logical pressures, middle-income countries are expected to spend more on health than their current commitment of some 6 percent of GDP.

Large out-of-pocket expenditures

As shown in chapter 1, out-of-pocket expenditures have contributed some 50 per-cent of total health spending in lower-middle-income countries and around 35 percent in upper-middle-income countries, considerably higher than in high-income countries. Out-of-pocket spending consists of official fees charged by ser-vice providers; user charges for publicly provided services and consumables, such as drugs and medical supplies; or under-the-table payments as gifts for services.

Out-of-pocket expenditures are estimated to be more than 50 percent of all health expenditures in Kazakhstan and the Arab Republic of Egypt (Langenbrun-ner 2005; WHO 2005), and approximately 40 percent in Latin America and the Caribbean (Baeza and Packard forthcoming). In East Asia and Pacific, such expen-ditures account for an even higher share of total health spending (Sekhri and Savedoff 2005; WHO data). The impoverishing effect of direct out-of-pocket spending for medical services has been described in recent country surveys, includ-ing Russia (2004), Kazakhstan (2004), Argentina (2004), Chile (2000), and Peru (2002) (Baeza and Packard forthcoming; Langenbrunner 2005). In Latin America, those relying heavily on out-of-pocket expenditures as the main source of health care financing have become poorer as a result of illnesses than those with any kind of health insurance.

Inequitable and ineffective financing systems

In middle-income countries the disparate expenditure patterns across income groups are as significant as the high proportion of out-of-pocket payments. Lower income groups pay more toward health care as a percentage of household resources than do high-income groups. They are more at risk of falling into poverty as a result of prolonged health events because they have fewer household resources and less safety net protection through private health insurance (Baeza and Packard forthcoming).

This biased distribution of household out-of-pocket spending on health care exposes the health financing systems' failure to provide adequate financial protec-tion to certain segments of the population in middle-income countries. Hence, the lack of universal coverage and financial protection are symptoms of ineffective financing instruments and the misalignment of policy incentives in these coun-tries. Furthermore, implementing universal coverage would require middle-income countries to increase health spending, demographically adjusted, to levels closer to those in OECD countries, most of which currently offer universal cover-age. To move beyond the status quo, middle-income countries need to better mobi-lize resources and use existing resources more efficiently.

System inefficiencies

Many financing systems in middle-income countries are fraught with duplication and inefficiencies. Fragmentation of health systems often precludes consistent policy focus and incentives for efficiency on both risk pooling and purchasing grounds. From Latin America to the Middle East and Eastern Europe, there are many organizations pooling resources and allocating health spending. The list of actors includes social health insurance organizations, central and local governments, health authorities, the military and security agencies, and commercial insurers. For example, there are 29 public agencies in Egypt managing health financing with service provisions linked to specific schemes.

Often, the efficiency of public providers is also problematic. Many local hospitals have occupancy rates below 50 percent (Gericke 2004). Similarly, post-Communist countries inherited excess capacity in health care facilities and personnel, as well as rigid budget allocation processes. Many countries have not been able to redesign essential benefits and streamline service delivery (Langenbrunner 2005). Although the region has had many financing reforms, a fragmented incentive structure has undermined the outcomes and the effectiveness of health care delivery systems (Langenbrunner 2005).

Revenue mobilization

As middle-income countries attempt to strengthen financing instruments for better revenue mobilization, risk pooling, and purchasing of services, they will have to overcome many structural and implementation obstacles. Challenges include insufficient public resources allocated to health and limits on the government's ability to increase the amount and share of public revenues devoted to health, together with a lack of sustainable financing sources, thereby affecting fiscal sustainability. Risks also need to be pooled more effectively. This could be done by expanding the size of the pool and reducing fragmentation across the system, for example, or by other means. Finally, to improve service purchasing, countries will need to improve the structure of their defined benefit package or covered services and implement appropriate provider payment incentives. In evaluating the array of possible solutions to financing issues, the merits and drawbacks of each option are reviewed in detail.

Allocating more public resources to health

Compared with high-income countries, most middle-income countries devote far fewer resources to health care and more of what they do spend comes from non-public sources. As discussed in chapter 1, high-income countries spend about $3,000 per capita (population-weighted) on health each year, almost 10 times as much as upper-middle-income countries (which spend $309) and more than 36 times as much as lower-middle-income countries (which spend $82). At the same time, public sources account for 65 percent of health expenditures in high-income countries, but 56 percent in upper-middle-income countries and 42 percent in lower-middle-income countries. The high level of out-of-pocket spending by average households, a phenomenon found in most Latin American, East Asian, Middle Eastern, and Central Asian countries, is another sign of insufficient risk pooling and public funding for health.

Why is public funding allocated to health care insufficient in these countries? A primary reason is the state of the economy. For instance, Georgia, Kazakhstan, Poland, and Russia have seen their overall public funding for health decrease during the 1990s, as the Eastern Europe and Central Asia region as a whole suffered an economic downturn (Langenbrunner 2005). In countries where GDP growth is slow, such as Ecuador and Peru, public spending on health is understandably limited. By contrast, in the East Asia and the Pacific region, where economic growth has been very strong, some economies have been able to fund social health insurance through general revenues and expand coverage to the entire population (Republic of Korea and Taiwan, China).

Other factors contributing to the lack of public resources are weak or inefficient revenue collection systems and a heavy reliance on payroll taxes, which present many challenges, as discussed below. In a number of countries, the government also offers guarantees for the debt of health insurance funds. Thus, when health insurance runs a deficit or becomes insolvent, as in Argentina or Russia, governments must cover the costs. Given that low-income people generally do not have social health insurance, subsidizing social insurance with general revenues in this fashion may prove regressive.

Finding new sources of financing

Like low- and high-income countries, middle-income countries may choose from or combine the revenue sources of payroll taxes, general taxation, and even to some extent private insurance to fund their health financing systems. The question of which source is most appropriate depends on a country's infrastructure, socioeconomic situation, and political context. Policy makers should assess the strengths and weaknesses of each source and determine whether their country meets or is capable of meeting the enabling conditions for each option (chapter 3).

Payroll contributions. Compulsory payroll contribution systems were introduced at the end of the nineteenth century, along with social health insurance schemes. These contributions are generally shared between employers and employees, with some variation in the distribution. Contribution rates in middle-income countries fall within a wide range, from as low as 2 percent to as high as 18 percent.[1] In general, rates tend to be higher in Eastern Europe than elsewhere (Langenbrunner and Adeyi 2004).

In addition to weighing the pros and cons of a payroll-based revenue source, as discussed in depth in chapters 2 and 3, middle-income countries must also assess the feasibility of implementing such a system. Experiences from countries relying on payroll taxes suggest that the following enabling conditions are necessary: a growing economy, a large formal labor market, an administrative capacity for collection, a good regulatory and oversight structure, and an appropriate incentive structure.

The middle-income countries that chose payroll taxes as the primary funding source have a large percentage of their working-age population employed in the formal sector, which constitutes the government's revenue base (Ensor and Thompson 1998). In Eastern Europe, payroll taxes are the predominant source of funding, financing much of the health care costs in Estonia, the Czech Republic, Hungary, and Slovakia (Langenbrunner 2005). In these countries, state enterprises and civil service institutions are large formal sector employers and are a reliable source of payroll contributions. In addition, the shift to payroll contributions (away from general revenue-based funding) offered a way for these countries to break with their Soviet-era past and reduce the role of the state. Payroll taxes also play a prominent role in Argentina, Chile, and the Republic of Korea. In Latin America and the Caribbean, labor unions representing a large share of the formal workforce are actively involved in collecting and managing health insurance contributions, as seen in Argentina's Obras Sociales (ILO 2001).

Middle-income countries that have successfully used payroll taxes also share the structural characteristics of strong administrative and regulatory oversight, which facilitate collection. For instance, good record-keeping systems are available to register workers and to enforce collection, especially in the former communist states. As a group, these countries tend to have greater bureaucratic institutional capacity than many lower-middle-income countries. Therefore, collection rates are higher, and the related processes are more efficient in these countries.

Finally, middle-income countries choosing the payroll option must have reasonable rates of contribution and incentives for a majority of the population to participate in payroll contribution mechanisms. Despite their significant payroll deductions for social security and health insurance, the Eastern European countries are committed to the system of universal coverage and continue to value solidarity.

Countries that have difficulties meeting the enabling conditions for successful implementation of payroll contributions may need to reconsider plans to rely heavily on such payments. Middle-income countries in the lower income group, such as Ecuador and Peru, may not have a large enough economy or enough growth to support the expansion of health coverage beyond basic services. In Latin American countries where the informal segment of the labor market is growing, a largely payroll-based system is not likely to be feasible or sustainable. The revenue base is too small to be the sole source of health funding for the entire population. In such circumstances, many countries use general taxes to subsidize or supplement payroll sources.

Similarly, studies have shown that payroll contributions have a negative impact on the labor market in Latin America and the Caribbean by increasing tax evasion and reducing the size of formal labor market (Baeza and Packard forthcoming). Finally, experiences from Albania, Kazakhstan, Romania, and Russia show that payroll-based revenues fell short of expectations because of common operational challenges, weak tax collection systems, and less developed regulatory capacity (Langenbrunner 2005). Unless these middle-income countries expand revenue collection efforts into the informal sectors and improve their administrative capacity, they may be better off pursuing alternative sources for health financing.

General taxation. Many of the pros and cons of this revenue source were discussed in chapters 2 and 3. Countries relying on general taxation, or wishing to rely on it more heavily, in funding their health systems must consider whether they have some key enabling conditions that facilitate revenue mobilization through general taxation: a growing economy, sound administrative capacity, and an appropriate tax structure and incentives.

A growing economy is important for general revenue collection, as it is for payroll contributions, because as income levels improve, so do tax contributions. But more important, the administrative capacity to raise taxes is crucial for sustainability. For instance, middle-income countries in Latin America and the Caribbean have collected much less in total taxes, relative to their per capita income, than the European countries (Baeza and Packard forthcoming, figure 5.5). These countries also need appropriate tax structures and incentives, including clear rules and transparency. There is a high level of inequality in wealth and power within middle-income countries (Anderson and others 2003). Many governments have been unable to sufficiently tax the wealthy elites in their societies, as is also the case in low-income countries. Furthermore, the growing informal sector in some middle-income countries complicates efforts to collect both general taxes and payroll taxes. In countries that increasingly rely on indirect taxes, the system is generally regressive and hurts the poor. Thus, tax reforms may be necessary to introduce a progressive structure and the right incentives for participation.

A number of middle-income countries, such as Ecuador, Kazakhstan, Lithuania, Malaysia, and Ukraine, rely primarily on general revenue as their health financing source. Others are contemplating shifting to general revenues, including Chile, Mexico, and Russia. Among the high-income countries, Spain has changed to general revenues. Most middle-income countries have the infrastructure to raise general taxes, although some countries have more capacity than others. Yet, they must first improve the tax structure and the efficiency of collection.

For countries using a mixed funding base or contemplating a switch to general revenue funding, an incremental approach may be in order. Countries such as Argentina, Colombia, and Mexico, where less than 15 percent of health expenditures are financed through general revenues, may want to build up the tax base first by increasing collections from nonpoor informal workers and the wealthy (Baeza and Packard forthcoming).

Private health insurance premiums. Private health insurance premiums are increasingly becoming an alternative source of financing in developing countries. As with all funding sources, countries must carefully weigh the advantages and drawbacks of this approach. To take advantage of private resources alongside government funding for health care, middle-income countries should consider the following enabling conditions: a substantial middle-class population, a capacity for regulatory oversight and management, viable financial markets and institutions to invest reserves, and the availability of other funding sources for health care.

Since private health insurance caters primarily to paying customers, the existence of a middle class is a prerequisite to its development. In East Asia, Latin America, and the Middle East, where the level of out-of-pocket health payments is substantial and where middle-class populations are growing, private health insurance is becoming more popular (Sekhri and Savedoff 2005). With the exception of the Eastern Europe and Central Asian region, private health insurance accounts for more than 5 percent of health expenditures in 19 middle-income countries. In Brazil, Chile, Namibia, South Africa, and Uruguay, it exceeds 20 percent of total health spending (Sekhri and Savedoff 2005). Nonetheless, it still remains a minority source of health funding in all countries across the world, except for the United States (Tapay and Colombo 2004).

Regulatory oversight and management skills are necessary to ensure that all parties in private health insurance systems carry out their fiduciary responsibilities. Despite their significant presence in many middle-income countries, private health insurance markets are still largely unregulated. The lack of regulation, management skill, and actuarial sophistication contributed to the failures of private sector–based reforms in Latin America and Eastern Europe. The extent of and possibility for risk selection within private insurance markets is less studied in developing countries, although it is already well documented in several high-income countries (Newhouse 1998).

A viable financial market is also a precondition to the development of private insurance entities. The reserves from premiums collected must be invested to ensure profits over resource outlays; this profit stream is critical for the sustainability of private entities. In East Asia and the Middle East, a growing private insurance market parallels healthy development in the financial sector over the past decade (World Bank 2005). In Latin America and Eastern Europe, weaker financial markets hinder the development of a private insurance industry.

Of course, middle-income countries cannot rely solely on private health insurance premiums to fund their health systems. Other publicly funded insurance programs must be available to serve as a safety net for those who cannot afford private insurance. Across the world, the most common forms of private insurance serve a supplementary or complementary coverage role. In most countries where private health insurance flourishes, social health insurance or national health services have the prominent roles. A number of middle-income countries, including

Brazil, Chile, Indonesia, Mexico, the Philippines, and Uruguay, have integrated private insurance into their health financing systems (Sekhri and Savedoff 2005).

Risk pooling

Regardless of funding sources, governments also need effective methods to pool risks (see chapters 2 and 3). Currently, risk pooling arrangements are imperfect, with segmented or fragmented risk pools. Although debates continue about the most appropriate risk pooling arrangements, the experiences of countries that were able to expand coverage suggest that increased risk pooling and better equity-related, distributional subsidies are critical to success.

Expanding coverage and resources

Many middle-income countries are concerned about the failure of their pooling arrangements to cover vulnerable and disadvantaged groups. Furthermore, the failure to pool out-of-pocket payments has prevented middle-income countries from harnessing the substantial private resources that are needed to extend risk pooling and provide improved financial protection.

Reducing risk segmentation

An important concern with current pooling arrangements is risk segmentation, whereby health risks are spread unevenly across different pools.[2] Without the ability to cross-subsidize across pools, segmentation can result in an excess of financial resources for some pools and less than adequate funding for others. Transferring funds between pools can help adjust for potential shortfalls in each fund. However, this procedure substantially increases administrative costs and inefficiencies. Furthermore, those who are not covered by social insurance pools typically have higher health risks than those who have insurance, as many studies have found in high-income countries (Newhouse 1998). These uninsured populations tend to use national health service delivery systems, so that the government often finances the health care of a higher proportion of high-risk individuals than do the other financing mechanisms.

The sheer number of pools and the complexities involved in cross-subsidies often contribute to regional inequities in funding levels, as in Bosnia and Herzegovina, Poland, Romania, and Russia, where revenue collection processes for health are decentralized. Most funds are collected and allocated by local governments, and risk pooling rests at the local level. As a result, thousands of risk pools coexist.

Furthermore, most middle-income countries do not have the regulatory capacity to ensure transparency of fund transfers. Without such oversight, mismanagement and misallocation of resources are likely. In Kazakhstan, corruption resulted in the disappearance of millions of dollars in health insurance funds. Because of such corruption and other mismanagement issues, Kazakhstan's payroll revenue system was replaced in 1999 by general budget financing, a simpler process.

Changing risk pooling arrangements

Many recent reforms of risk pooling arrangements occurred in response to challenges relating to risk selection and lack of financial protection. Box 8.1 describes successful reforms in the Republic of Korea and Taiwan, China. Most of the innovations that are suitable for middle-income countries are built on three basic mechanisms: creating a single pool through a national health service system, expanding pooling through social health insurance reforms and payroll contribution, and reducing the fragmentation of pools.

Creating a single pool through a national health service system. Some countries are considering shifting from a social health insurance model to a general tax–funded national health service system, as Spain did in the mid-1990s. This trend is facilitated by some countries' desire to use public financing instruments that are more broadly based than payroll taxes. Among middle-income countries, Costa Rica successfully merged its national health service and social health insurance systems in the mid-1990s.

Policy makers considering such a shift, however, will likely need to convince the public that the quality of the services provided under a national health service system will match that of the current social health insurance system or private health insurance plans. It will also be more feasible if there is fiscal, technical, and political support. Consequently, many reforms of national health services have concentrated on improving the efficiency of service delivery and deepening the benefit package, rather than on enlarging the pool or reducing fragmentation of the pools.

Expanding pooling through social health insurance reforms and payroll contributions. Social health insurance is the main risk pooling arrangement in many middle-income countries in Latin America, Eastern Europe, and the Middle East. One of the most important advantages underlying social health insurance reforms for expanding universal coverage is the existence of pooling funds (sometimes a single large fund) that allow newly enrolled individuals and groups to take advantage of existing risk and income cross-subsidization mechanisms (chapter 3) rather than creating new pools. The organizational and institutional capacity in social health insurance systems also provides an important foundation from which countries can expand coverage to new populations. The reality, however, is that social health insurance schemes usually cover a relatively small proportion of the total population in these countries. Their structural capacity to reach the informal sector and the poor are limited because of their link with formal employment. Therefore, specific reforms and innovations in middle-income countries have focused on expanding coverage to informal sector workers and the poor.

Innovations to extend social protection in health include: opening voluntary affiliation to self-employed and informal workers; providing public subsidies to

BOX 8.1 *Republic of Korea and Taiwan, China—from fragmentation to universal coverage through social health insurance reforms*

The Republic of Korea and Taiwan, China are models of social health insurance reform successfully implemented to achieve universal coverage.

Republic of Korea

In 1989 the Republic of Korea legislated universal health insurance, successfully completing a health care reform process that took more than a decade. At the core of this process was the introduction of progressive innovations in the initially small and shallow social security–based health coverage system to extend its reach to all workers and their families, in both the formal and the informal sector. The process was greatly facilitated by a period of important economic growth.

In 1977, Korea had only 8.8 percent of the population covered by formal social security insurance (Peabody, Lee, and Bickel 1995). That year two programs were established: the Free and Subsidized Medical Aid Program, for people whose income was below a certain level, and a medical insurance program that provided coverage for individuals and their immediate families working in enterprises of 500 people or more. In the next major step two years later, coverage was expanded to enterprises with 300 or more people and to civil servants and teachers in private schools. In 1981, coverage was extended to enterprises employing 100 or more people and in the following three years to firms with as few as 16 employees. This process was largely made feasible by an unprecedented period of prosperity for the smaller businesses that were directly and indirectly benefiting from an economic process of clear expansion and macroeconomic stability.

By the end of 1984, 16.7 million people, or 41.3 percent of the population, had medical insurance. By 1988, the government had expanded medical insurance coverage in rural areas to almost 7.5 million more people. Ten years after beginning the first reforms, approximately 33.1 million people, or almost 79 percent of the population, received medical insurance benefits. At that time, the number of those not receiving medical insurance benefits totaled almost 9 million people, mostly independent small business owners in urban areas. In July 1989, however, Seoul extended medical insurance to cover these self-employed urban workers, so that the medical insurance system extended to almost all Koreans.

Taiwan, China

In 1995 Taiwan's public authorities introduced legislation to create a mandatory national health insurance scheme. At the time only half of the population was covered by a social security scheme. At first, the process seemed extremely rapid, given the fact that one year later 92 percent of the population was covered. However, the process had started more than a decade before through the Council for Economic Planning and Development (CEPD). The first planning stage took two years of studies and the original proposal included a project to phase in the nationwide insurance program progressively until reaching universal coverage by 2000.

The first pilot project for the expansion started with well-organized farmers' groups in 1987. Political events in the first half of the 1990s created a strong political incentive to give priority to the fast expansion of social security to the whole population. A careful analysis of the pilot projects and the lessons learned from the farmers' experiences and studies on trends of health expenditures allowed for the legislation to be introduced in 1995 (ILO/STEP 2002).

social health insurance systems to enroll the poor, or subsidizing premiums for poor self-employed or informal workers; mandatory universal participation; and expanding the pool through the integration of private health insurance.

- *Opening coverage to self-employed and informal workers through voluntary affiliation.* This innovative method has been tried by the Mexican Social Security Institute (IMSS) in Mexico, the National Health Fund (FONASA) in Chile, and by many others, but has met with limited success (Bitran and others 2000; IMSS 2003). There are some major obstacles to this innovation. Its voluntary nature, together with a typically flat rate contribution, may encourage more high-risk enrollees to join, resulting in adverse selection and potential financial loss for the social insurance system. Another issue particular to Latin America and the Caribbean is the high cost of "bundled" contributions (payment of joint contributions for pension and health)—and consequently the perceived gap between benefits and contributions—which may drive away potential participants. Moreover, even if enrollment is opened to informal and self-employed workers, the poorest among them may not be able to afford the contributions and therefore will not join.

- *Subsidizing the social health insurance systems to help the poor pay premiums.* Some reforms aim at assisting the self-employed and informal sector workers to join the existing social health insurance schemes by helping them overcome financial obstacles. Government subsidies have been granted to FONASA in Chile and the Costa Rican Social Security Organization for this reason. In another approach, the Colombia Subsidized Mandatory Health Plan (POS-S; see box 8.2) and the Indigent Program[3] of PhilHealth in the Philippines provided premium subsidies to the poor (Alamiro and Weber 2002).

- *Implementing mandatory universal participation.* Some middle-income countries have passed laws requiring mandatory universal participation. Successful cases include gradual expansion to the whole population in the Republic of Korea and the Samara region within the Russian Federation, as well as in Taiwan, China, and less ambitious programs such as an incremental expansion to cover more dependants of the contributing members in Panama (see box 8.1 for more details on the Republic of Korea and Taiwan, China).

- *Expanding the pool through the integration of private health insurance.* In the past 20 years middle-income countries have seen two main reforms of private health insurance: facilitation and promotion of voluntary health insurance, including formalized competition, and integration of regulated private insurance into the social security system.

The debate on whether harnessing private health insurance contributes to or damages middle-income countries' chances of achieving universal coverage has focused on whether countries can take advantage of the benefits of health insurance competition and avoid the associated efficiency and equity problems. The technical and institutional feasibility of specific financial, regulatory, and organizational reforms (risk adjustment mechanisms, risk equalization, and solidarity funds, among others) is at the core of this debate. Such reforms can be implemented only if the transaction costs do not offset the benefits of competition and privatization (Coase 1937; Williamson 1985; Baeza and Cabezas 1998; Newhouse 1998).

The literature provides some evidence of problems that have followed the introduction of private health insurance and competition in the insurance market in some countries (Londoño and Frenk Mora 1997; Sheshinski and López-Calva 1998). Problems such as risk selection and underservice have been studied intensively and have been discussed in previous chapters (Arrow 1963; Rothschild and Stiglitz 1976; Laffont 1990; Milgrom and Roberts 1992; Hsiao 1994, 1995).

It is not clear whether middle-income countries can reduce—or eliminate—risk selection, segmentation, and equity problems within systems with competing multiple health insurers. Although there is not enough evidence on the effectiveness of introducing competition when coupled with adequate regulation and incentive frameworks, it is clear that introducing private health insurance competition within social health insurance systems without the necessary regulations, solidarity, and risk adjustment mechanisms can have severe negative consequences. Efficiency and equity may suffer, as evidenced in the health insurance reforms in Chile in the early 1980s (Baeza and Muñoz 1999).

Reducing the fragmentation of pools. To reduce the risk fragmentation and segmentation presented by multiple pools, middle-income countries face the strategic decision of whether to pursue a single or a "virtual" pooling arrangement. Although in reality there are multiple pools, a "virtual pool" system functions like a single pool by allowing cross-subsidization among member pools and subjecting them to the same rules. More efficient cross-subsidies across income groups and health risks can be achieved by merging smaller pools into larger pools or, in some cases, into a national pool. Creating a single large risk pool is ultimately better than multiple pools for spreading risk and improving equity through subsidies, as explained previously. Disadvantages of the virtual pool arrangement, when compared with a single pool, include the more complex regulations and incentives needed to counterbalance adverse selection. Such procedures can result in high transaction costs to society, but most of all, many middle-income countries are not well-equipped technologically or institutionally to deal with the challenge.

Some countries have a single pool arrangement and others have the virtual pool or multipool arrangement. Those with a single pool include Costa Rica and Poland. These middle-income countries have expanded risk pools to include the entire population, independent of the type of insurance schemes employed. Middle-income countries that have virtual pools include Brazil, Chile (virtual pool integration), and Colombia (comprehensive multipool, as described in box 8.2) (Londoño 1996; Bitran and others 2000).

BOX 8.2 *Colombia—reducing fragmentation among health coverage schemes*

Colombia is by far the best example among middle-income countries of the integration of private sector participation into the social health insurance system. Its 1993 reform mandated radical changes in risk pooling and health insurance, including participation of private sector entities in social health insurance and demand-side subsidization of social health insurance contributions. The new law separated the financing and provision of services across the health sector (except in the publicly managed fund). Private entities and providers are able, together with their public counterparts, to provide services for payroll-tax contributors (who pay 11 percent of their salary) and subsidy-eligible citizens. Participants can select their health insurer and providers.

The law also established mandatory universal coverage for the population, which receives two kinds of basic coverage, depending on their income. Payroll-tax contributors have access to a minimum level of coverage, defined as the Contributive Mandatory Health Plan (*Plan Obligatorio de Salud—POS*) and nonpayroll-tax contributors, or subsidy-eligible citizens, have access to the Subsidized Mandatory Health Plan (*Plan Obligatorio Subsidiado de Salud—POS-S*). Payroll-tax contributors can purchase additional coverage from for-profit health insurance institutions (*Empresas Promotoras de Salud—EPS*) (Yepes 2001). The new system creates solidarity among payroll-tax payers through a fund that collects all payroll-tax contributions and then distributes resources on a per capita basis using a demographic risk adjustment mechanism (based on age and sex). The system is regulated through a regulatory agency under the Ministry of Health (Londoño 1996; Restrepo Trujillo 1997).

A main objective was to maintain solidarity and equity within the system while introducing competition and choice. The system has a redistribution fund, which uses a demographically based risk-adjusted capitation. The fund collects all contributions from payroll and general taxes and distributes the capitation to all insurance agencies. There are strong conceptual and empirical reasons to believe that the risk adjustment mechanism does not prevent enough selection behavior on the part of insurers and that the specific design of the package and the solidarity fund provides strong incentives for participants to avoid contributing or to contribute below the desired levels.

Unfortunately, there has been little evaluation of the potential or current selection problems in the Colombian system. There is some evidence that the subsidized portion of the system positively affected financial protection for the covered population. Yet, there is no evidence regarding the impact on health status and utilization of services. However, there is ample evidence of significant fiscal sustainability problems, due mostly to declining contributions resulting from perverse incentives relating to contributions and significant difficulties in transitioning from historical supply financing to demand-side financing within the public sector. At the core of the transition problem has been the great difficulty in overcoming the rigidities of public providers and ensuring their financial sustainability in the presence of the demand-side subsidy.

Colombians are on the brink of a major restructuring of their previous reforms in an effort to resolve the perverse incentives affecting contribution levels and to encourage public providers to be more flexible in the way they manage resources. Expected savings should make it possible to adjust the cost structure in the way needed to accommodate demand-side financing.

Yet, policy debates on alternatives in this area tend to go beyond technical issues to reflect cultural and historic backgrounds of a country. The virtual pool strategy is more feasible in middle-income countries with coexisting, multiple coverage pools. It is difficult, especially from a political perspective, to merge all the pools and restructure the associated and distinctive collection and distribution systems.

For example, local governments in Kazakhstan and Russia have been unwilling to transfer funds to a health insurance system and lose control of a large portion of their health budget. Furthermore, a single pool, in particular a national pool in the form of national health service, would introduce a type of "public monopoly" in health, which may not be palatable in countries struggling to move away from the centralized public systems of the Soviet era. National health service systems typically confront significant efficiency problems, including governance challenges and problems relating to capture by health sector unions, because of their role in the direct provision of services. Thus, a debate on the efficiency of single pooling versus virtual pooling schemes ought to include consideration of the microefficiency limitations of public monopolies (Schieber and others forthcoming).

Although the performance of the two approaches has not been assessed, the trend among middle-income countries is to enlarge the risk pool size and reduce the number of pools. There have been recent initiatives in Eastern Europe and Central Asia to merge risk pools. Estonia has consolidated the number of pools from 22 to 7, while Romania has reduced them from 14 to 6. Russia is deliberating on a federally pooled health insurance system, while Kazakhstan and Uzbekistan are pooling general revenues at the territorial level, similar to the Canadian system. In the Baltic states, the Czech Republic, Hungary, Slovakia, and Slovenia, risk pooling is even more consolidated, with social health insurers controlling more than 70 percent of public health care funds (Langenbrunner 2005).

Purchasing services

The World Health Organization (WHO 2000) identified strategic purchasing as a central function for improving health system performance, and many countries have embraced the general principles of strategic purchasing in their health reforms. Yet, among middle-income countries, the progression from a simple, retrospective provider payment system toward strategic purchasing arrangements has been slow and uneven. In most developing countries, including middle-income countries, elements of passive purchasing still dominate and present challenges to financial protection and health care service efficiency.

Making purchasing strategic

Reforms in health service purchasing generally seek to address some of the following: the design of the standard benefit package, the fragmented pooling system, and the organizational incentives. Some reforms, particularly in Eastern Europe, have improved the health care service purchasing function as it relates to the incentives under provider payment schemes and the quality of services.

Benefit package affects purchasing efficiency and financial protection. A benefit package—a set of services covered by health insurance under specified conditions—sets the risk limits and standards for adequate financial protection. Experiences from economies that have successfully expanded risk pooling, such as Costa Rica, the Republic of Korea, and Taiwan, China demonstrate that it is important to develop an explicit benefit package, regardless of the kind of insurance model.

For most middle-income countries in Eastern Europe and Latin America, concerns about the design of the health care benefits package relate more to the depth of the coverage than to its breadth. A direct comparison between two government insurance programs in Chile indicates that the National Health Fund (FONASA), which concentrates on insuring impoverishing events, provides better financial protection for low-income populations than Institute of Public Health and Preventive Medicine (ISAPRE), which insures mostly frequent and low-cost events, has high deductibles, and excludes preexisting conditions (Baeza and Packard forthcoming). Those who are covered by a "deeper" package do not fall into poverty as often as those with the "shallower" package. And as people have become impoverished, they have had to disenroll from ISAPRE, undermining the objective of social insurance. In Latin American health reforms, there is therefore an increasing push to establish an explicit entitlement to a specific benefit package. Colombia (1994), Chile (1996 and 2003), Mexico (2003), and Argentina (2003) have introduced a standard benefit package as an entitlement even for services covered under the national health service.

By contrast, efforts in Eastern Europe and Central Asia to define a basic benefit package have been largely unsuccessful. The difficulties are often related to lack of expertise, information, or political will (Langenbrunner 2005).

Low risk pooling and fragmentation affect purchasing efficiency. Another factor affecting efficiency at the purchasing level is the low level of risk pooling in middle-income countries. Without pooling, a government has less control over service delivery strategy, and less purchasing power with which to negotiate with providers. In addition, a fragmented system may subject different services or delivery mechanisms to different and possibly conflicting incentives, distorting the health services market. For example, the former Soviet states did not start out with a pooling mechanism when their centralized model changed to social insurance. Revenues from general, payroll, and other taxation flowed down directly to providers and purchasers at the local level through the previous line-item budget allocation process (Langenbrunner 2005). Adding to the complexity, different funding sources financed different functional categories of expenditures; for example, there were different funding sources for capital investments and operational costs. Such a disjointed approach prevents transparency, reduces efficiency gains at the service purchasing level, and raises transaction costs.

Organizational issues affect purchasing efficiency. Organizational and management problems also contribute to inefficiencies in service purchasing. The most apparent problems have been associated with a lack of adequate and predictable funding, autonomy for providers, timely information, and technical and managerial skills. Countries in Eastern Europe and Central Asia often prefer highly technical solutions, which can add to, rather than ameliorate, existing challenges. For example, Kazakhstan has geographic resource allocation formulas with 100 or more variables, and some countries have complex provider payment systems (some regions in Russia have 55,000 diagnostic payment groups), some of which are even more complicated than those in OECD countries (Zhuganov, Vagner, and Zhuganov 1994). These systems suffer from new administrative burdens, and the signals they send to providers are often too complicated to achieve a meaningful behavioral response.

Changing service purchasing arrangements

There is no comprehensive account of the types of purchasing entities in place in middle-income countries, nor of their impact. There are examples of single-payer mandatory health insurance funds acting as sole purchasers (Baltic states, Bulgaria, Costa Rica, Hungary, the Kyrgyz Republic, Romania, and Slovenia) or multiple health insurers acting as third-party payers (Argentina, Colombia, Czech Republic, Russia, and Slovakia). There are also examples of contracting taking place without a new separate third-party purchaser apart from the ministry of health. In Kazakhstan, the law requires that all levels of government contract with providers through special units ("Densaolik") that are inheritors of the collapsed mandatory health insurance fund (Duran, Sheiman, and Schneider 2004). Detailed accounts of the reform experiences in Estonia and Slovenia are described in boxes 8.3 and 8.4.

Reforms to separate purchasers from providers. Some middle-income countries have undertaken initiatives to separate purchasers from providers, improve services by linking plans and priorities to resource allocations, shift to more cost-effective interventions, and move care across boundaries (such as, from in-patient to out-patient care). Purchasing, in this sense, is an alternative way to plan and better meet population health needs and consumer expectations. It seeks to improve providers' performance by giving purchasers financial incentives and monitoring tools to increase provider responsiveness and efficiency, facilitate decentralization of management and the devolution of decision making, allow providers to focus on the efficient production of services as determined by the purchaser, introduce competition among providers, and use market mechanisms

BOX 8.3 *Estonia—successful reform in financing, purchasing, and payment methods*

Estonia's reform of its health financing and delivery systems during the transition of the early 1990s is perhaps the most successful in the Eastern Europe and Central Asia region over that period. Success is attributed to two measures: institutional capacity and government commitment.

The government established a national health insurance in 1991, financed through a 13 percent wage tax that includes sick and disability funding (Jesse 2000). The initial insurance law established semi-autonomous funds in each county (district). Estonia consolidated 22 pools into 7 over time, and in 2000, created the unitary Central Health Insurance Agency. The fund is now adequately staffed and equipped and has a full-range of planning and operating systems. Responsibility for revenue collection has been transferred to the government's tax bureau, and compliance is high, thanks largely to a relatively small informal sector. The health insurance fund functions like public insurance funds in many OECD countries and serves as an example for other countries in the region.

Purchasing reforms were also initiated, particularly in the areas of provider payment and service contracting. Payments for family doctors are based on a mix of capitation and fees for priority services such as immunization. The capitation payment constitutes more than 70 percent of the total payment and is adjusted by age groups. There is also an allowance for capital investments and for distance from hospitals. Outpatient specialists are subject to a fee schedule with an overall cap.

Family practitioners have undertaken limited fund-holding functions since 1998. In 2002 they received a virtual budget representing just under 20 percent of the total capitation fee, with which they can purchase selected clinical and diagnostic services. These include minor surgery and physiotherapy, common endoscopic procedures, x-rays, and biochemical tests. Parts of family practice and some other system features were privatized.

Contracts with hospitals are capped, and case-mix adjusters have been developed. The hospital payment system evolved from line-item budgets, to per diem, to simple case-mix adjusters with fee-for-service for some services, and most recently diagnostic-related groups.[1] The diagnostic-related groups are scheduled to

(Continues)

to increase efficiency (Figueras, Jakubowski, and Robinson 2001). Since 1990, most health reforms in Latin America, including those in Argentina, Brazil, Chile (FONASA), Colombia, Costa Rica (Social Security reform), Mexico, and Peru (Baeza and Packard forthcoming), have included some elements that sought to strengthen the purchaser-provider compact.

Innovations in contracting. There have also been innovations in purchasing methods. Over the past decade, a wide range of contract-like models for purchasing services have been developed in several middle-income countries in Eastern Europe, Latin America, and the Middle East. The rationale of such a "contract" is to introduce some form of accountability that is often lacking under state-run or public sector entities. Contracting is applied to a selection of providers (hospitals and clinics), staffing of physicians and nurses, and individual services or benefit packages, and it often includes terms relating to quality assurance programs and performance enhancement. However, the countries in Eastern Europe and Central be phased in over several years to achieve 30 percent phase-in by 2005. Payment methods for capital and long-term care are also being developed. From 1990 to 2000, average length of stay decreased a significant 47 percent to less than seven days, but admissions rose 10 percent because of payment incentives.

An aggressive rationalization strategy of hospitals also played an important role. A facility master plan was developed in the 1990s to consolidate vertical specialty hospitals under the old Soviet model into larger network facilities with autonomy to develop community governing boards. The networks progressively downsized within their own capacities and budgets. The total number of facilities was reduced from 115 to 67 between 1993 and 2001, with the target of 13 regional hospitals by 2015. Overall, beds decreased 38 percent between 1990 and 2000.

Estonia benefited from a cadre of well-trained and enthusiastic leaders who pushed for sweeping reforms. Donor countries such as Finland and Sweden appeared to have positively influenced Estonia in developing a reform agenda and provided blueprints for delivery system planning. Furthermore, the World Bank's Estonia health project supported staff training and development, improved accounting and management information systems, and contributed to further refinements in the payment system to stronger incentives for efficiency and quality of care.

Improvements in the economy and employment and the implementation of new regulations seemed to have contributed to the success. Continued macroeconomic stability plus further efforts to improve efficiency bode well for the system's financial sustainability.

[1] Diagnosis-related groups (DRGs) are a classification of the types of hospital cases into groups expected to use similar levels of hospital resources. The U.S. Medicare system uses this classification to pay for in-patient hospital care. The groups are based on diagnoses, procedures, age, sex, and the presence of complications or comorbidities. Comparisons among different DRG versions should be made with caution because criteria are revised periodically (Agency for Health Care Research and Quality 2004).

Asia use contracting primarily to encourage new directions and delivery targets, not as a legal covenant. As such, these contracts tended to be "soft" agreements, rather than legally binding documents. Nevertheless, many countries continue to push for more performance-based contracting, as Romania has with primary care physicians (Vladescu and Radulescu 2001).

Innovations with provider payment mechanisms. There have also been innovations in provider payments, mainly by changing incentives for hospitals and physicians. Traditional hospital provider payment mechanisms are being converted to different methods, such as per diem, per case, or diagnostic-related groups (DRGs) for hospitals. Similarly, in several Baltic states, primary-care fund-holding arrangements and physician capitation have evolved to include a variety of models, such as direct payment to doctors or payment through facilities, "carving-out" priority services, or bonus add-ons for specific purposes. Specialist payments are managed through a separate insurance fund.

BOX 8.4 *Slovenia—improvement in financing, payment methods, and quality of care*

Slovenia established a national health insurance scheme in 1993, with a payroll tax rate of 13.25 percent. Since 2000 Slovenia has been engaged in reforms aiming at cost-containment, access, and quality of care. Improvements have included health financing reforms such as changes in the coverage and structure of copayments under the Basic Benefits Package and the introduction and management of supplementary health insurance; payment reforms covering primary, secondary, tertiary, long-term, and palliative care; and quality of care improvements. An evidence-based approach was adopted in the design of the reforms, and implementation was assisted by the World Bank–financed health sector management project (2000–4).

Voluntary supplementary insurance was introduced to cover copayments for mandatory social health insurance. Because the flat contribution rate for the supplementary insurance is relatively low and the copayments for many items in the mandatory package are quite high (such as, for pharmaceuticals), most citizens (more then 90 percent) have purchased supplementary insurance. As such, it is a steady and secure form of extra income for the health sector. But supplementary health insurance is beginning to show some drawbacks. It is somewhat regressive due to the flat rate premiums, and it has diminished the utilization control mechanism inherent in co-payments. Supplementary health insurance covering copayments has been found to increase patient utilization of discretionary services and publicly funded services, as in France and the United States.

Slovenia has accomplished major reforms in its health information systems, which provide a building block for developing more sophisticated payment and utilization management systems. The system uses smart cards that collect health information at the individual level. The creation of minimum standards on information architecture and datasets may have benefited from the European Union (EU) standards. The next step is diagnosis data linking use with data for providers, facilities, and costs. Such a comprehensive system will help to improve the process for payment, quality, and management.

As part of the reform to improve the quality of care, Slovenia has involved its medical community in developing clinical pathways or standard-of-care guidelines. A comprehensive system for quality improvement of health services is also under way. Some examples include voluntary reporting of sentinel events at the national level; a national manual on the methodology of clinical practice guidelines development; and (within the hospital setting) clinical pathways development, facility accreditation, a manual for self-assessment, indicators development, and health promotion projects in collaboration with WHO.

Slovenia has achieved reform success due to several favorable factors. It has been aided by excellent institutional, managerial, and administrative capacity within the Slovenian Ministry of Health, which led the process and mastered the difficult technical aspects of the process. The country's impending EU membership also helped promote a results orientation and ensure sustainability. Finally, the country has involved stakeholders in quality standards agreements and in the evaluation and updating of health systems.

Strategic purchasing coupled with new provider payment incentives has increased efficiency to some extent, but there are unintended consequences. Strict capitation models have been shown to decrease use of preventive services and cause providers to underserve patients, as seen in Kazakhstan (Langenbrunner and Adeyi 2004). Per diem and per case payments have been known to induce excess service consumption and cost increases by driving up the volume of cases.

Some middle-income countries in Eastern Europe and the former Soviet Union are shifting their focus to the next financing challenges: cost containment.

Reforms to introduce internal markets. These include introduction of purchasing-provider splits, public-private purchasing, provider payment reform, and decentralization. These reforms attempt to address barriers to the extension of coverage that stem mainly from microinefficiency problems in public providers' production of services and seek to establish a more user-oriented incentive framework for providers (Enthoven 1985).

Along with purchasing reforms occurring within the social insurance systems, three key elements seem to be common to the introduction of internal markets. First, a new relationship between the purchasing organization and individual providers or networks of providers must be established. In this relationship the demand for health services is separated from supply using price mechanisms, provider payment mechanisms, or contractual and quasi-contractual arrangements. Second, the correct incentive environment for providers, especially the correct price signals, must be set. This environment includes provider payment reforms shifting historical supply-side financing of line-item budgets to more mixed demand and supply-side financing payment mechanisms (or at least "money follows the patient" mechanisms) linked to the production of services, but also containing elements of risk sharing between purchasers and providers through mechanisms such as global budgets, capitation, or DRGs. Third, successful implementation of provider payment reforms will necessitate significant flexibility in resource management by public service providers. They need to be able to adapt their service production functions and cost structures to the continuing evolution of price signals determined by the new payment mechanisms and competition with private providers. This includes diverse forms of hospital autonomy, including corporatization and privatization.

Evidence on the impact of provider-purchaser splits on microefficiency in low- and middle-income countries is still evolving, as there have been significant restrictions on the full implementation and functioning of such splits. This is often due to the difficulties public providers face in adjusting their cost structures without major, accompanying reforms to public sector management, particularly personnel management.

Initial provider payment reforms assumed that managers of public providers would receive and understand the price signals in the new payment mechanisms; know how to respond and be willing to act accordingly, despite other organizational and institutional incentives; and have adequate legal and administrative flexibility to make the right changes. It also assumed that political authorities in the sector and the government would be willing and able to deal with the political problems associated with such flexibility (Baeza 1998). Experience over the past 15 years has increasingly demonstrated that these conditions have often been missing. Effective institutional reforms must be implemented in tandem with purchasing reforms, particularly those providing increased flexibility to manage personnel. In addition, a necessary condition for provider payment reforms—effective modernization of the public sector management and civil services statutes—has been missing from most health sector reform efforts.

Other considerations

In addition to the three financing functions previously discussed, middle-income countries are well aware that other institutional considerations are essential to the success of their health financing systems: strengthened health care provider infrastructure, timely information to the public, improved governance through policy incentives to insurers and providers, and strong regulatory oversight of private sector insurance and delivery. These issues are explored and discussed in other chapters.

The success stories described in this chapter suggest that a clearly defined benefit package, in concert with reforms aimed at enlarging risk pools, plays a critical role in achieving greater inclusion through solidarity in health care financing (potentially increasing financial protection) and in increasing access to needed health care services. Improving provider incentives through effective purchasing arrangements is also an important part of successful reforms.

Annex 8.1   Summary of recent health reforms in middle-income countries

TABLE A8.1   Summary of recent health reforms in middle-income countries

Type of reform	Specific reform	Country	Features
Strengthening the purchaser-provider compact in national health service and social security	Purchasing-provider split	Uruguay (1998)	Strengthening of ASSE (State Health Services Administration) as the purchasing agency
		Argentina (1997)	Salta and Mendoza health sector reforms in the late 1990s
		Chile (1981–97)	Creation of *FONASA* in the early 1980s and its consolidation as the public sector purchasing agency in the late 1990s
		Colombia (1994)	
		Slovenia	
		Estonia	
	Public provider payment reforms	Costa Rica (1995)	Payment reforms within the *Caja Costarricense de Seguro Social*
		Chile (1985–92)	Municipal primary health care capitation and FONASA-NHSS payment reforms
		Brazil (1985)	Contracting and payment reforms for contracting with private providers
		Nicaragua (1998)	Budget decentralization and performance agreements
Introducing public-private competition	Private-public competition for mandated health insurance	Chile (1985)	ISAPREs
		Colombia (1994)	EPSs
		Estonia	
	Demand-side subsidy for insurance	Colombia (1994)	Subsidized modality in the social health insurance reform
	Public–private competition for the provision of publicly financed health services	Chile (1985)	FONASA voucher system
		Argentina (Salta, 2001)	Outsourcing public hospital management to the private sector (Hospital Materno-Infantil)
Re-converting public providers	Direct community participation in governance of public providers	Panama (1999)	San Miguelito Hospital
		Perú (1994)	CLASS
		Bolivia (1994)	Decentralization to municipal level for maternal and child insurance
	Public hospital autonomy	Argentina (1994)	
		Colombia (1994)	
		Uruguay (1998)	
		Panama (1999)	
		Chile (2003)	

(Continues)

TABLE A8.1 Summary of recent health reforms in middle-income countries *(Continued)*

Type of reform	Specific reform	Country	Features
Enlarge risk pools		Costa Rica	
		Chile	
		Poland	
		Estonia	
		Czech Republic	
		Brazil	
		Egypt, Arab Rep. of	
		Taiwan, China	
		Korea, Rep.	
Define benefit package		Colombia	
		Argentina	
		Chile	
		Mexico	
		Uruguay	
		Bolivia	
		Brazil	
Integrate private insurance		Philippines	
		Colombia	
		Chile	
		Slovenia	
Revenue base shift		Kazakhstan	
		Russia	
Universal coverage		Chile	
		Peru	
		Ecuador	
		Costa Rica	
		Argentina	
		Bolivia	
		Uruguay	
		Russia (Samara Region)	
Expand national health service		Brazil	
		Mexico	

Source: Authors' compilation.

Endnotes

1. Because of the bundling of pension and health insurance premiums, contributions can amount to as much as 40 percent of total wages, as in Argentina.

2. This chapter uses the terms "risk fragmentation" and "risk segmentation." In the literature, these terms sometimes have somewhat different meanings; risk fragmentation is often used to refer to the existence of multiple risk pools, whereas risk segmentation is used to refer to the existence of uneven risk distributions between or among pools. The use of the terms in this chapter seeks to mirror the common usage in the literature.

3. "The main pro-poor program of PhilHealth is the Indigent Program ('IP') or 'Medicare para sa Masa'(MpM)." (Almario and others 2002).

References

Agency for Health Care Research and Quality. 2004. [www.ahrq.gov/data/hcup/94drga.htm#TOC].

Alamiro, E. S., C. Soriano, J. M. Ochave, M. T. de los Angeles, and R. V. Macalintal. 2002. *Alternative Financing Sources for PhilHealth's Indigent Program.* Washington, D.C.: Health Sector Reform Technical Assistance Project, Management Sciences for Health.

Alamiro, E. S., and A. Weber. 2002. *Making PhilHealth Policies More Pro-Poor.* Eschborn: GTZ (Deutsche Gesellschaft für Zusammenarbeit).

Anderson, E., T. Conway, A. McKay, J. Moncrieffe, T. O'Neil, and L. H. Piron. 2003. "Inequality in Middle Income Countries: Key Conceptual Issues." Overseas Development Institute, Poverty and Public Policy Group, London.

Arrow, K. 1963. "Uncertainty and the Welfare Economics of Medical Care." *American Economic Review* 53 (5): 851–83.

Baeza, C. 1998. *Taking Stock of Health Sector Reform in Latin America.* Washington, D.C.: World Bank.

Baeza, C., and M. Cabezas. 1998. *Is There a Need for Risk Adjustment in Health Insurance Competition in Latin America?* Washington, D.C.: World Bank.

Baeza, C., and F. Muñoz. 1999. "Problemas y desafíos para el sistema de salud chileno en el siglo XXI." *Documentos para el Diálogo en Salud* 3. Centro Latinoamericano de Investigación en Sistema de Salud, Santiago.

Baeza, C., and T. Packard. Forthcoming. "Beyond Survival: Protecting Households from the Impoverishing Effects of Health Shocks. A Regional Study." World Bank, Washington, D.C.

Bitran, R., M. Munoz, P. Aguad, M. Navarrete, and G. Ubilla. 2000. "Equity in the Financing of Social Security for Health in Chile." *Health Policy* 50 (3): 171–96.

Coase, R. 1937. *The Nature of the Firm.* [http://people.bu.edu/vaguirre/courses/bu332/nature_firm.pdf].

Duran, A., I. Sheiman, and M. Schneider. 2004. "Contracting in Eastern and Central Europe." In J. Figueras, E. Jakubowski, and R. Robinson, eds., *Purchasing for Health Gain.* European Observatory on Health Systems and Policies. Berkshire, U.K.: Open University Press.

Ensor, T., and R. Thompson. 1998. "Health Insurance as a Catalyst to Change in Former Communist Countries?" *Health Policy* 43 (3): 203–18.

Enthoven, A. 1985. *Reflections on the Management of the National Health Service.* London: Nuffield Provincial Hospitals Trust.

European Observatory on Health Care Systems. 2002. "Health Care in Central Asia." Policy Brief, Brussels.

Figueras, J., E. Jakubowski, and R. Robinson. 2001. "Purchasing for Health Gain in Europe." Concept note, February draft, European Observatory on Health Systems and Policies. Brussels.

Gericke, C. 2004. "Financing Health Care in Egypt: Current Issues and Options for Reform." Paper presented at Global Medical Forum Middle East Summit, Beirut, May 11–13.

Hsiao, W. C. 1994. "'Marketization'—the Illusory Magic Pill." *Health Economics* 3 (6): 351–7.

———. 1995. "Abnormal Economics in the Health Sector." *Health Policy* 32 (1–3): 125–39.

ILO (International Labour Office). 2001. *Social Security: A New Consensus.* Geneva.

ILO/STEP (International Labour Office/Strategies and Tools against Social Exclusion and Poverty). 2002. *Towards Decent Work: Social Protection for Health for All Workers and Their Families.* Geneva.

IMSS (Instituto Mexicano del Seguro Social). 2003. Informe al Ejecutivo Federal y al Congreso de la Union sobre la situacion financiera y los riesgos del Instituto Mexicano del Seguro Social, Mexico City.

Jesse, M. 2000. "Health Care Systems in Transition: Estonia." European Observatory on Health Systems and Policies. Brussels.

Laffont, J.-J. 1990. *The Economics of Uncertainty and Information.* Cambridge, Mass.: MIT Press.

Langenbrunner, J. C. 2005. "Health Care Financing and Purchasing in ECA: An Overview of Issues and Reforms." Draft, World Bank, Washington, D.C.

Langenbrunner, J. C., and O. Adeyi, eds. 2004. *Ten Years of Transition in ECA HNP: Experiences, Lessons Learned, and Implications.* Washington, D.C.: World Bank

Linn, J. F. 2001. "Attacking Poverty in Middle-Income Countries: Tensions and Strategies." Closing statement at XIII Malente Symposium, Luebeck, Germany, June 26–27.

Londoño, J. 1996. "Estructurando pluralismo en los servicios de salud: la experiencia colombiana." *Revista de análisis económico* 11 (2): 37–60.

Londoño, J., and J. Frenk Mora. 1997. "Structured Pluralism: Towards an Innovative Model for Health System Reform in Latin America." *Health Policy* 41 (1): 1–36.

Milgrom, R., and J. Roberts. 1992. *Economics, Organization, and Management.* Englewood Cliffs, N.J.: Prentice Hall.

Newhouse, J. 1998. "Risk Adjustment: Where Are We Now?" *Inquiry* 35 (2): 122–31.

Peabody, J. W., S. Lee, and S. R. Bickel. 1995. "Health for All in the Republic of Korea: One Country's Experience with Implementing Universal Health Care." *Health Policy* 31 (1): 29–42.

Raad, F. 2005. "Health Reform in MENA." Presentation at Health Sector Retreat, Washington, D.C., January.

Restrepo Trujillo, M. 1997. "La reforma a la seguridad social en salud de Colombia y la teoría de la competencia regulada." Comisión Económica para América Latina y el Caribe (CEPAL), Santiago.

Rothschild, M., and J. Stiglitz. 1976. "Equilibrium in Competitive Insurance Markets: An Essay on the Economics of Imperfect Information." *Quarterly Journal of Economics* 90 (4): 630–49.

Saadah, F. 2005. "Health Reform in EAP." Presentation at Health Sector Retreat, Washington, D.C., January.

Savedoff, W. D. 2005. "Mandatory Health Insurance in Developing Countries: Overview, Framework, and Research Program." Unpublished paper, World Bank, Washington, D.C.

Schieber, G. 2004. "Health Reform in MENA: The Future Is Now." Presentation at Global Medical Forum Middle East Summit, Beirut, May 11–13.

Schieber, G., C. Baeza, D. Kress, and M. Maier. Forthcoming. "Financing Health Systems in the 21st Century." In D. Jamison, J. Berman, A. Meacham, G. Alleyne, M. Claeson, D. Evans, P. Jha, A. Mills, and P. Musgrove, eds., *Disease Control in Developing Countries,* 2nd ed. Forthcoming. Disease Control Priorities Project. Washington, D.C.: World Bank; New York: Oxford University Press.

Sekhri, N., and W. Savedoff. 2005. "Private Health Insurance: Implications for Developing Countries." *Bulletin of the World Health Organization* 83 (2): 127–34.

Sheshinski, E., and L. F. López-Calva. 1998. *Privatization and Its Benefits: Theory and Evidence.* Cambridge, Mass.: Harvard Institute of International Development.

Tapay, N., and F. Colombo. 2004. "Private Health Insurance in OECD Countries: The Benefits and Costs for Individuals and Health Systems." In *Towards High-Performing Health Systems: Policy Studies.* OECD Health Project. Paris: Organisation for Economic Co-operation and Development.

Vladescu, C., and S. Radulescu. 2001. "Improving Primary Health Care: Output-Based Contracting in Romania." In P. Brook and S. Smith, eds., *Contracting for Public Services.* Washington, D.C.: World Bank.

WHO (World Health Organization). 2000. *Health Systems: Measuring Performance.* Geneva.

———. 2003. *The World Health Report 2003: Shaping the Future.* Geneva.

———. 2005. *World Health Report Statistical Annex.* Geneva.

Williamson, O. 1985. *The Economic Institutions of Capitalism.* New York: Free Press.

World Bank. 2004. *World Development Indicators 2004.* Washington, D.C.

———. 2005. *World Development Report.* Washington, D.C.

Yepes, F. 2001. "Health Reform in Colombia." In P. Lloyd-Sherlock, ed., *Health Care Reform and Poverty in Latin America.* Washington, D.C.: London & Brookings Institute Press.

Zhuganov, O. T., A. V. Vagner, and N. O. Zhuganov. 1994. *The System of Health Finance Allocation.* Almaty, Kazakhstan: Institute of Medical Sciences.

Financing health in high-income countries

The main lesson from the experience of high-income countries with health care financing is a simple one: financing reforms should support the ultimate goal of universal coverage. Most high-income countries started with voluntary health insurance systems, which were then gradually extended to compulsory social insurance for certain groups and finally reached universal coverage, either as nationwide social health insurance schemes or as tax-financed national health services. The risk pooling and prepayment functions are essential. Moreover, the revenue collection mechanisms, whether as general tax revenues or payroll taxes, are secondary to the basic object of providing financial protection through effective risk pooling mechanisms. The experience of high-income countries indicates that private health insurance, medical savings accounts, and other forms of private resource collection are supplementary methods for increasing universal coverage.

Low- and middle-income countries can draw six lessons from the experience of high-income countries:

- *Facilitate steady economic growth.* Most important for speeding up the transition to universal coverage is raising the level of GDP per capita. An increasing GDP per capita enables individuals and employers to make contributions or pay taxes to support the health system. As health preferences change as income rises, boosting demand for benefits, steady economic growth and its multiplier effects are needed to facilitate universal coverage.

- *Initiate pilot projects for voluntary health insurance.* The development of financing schemes seems to roughly follow a standardized path, beginning with voluntary health insurance, often in the form of community-financed schemes. Such pilot projects play a vital role in building public confidence in prepaid schemes. For example, voluntary health insurance clearly helped Germany and Japan develop skills in administering funds and provided skilled staff for the later introduction of compulsory schemes (Bärnighausen and Sauerborn 2002).

- *Foster administrative ability.* Evidence shows that ability to administer complex programs is essential for the survival of health financing schemes. In the Republic of Korea, the availability of well-trained middle-management administrators was instrumental in expanding the social health insurance system (Carrin and James 2004).

- *Ensure political commitment to expand population coverage.* Voluntary health insurance was usually followed by the introduction of compulsory social health insurance for certain groups. The experience of Germany and Japan shows that economic prosperity is not a precondition for this essential step, as both countries were still "poor" when compulsory social health insurance was introduced. The further development of financing schemes toward full coverage, however, does require economic development. It is striking that—after the introduction of social health insurance—most of the studied countries gradually integrated more and more groups, extending coverage from the employees of larger companies to those of medium-size and small companies as economic prosperity increased and the middle class started to grow (OECD 2003). The gradual expansion of coverage was essential in training administrators and staff. Whereas a formal sector—an achievement of economic growth—is relevant for the systematic expansion of social health insurance, a clear political commitment to expand population coverage is crucial, as Germany demonstrated.

- *Combine expansion of population coverage with risk pooling.* As coverage is expanded, reliance on small, fragmented risk pools (such as community schemes in each village) will be insufficient. Such small insurers are at high risk of insolvency, because their income and expenditures are unstable. Furthermore, the insured in those small pools are at high risk of paying inequitable premiums, because their health risks are unevenly distributed. These problems can be countered by increasing the size of each insurer (to more than a few thousand), by introducing reinsurance, and ultimately by introducing a more encompassing risk pooling mechanism, optimally including the total population. Such mechanisms can be initially relatively simple and administratively easy to handle.

- *Ensure evaluation of products and services at each stage.* No matter how small the initial budget for health care, it should include a system to evaluate the effects of the products and services financed. Only technologies that have proved their effectiveness under the circumstances of the particular countries should be included in the benefit package.

Main reform trends in high-income countries

This chapter defines high-income countries as having a per capita gross domestic product (GDP) of more than $16,000 in purchasing power parities. That encompasses all established market economies within the Organisation for Economic Co-operation and Development (OECD), except for Mexico, Turkey, and the countries of Central and Eastern Europe, and including Singapore. These 25 countries include 18 within Europe (the EU-15 countries plus Iceland, Norway, and Switzerland), 2 in North America (Canada and the United States), and 5 in East Asia and the Pacific (Australia, Japan, the Republic of Korea, New Zealand, and Singapore). Countries are divided into three groups on the basis of their main mechanism of health care financing (table 9.1). Where appropriate, the degree of private financing as a percentage of total health expenditure is also used for groupings.

Since the late 1970s, much political and scientific attention in high-income countries has focused on the "financial" aspects of their health care systems. This attention has been driven by concern for containing costs and, to a lesser degree, increasing efficiency. At the same time, health care systems were substantially— albeit often publicly less visibly—reformed in pursuit of nonfinancial objectives, such as greater coverage and comprehensiveness, to increase access and equity.

Most notably, Australia (in 1975), Portugal (1978), Ireland (1980), Greece (1984), Spain (late 1980s), and Korea (1989) introduced mandatory universal

TABLE 9.1   High-income country groups by health financing mechanism, 2002

Mainly tax-financed systems	Systems financed mainly through social security contributions	Mixed, mainly private financing
High public share (more than 70 percent)		
Denmark	Belgium	
Finland	France	
Iceland	Germany	
Ireland	Japan	
Italy	Luxembourg	
New Zealand	Netherlands	
Norway		
Spain		
Sweden		
United Kingdom		
Relatively high private share (more than 30 percent)		
Australia	Austria	Greece
Canada	Korea, Rep. of[a]	Singapore
Portugal	Switzerland	United States
13 countries	9 countries	3 countries

a. Strictly speaking, private expenditure constitutes a majority of the total, but due to the dominance of the social security mechanisms in its whole health care system, Korea has been grouped here.

coverage. Belgium (1998) and France (2000) followed by extending their social health insurance systems to parts of the population that were still uninsured because of the prevailing principle of present or past professional status as the basis for sickness fund enrollment.

The most important expansions of coverage occurred in long-term care, as in Austria (1993), Germany (1996), Luxembourg (1998), and Japan (2000). Developments differed for dental care and pharmaceuticals; some countries restricted coverage in these areas, whereas others included them.

The organization of pooling and purchasing arrangements has seen changes in many high-income countries. Pooling has generally—at least in social health insurance countries—become more centralized, while purchasing—at least in most tax-financed systems—has generally become more decentralized. Social health insurance systems pursued this road to achieve more equity among their often small and fragmented sickness funds, often further burdened by very differing risk structures. In some countries, such centralization was combined with both more state intervention (into the pooling mechanism and the allocation formula) and free choice among sickness funds for those insured. In tax-financed countries, decentralization of the purchasing function is thought to increase accountability to the public, as well as the efficiency of care provision (and, in some countries, choice of provider). Whether this decentralization of purchasing—and concurrently provision of services—will be followed by similar trends on the collection and pooling side is subject to debate—most notably in Italy.

In addition to spending controls through budgets or caps, cost containment efforts have included increased reliance on out-of-pocket payments by patients at the point of service, albeit not in all countries. Such payments can be regressive and are not considered to be clinically appropriate tools for moderating demand, but they can increase allocative efficiency if carefully designed. For example, a copayment scheme with income limits, recently introduced in Germany, led to significantly less physician contacts without discouraging either low-income groups or persons with bad health. As the importance of copayment mechanisms grows, policy makers are increasingly aware of their problems of regressivity. In the Netherlands, for example, dental care for adults was excluded, then partly reintroduced out of fear of uncovered parts of the population—but then again excluded. In Japan, the last big increase in coinsurance rates from 20 to 30 percent in the employees' health insurance in April 2003 was politically sold as increasing equity, because the national health insurance rate was already at that level. At the same time, policy makers added a clause to the law that cost sharing would never exceed that level.

Coverage decisions and benefit entitlements

Coverage entails the extent of the covered population, the range of covered services, and the extent to which costs of the defined services are covered by prepaid finances rather than cost-sharing requirements. The aspiration of fulfilling these three dimensions of coverage as completely as possible can be best described by the founding principles of the British National Health Service in 1948: "universal, comprehensive, and free at the point of delivery."

Who is covered?

Improving access to health care services has been a fundamental objective of health policy making in OECD countries in the past 30 years. With the exception of the United States, all countries reviewed here had achieved universal or nearly universal coverage of their populations in the 1990s (Docteur and Oxley 2003). The criteria for entitlement to coverage differ markedly among social health insurance countries, tax-financed countries, and countries where a large part of health care is financed through private health insurance or medical savings accounts.

Social health insurance system countries. Because historically social health insurance systems are work-related insurance programs, universal coverage was not their original intention. Although coverage has been gradually expanded to non-working parts of the population in all social health insurance countries, universal coverage is a recent phenomenon. Switzerland achieved universal coverage in 1996, Belgium in 1998, and France as late as 2000. A notable exception in Europe was the Netherlands, which introduced its long-term care insurance (AWBZ) on a full-population basis as early as 1968. Even earlier, the Japanese social health insurance system achieved universal coverage with an amendment of the 1938 National Insurance Act in 1961. Since then, membership in one of the 5,124 sickness funds (as of 2002) is compulsory for the entire population.

The government of the Republic of Korea introduced social health insurance in 1976 to relieve the excessive burden of household medical care expenses and to promote the health of its population. Initially, all companies with more than 500 employees were required to offer health insurance to their employees. Over the years, this obligation was gradually extended to companies of ever smaller size, reaching those with only five employees in 1988. At the beginning of the 1980s, insurance coverage was also gradually expanded to government and private school employees and the self-employed, including employees in companies with fewer than five employees. Universal coverage was thus achieved in 1989, when the urban self-employed were incorporated into the scheme (OECD 2003). At the end of the 1990s a convergence process started, leading in 2000 to the formation of the National Health Insurance Corporation which absorbed all 139 employee health insurance societies (OECD 2004a).

Tax-financed system countries. In contrast to most social health insurance countries, where the goal of universal coverage has been stated fairly recently, universal coverage has been a central feature of countries with tax-financed models. In New Zealand the main policy objective to provide "free care for all" dates to 1938. The

United Kingdom followed with the creation of its national health service in 1948. With the establishment of the Medicare Program in 1984, Australia reestablished a mandatory insurance scheme to obtain universal coverage (which had been introduced as Medibank in 1975, but which was then diluted through the subsequent addition of an opt-out option) (Hilless and Healy 2001).

In Northern European and Australasian tax-financed health care systems (such as in the United Kingdom, Australia, New Zealand, and the Scandinavian countries), entitlement to health care services is based on residence, independent of citizenship. The population not covered in these countries is accordingly very small and limited basically to illegal immigrants. Universal coverage is a more recent phenomenon in Southern European tax-financed countries, but by 2002 all countries with a national health service in Southern Europe had also achieved nearly universal coverage.

Italy introduced a national health service with the objective of universal coverage in 1978. Before 1978, 93 percent of the population was covered by public health insurance, although under markedly varying conditions. The 1978 reform changed the principle of health care financing: solidarity within professional categories was discarded in favor of intergenerational solidarity, which backed the introduction of universal, free coverage for all Italian citizens. Non-Italian residents were at first not included under this legislation. Since 1998, however, legal immigrants have had the same rights as Italian citizens. Measures were also taken to provide some care to illegal immigrants, who now have access to a limited range of health care services, in particular to treatment for infectious diseases and health care schemes for babies and pregnant women (Donatini and others 2001).

In Spain, access to health services is through ownership of an individual electronic health card (TSI). Since 2001, the TSI has been available for citizens and foreign residents. There is no difference between Spanish citizens and migrants, even if they are considered "illegal." A new initiative in Catalonia has broadened the group of migrants owning a TSI, irrespective of their legal status, thus enabling them to access the public health networks. By offering information about services included in the TSI and facilitating access, Spain's strategies for reaching marginalized populations will make coverage almost universal (Velasco Garrido and Busse 2005).

In Portugal, in addition to the national health service, which covers 83.5 percent of the population, private insurance schemes cover an additional 10 percent, and mutual funds cover 6.5 percent. Generally, the benefits received under private insurance or mutual fund schemes exceed those provided within the national health service. However, in both subsystems employer and employee contributions are often insufficient to cover the full costs of care, and consequently a significant proportion of costs are shifted onto the national health service. If enrollees in these funds do not declare their membership when receiving treatment within the national health service, the funds are exempted from responsibility for the full costs of the members' care. The relationship between the national health service and the subsystems was explicitly addressed by legislation in late 1998. Under an "opting-out" scheme, financial responsibility for personal care in the national health service could be transferred to public or private entities through a contribution established in a contract with the Ministry of Health (Bentes and others 2004).

In the U.S. health system, individuals are insured through a variety of schemes: employer-sponsored insurance, individual (nongroup) insurance, Medicare, Medicaid, the State Children's Health Insurance Program, and coverage offered by the military and the Veterans Administration. In 2002 an estimated 43.6 million people, 15.2 percent of the U.S. population, had no health coverage during the entire year (U.S. Census Bureau 2003). Health insurance coverage in the United States is more dynamic than in countries with less fragmented health systems because, for most people, it is closely linked to individual employers who negotiate and take out group insurance plans for their employees. This means that many people are uninsured, at least for part of the year (CBO 2003).

In summary, all high-income countries reviewed have achieved nearly universal coverage independently of the financing mechanism—with the exception of the United States. The difference in the speed of attaining universal coverage is linked to the choice of financing mechanism. In Northern European and Australasian tax-financed systems, universal coverage was a political goal from the start in the 1930s and 1940s, whereas in European social health insurance systems, universal coverage developed gradually over the past 100 years, and even the political discussion about universal coverage in these countries is fairly recent. Southern European tax-financed systems take an intermediate position. They have in common rapid economic growth in the second half of the twentieth century, paralleled by an expansion of tax-financed health coverage or, in Spain, by a shift from a fragmented social health insurance system to a tax-financed system. Likewise, Japan expanded coverage under its social health insurance system during a phase of rapid economic growth in the 1960s. Korea expanded coverage the fastest, increasing coverage from 15 percent to 100 percent within 10 years, again during a period of economic growth. This rapid expansion was facilitated by initially relatively high copayment levels and limited benefits.

The other crucial factor for attaining universal coverage is political will: clear legislation, either at the set-up or gradually to fill in coverage gaps, to achieve universal coverage. Such political will is best exemplified by recent Italian legislation that addresses health care for illegal immigrants. The United States, despite several attempts (most recently during the Clinton administration), has no political consensus to achieve universal coverage—a high-income country with sustained economic growth and no major changes in coverage levels over the past 30 years.

What is covered?

Social health insurance system countries. A central characteristic of social health insurance systems is the definition of the benefits to which the insured are entitled (Gibis, Koch-Wulkan, and Bultman 2004). This characteristic was recently reinforced in 2001 in the Netherlands, when a court ruled that entitlements (in this case, in AWBZ) had to be guaranteed irrespective of their costs. The contents of the benefits basket, as well as the processes applied to define them, range from a list of benefits decreed by law (as in the Netherlands) to negotiations between sickness funds and providers (as in Germany). Among the notable differences in contents are the inclusion of benefits outside acute curative care, especially health promotion measures and long-term care. For example, Germany introduced a separate social care insurance scheme to cover ambulatory long-term care in 1995. This scheme was rapidly expanded to cover institutional care in 1996.

Historically, European social health insurance systems, initially set up to regain and maintain the productivity capacity of diseased workers, focused on insuring curative hospital and ambulatory care (Kupsch and others 2000). To this day, preventive services are offered to a lesser extent by the social health insurance systems, compared with the British or Scandinavian tax-financed systems (McKee, Delnoij, and Brand 2004).

There are at least two ways to enhance the supply of preventive services in social health insurance schemes with multiple sickness funds. First, collective health services could be kept separate from the social health insurance scheme, as in the case of mammography in the Netherlands, where such services parallel the main social health insurance scheme. Second, incentives could be provided for sickness funds to invest in the future of their insured by offering certain prevention programs. Some social health insurance countries regulate preventive services by law. Germany, for example, has chosen to enhance preventive activities by direct regulation in a social health insurance system. Apart from enhancing public supply, increased use of preventive services can be stimulated through financial incentives for individuals. Bonus payments or similar instruments can be offered by sickness funds to increase the use of preventive services (for example, in Germany certain copayments can be lifted if individuals can prove they have made use of preventive services).

In almost all European social health insurance countries, ambulatory health care is provided by physicians operating mainly on a fee-for-service basis (Gibis, Koch-Wulkan, and Bultman 2004). Consequently, benefits catalogues had to be introduced—primarily as fee schedules. However, fee-for-service payments have evolved into quite elaborate remuneration schemes in some countries or have been limited to certain groups of doctors.

Hospital care is usually organized in a decentralized way, and hospitals have a high degree of autonomy. Benefits catalogues for hospital care are rare. Some social health insurance countries, such as France, Germany, and Switzerland, are implementing diagnosis-related group (DRG) payment systems. These systems could subsequently lead to benefits catalogues that list all approved interventions grouped around diagnoses. The government's role in defining such in-patient benefits catalogues is likely to be greater than its role in ambulatory care (Gibis, Koch-Wulkan, and Bultman 2004).

Coverage of pharmaceuticals differs considerably among the European social health insurance countries. In some countries, such as Germany or Switzerland, licensure by the European Medicines Evaluation Agency or the national equivalent allows reimbursement in the social health insurance system; other countries, such as France and the Netherlands, have established positive lists of covered drugs. This also applies to the amount of coverage. Dental coverage has been reduced or restricted (despite the technical progress in this field) in almost all European social health insurance systems (Kaufhold and Schneider 2000).

Tax-financed system countries. In most European tax-financed systems, benefits catalogues are not explicitly defined. For example, in the United Kingdom, the secretary of state for health is legally required to provide services "to such extent as he considers necessary to meet all reasonable requirements" (1977 Act). The secretary's duty is to arrange for practitioners to provide an acceptable level of service for the resident population. What constitutes an acceptable level of service remains vague, however.

Among Southern European tax-financed countries, Spain introduced the first explicit benefits catalogue in 1995. A list of benefits guaranteed by the public health system was drawn up under a royal decree, which maintained the benefits already available within the system and made those services universal (Rico, Sabes, and Wisbaum 2000). A number of services have been specifically excluded from the benefits catalogue, including psychoanalysis, sex-change surgery, spa treatments, cosmetic surgery, and all but the most basic dental care. In practice, however, the royal decree has never been fully implemented. Following regionalization of the national health service in January 2002, regional variations in covered benefits became more obvious: some regions cover dental care, whereas others have a smaller negative pharmaceutical list (cover drugs more generously).

In contrast to most European systems and the New Zealand tax-financed system, the Australian health system has an explicit benefits catalogue called the Medicare Benefits Schedule, which is constructed using an evidence-based approach. The Medicare Benefits Schedule sets out a schedule fee for medical services for which the commonwealth government will pay medical benefits. Covered items include consultation fees for doctors and specialists, radiology and pathology tests, eye tests by optometrists, and surgical and therapeutic procedures performed by doctors. Medicare does not cover dental treatment, ambulance services, home nursing, physiotherapy, occupational therapy, speech therapy, chiropractic and podiatry services, treatment by psychologists, visual and hearing aids and prostheses, medical services that are not clinically necessary, and cosmetic surgery (Hilless and Healy 2001).

In the United States, covered benefits vary widely across private health insurance plans—from the most basic to luxury care—depending on the level of premium and the employer. Medicare is the main insurance program for the population above 65 years old (as well as for the disabled and those with end-stage renal disease); it covers approximately 41 million people. The Medicare Coverage Database contains a detailed list of all benefits included on a national and a state-by-state basis. This list is continuously reviewed and amended. For example, the Medicare law (effective since January 1, 2005) expanded coverage to diabetic screening services, and the benefits catalogue had to be amended accordingly (for example, home blood glucose testing had to be added to the catalogue). The most important change in recent years was the inclusion of prescription drugs in the 2003 Medicare Modernization Act, which took effect in January 2006. Reimbursement is through a complex payment structure that covers an initial portion of drug costs, then includes a significant gap in coverage, and later picks up the costs of catastrophic drug coverage at a defined level.

Summary. Most tax-financed health systems do not have a defined benefits catalogue, whereas most social health insurance systems, which have fee-for-service payment mechanisms to remunerate providers, do. Lack of defined benefits leads to implicit addition of new services or technologies to the national health service benefits catalogue during the commissioning process, which can vary among geographic areas. The result can be what is called "postcode prescribing" in the United Kingdom. Such prescribing is considered to be inequitable. Most social health insurance systems need an explicit mechanism to include new technologies or to exclude those thought to be ineffective or inefficient from the explicit benefits catalogue. Inclusion and exclusion decisions are often difficult to make because good evidence is sparse and often costly to develop. Moreover, such decisions are subject to the threat of lawsuits by industry. Thus, many countries have set up capacity-building programs, such as the United Kingdom's national health service research and development evidence-base research program, and new agencies for health technology assessment to guide decision makers (Velasco Garrido and Busse 2005).

Paying for health services

All countries under review require some form of cost sharing from individuals. However, the amount of out-of-pocket payments for health services in high-income countries varies widely. In Europe, cost sharing has not followed a consistent trend from 1980 to 2001 (table 9.2). While in many countries cost sharing has increased during this period, it has decreased in others, such as in Ireland and the

TABLE 9.2   **Share of out-of-pocket and voluntary health insurance payments in total health expenditures in 12 European countries, 1980–2001**

Country and type of payments	1980 (% of total health expenditures)	1999–2001 (% of total health expenditures)	Percentage point change, 1980–2001
Austria			
Out of pocket	—	28.0	—
Voluntary health insurance	—	2.0	—
Belgium			
Out of pocket	—	19.0	—
Voluntary health insurance	—	—	—
Denmark			
Out of pocket	11.4	16.4	+5.0
Voluntary health insurance	0.8	1.6	+0.8
Finland			
Out of pocket	17.8	20.2	+2.4
Voluntary health insurance	0.8	2.0	+1.2
France			
Out of pocket	—	10.6	—
Voluntary health insurance	—	12.7	—
Germany			
Out of pocket	8.1	11.0	+2.9
Voluntary health insurance	7.4	7.7	+0.3
Greece			
Out of pocket	—	41.4[a]	—
Voluntary health insurance	—	3.2	—
Ireland			
Out of pocket	14.3	9.1	−5.2
Voluntary health insurance	3.5	6.4	+2.9
Italy			
Out of pocket	—	22.0	—
Voluntary health insurance	—	0.9	—
Netherlands			
Out of pocket	7.0	6.3	−0.7
Voluntary health insurance	24.0	14.0	−10.0
Spain			
Out of pocket	21.3	22.0	+0.7
Voluntary health insurance	2.9	6.0	+3.1
Sweden			
Out of pocket	—	16.0	—
Voluntary health insurance	—	—	—

Source: Adapted from Thomson, Mossialos, and Jemiai 2003 on the basis of national statistics.

— is not available.

a. Including an estimated 16 percent in informal payments.

Netherlands. Outside of Europe, New Zealand saw a steep rise in out-of-pocket payments between 1980 and 1999, from 10 to 16 percent of total health expenditure, corresponding to a 6.2 percent yearly increase in real terms (French, Old, and Healy 2001).

All high-income countries reviewed here levy some form of user charges and have significant out-of-pocket payments. With the exception of Austria, Greece, and the United States, however, out-of-pocket payments represent less then 22 percent of total health expenditure and often less than 10 percent. There is no clear trend in tax-financed or social health insurance systems toward increases or decreases in cost sharing, and a great variety of cost sharing and protection mechanisms are employed. Decisions on the extent and type of cost-sharing mechanism seem more often guided by political opportunism than by rational arguments regarding technical efficiency (Thomson, Mossialos, and Jemiai 2003; Gericke, Wismar, and Busse 2004).

Collection of funds

The total amount of resources collected is usually not available in international databases. Health expenditure is most often used instead, although the amount of resources collected is in many cases higher. National health service countries are often claimed to be more successful in cost containment and therefore are thought to collect fewer resources, but Greece, Iceland, Norway, and Portugal are among the countries with the highest increase in health expenditure as a percentage of GDP. High economic growth rates contributed to low or even decreasing shares of health expenditure as a percentage of GDP in the Republic of Korea, Singapore, and Ireland. Norway and the United States, with similar high economic growth rates, have experienced large increases. Thus, health expenditure and the amount of resources collected in each country obviously depend on the individual preferences of each country.

Sources of financing

High-income countries rely mainly on individuals, firms, and corporate entities as sources of health care financing and to a very small extent on nongovernmental organizations or charities. It is generally difficult to determine the exact amount firms or corporate entities contribute to health financing, especially regarding tax payments for general revenue. However, in countries that finance their health expenditure mainly by social health insurance, the ratio of contributions of employers to those of employees provides some information on the employers' contribution as a source of financing. There is a slight trend in certain social health insurance countries toward shifting a portion from the employers' contribution to the employees' contribution, as in Germany and the Netherlands. However, a systematic change in the financing ratio could not be identified across countries over the past 30 years.

Financing mechanisms

Apart from the United States, all of the countries examined derive the main part of their health care resources either through social security contributions (or similarly termed social health insurance arrangements) or through direct and indirect tax payments in national health services. Currently 9 of the 25 countries studied finance their health care system mainly by social health insurance contributions, while 13 countries use mainly tax payments (figure 9.1). Singapore[1] and the United States fit neither of these classifications, since they finance more than half of their health expenditure through other mechanisms, such as voluntary insurance premiums and out-of-pocket payments. Nor does Greece, where private expenditure finances slightly less than 50 percent of the total, and neither of the two main public financing mechanisms dominates.[2]

The relative importance of the various financing mechanisms has changed somewhat in most countries since 1975. However, in only 9 of 23 countries (data were not available for Belgium and Greece) did the relative importance of one of the two main public financing mechanisms change by more than 5 percentage points.

Compulsory social health insurance contributions. Eight of the nine countries that predominantly rely on compulsory social insurance contributions can look back on years of experience with social health insurance. Korea represents a special

FIGURE 9.1   Share of tax and social health insurance revenues in total health expenditures in high-income countries, 2002

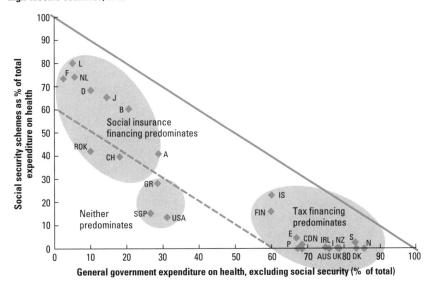

Source: OECD 2004a or national data.
Note: A = Austria; AUS = Australia; B = Belgium; CDN = Canada; CH = Switzerland; D = Germany; DK = Denmark; E = Spain; F = France; FIN = Finland; GR = Greece; I = Italy; IRL = Ireland; IS = Iceland; J = Japan; L = Luxembourg; N = Norway; NL = Netherlands; NZ = New Zealand; P = Portugal; ROK = Republic of Korea; S = Sweden; SGP = Singapore; UK = United Kingdom; USA = United States of America.

case, since it moved from a predominantly privately financed system with taxes as the second most important financing mechanism in the 1970s to a system based to a considerable degree on compulsory social health insurance contributions. As in many other countries, such as Germany, social health insurance in Korea started with a small scheme for industrial workers in 1977 and was gradually extended to other population groups. In 2002, 42.2 percent of total health expenditure was financed by compulsory insurance contributions.

The main part of the collected health care resources in countries with social health insurance is raised through wage-related contributions, which are shared between employers and employees. Nonetheless, arrangements differ among countries, and changes have taken place over the past three decades.

All insured, regardless of their sickness fund and membership status, contribute at a uniform rate in Belgium, France, Korea, Luxembourg, and the Netherlands. In Austria, as of 2003, rates varied between 6.9 percent and 9.1 percent, according to employment status but not between funds. In 2004, a reform equalized contribution rates among different employment groups. In Japan, rates differ according to employment status, and in the municipal health insurance scheme rates also differ among sickness funds of each municipality. In Germany, the contribution rates differ among funds but not by employment status. Germany is also the only country (since 1996) that uses the variability of contribution rates among sickness funds as a parameter for competition among funds. However, in Switzerland differing per capita premiums are used in a similar way.[3]

In Belgium and the Netherlands, a nonincome-related per capita premium on top of the contributions was introduced in the 1990s. Premiums differ among sickness funds in the Netherlands, but have remained mostly uniform in Belgium. Like the contribution rate in Germany, this mechanism allows varying contributions among sickness funds to be used as a parameter for competition among them. In contrast, in France and Korea, nonwage-related components were introduced to enlarge the financial base for sickness funds and thus increase overall revenue. In addition, contributions became less vulnerable to wage and employment fluctuations (Sandier and others 2004). Since 1998, France has replaced the solely wage-related contributions of employees with a general social contribution of 5.25 percent that, apart from wages, also includes such nonwage-related income as capital gains and interest; 3.25 percent is charged on benefits and allowances.

Direct and indirect taxes.   Spain and Iceland have moved away from social health insurance and managed the transition to tax payments as the main financing mechanism (box 9.1). In both countries this change was motivated by the perception that the tax payment mechanism was less regressive, although social health insurance contributions, if designed appropriately, might have achieved a level of progressivity similar to that achieved in Spain, which transformed its system from a regressive one in 1980 to a neutral one in 1990.

BOX 9.1 *The transition from social health insurance to tax financing in Iceland and Spain*

In Iceland, more than 60 percent of health expenditures were financed by flat-rate insurance contributions to sickness funds until 1972. Because these contributions were perceived to be too regressive and because health expenditures were rapidly rising, it was decided to shift to tax payments. In the transition period from 1972 to 1989, sickness funds were retained but received their funding completely from tax payments, 80 percent from the state and 20 percent from local governments (Halldorsson and Bankauskaite 2003).

Spain also relied mainly on social health insurance contributions. In the mid-1970s, the social health insurance contributions made up about two-thirds of total health care expenditures, and tax payments covered the rest. In 1986 the introduction of a national health service initiated a major shift toward tax funding. By 1989 the previous pattern was reversed for the first time; tax payments constituted 70 percent and social health insurance contributions dropped to about 30 percent of the total. Throughout the 1990s, the role of social health insurance contributions has been steadily decreasing (Rico, Sabes, and Wisbaum 2000).

In contrast to Spain and Iceland, Finland decreased the level of tax financing, which led to a relative (albeit minor) increase in the percentage of social security contributions. The share of tax payments decreased from 66.1 percent of total health expenditure in 1975 to 59.7 percent in 2002, while social security contributions increased from 12.6 percent in 1975 to 15.9 percent in 2002 (Järvelin, Rico, and Cetani 2002). Canada and Norway experienced even more dramatic slashes in the share of taxes in health expenditures in favor of more private financing mechanisms. However, this development did not reflect a decrease in available taxes (as in Finland), but rather a massive cut in health spending from general revenue, revealing the vulnerability of tax payments to changes in political priorities.

Instead of getting resources for health from general revenue, some suggest earmarking taxes for health expenditure, a move not even undertaken in countries whose health expenditures are mainly tax financed (though in the case of Sweden it could be argued that provincial taxes are de facto earmarked as the vast majority are used for health care). Instead, earmarked taxes have been introduced as a source of complementary financing in countries with mainly social security financing: in France, 3.3 percent of the total health revenue is raised as earmarked taxes on car usage, tobacco, and alcohol consumption. In addition, the pharmaceutical industry is required to pay an earmarked tax on advertising, accounting for 0.8 percent of total health revenue (Sandier and others 2004).

Voluntary insurance premiums. Voluntary health insurance can be classified into various forms that, depending on the definition, partly overlap: *substitute health insurance* as an alternative to statutory schemes; *supplementary health insurance* to cover services not included in the benefits basket of statutory schemes and to provide superior amenities; *duplicate health insurance,* which provides people already covered by a given public health system with private alternative coverage for the same sets of services, often furnished by different providers; and *complementary health insurance* covering copayments or deductibles applicable to public health systems (OECD 2004b).

Small markets for supplementary health insurance occur in all included countries, but Canada represents a special case because 65 percent of its population is covered by this kind of voluntary health insurance. Voluntary health insurance is allowed to cover only services not covered under the public system. Such additional benefits include mainly drugs and certain dental services, long-term care, rehabilitative care, and home care. Switzerland is by far the largest market for supplementary voluntary health insurance (OECD 2004b).

Duplicate voluntary health insurance is typically available in countries with tax-financed national health services, where amounts or quality of publicly provided health services are perceived to be insufficient or inappropriate. The main drivers are the length of waiting lists and the desire to choose providers. Large parts of the population are covered by duplicate voluntary health insurance in Australia (more than 40 percent), Ireland (also more than 40 percent), and New Zealand (35 percent) (OECD 2004b). While the share of voluntary health insurance increased in New Zealand over the last decade, it decreased in Australia, perhaps because of improved public services, among other factors. However, the Australian government has repeatedly tried to reverse this decline in voluntary plans (box 9.2).

Many high-income countries have markets for complementary voluntary health insurance; France and the United States (Medicare only) are the most relevant cases. In France, voluntary health insurance is purchased to cover coinsurance rates ranging from 20 percent for in-patient treatment and 30 percent for

---

BOX 9.2 *Tax subsidization of duplicate private health insurance in Australia*

Since 1997 in Australia, individuals receive a tax-subsidized rebate of 30 percent on health insurance premiums, and out-of-pocket payments have been increased for persons using medical services in private hospitals. In 2000, lifetime coverage was introduced, and private health insurers are allowed to vary premiums for persons older than 30, according to age at entry, to provide financial incentives for joining a voluntary health insurance plan before the age of 30. These measures aim mainly at bringing more people into private health insurance to relieve the pressures on the public system (Busse and Schlette 2003; Colombo and Tapay 2003). Although population coverage in voluntary health insurance increased from 31 percent in 1996 to 45.3 percent in 2001 after those measures were introduced, it is questionable whether the whole strategy has been very successful. Health expenditure rose even faster in the second half of the 1990s than it had before (from 8.5 percent to 9.0 percent of GDP between 1995 and 2000).

physician fees to 65 percent for certain drugs (OECD 2004b). The main motivation is therefore to limit the financial risk posed by high utilization of services. This kind of insurance, which increased over the last decade, accounts for most of the large per capita spending on private health insurance.

Medical savings accounts. The medical savings account, first developed in Singapore in the 1980s (box 9.3), has also been adopted in the United States. Unlike in Singapore, the objectives in the United States are cost containment and expansion of insurance coverage to include the uninsured (15 percent of the population). Medical savings accounts serve primarily to finance a high deductible in order to reduce premium payments. Medical savings accounts were tested during the 1996–2003 period in a pilot project for a limited sample of insured persons (750,000 accounts) in the private health insurance market. Depending on the insurance contract, either the employer or the employee was allowed to make tax-exempt payments into medical savings accounts within a given year. The payment of interest on capital stocks accumulated in accounts was a matter for the individual insurance companies to decide (Public Law 104-191, August 21, 1996). Although 4 of 10 participants had not previously been insured (U.S. GAO 1998), total

---

BOX 9.3 *Health financing with medical savings accounts in Singapore*

In 1984 Singapore introduced a system of medical savings accounts, called Medisave. Every employed citizen is obliged to pay a 6–8 percent share of income—according to age—into an individual account managed by the state. Funds in the accounts are invested in the capital market by the government, and interest is paid at the current market rate (Asher 2002). Savings in the individual medical savings account can be used to pay for hospital costs and certain selected out-patient costs approved by the state in a catalogue of services. This system was supplemented by a high-risk health insurance scheme (called Medishield), which is paid from contributions depending on age and which can be financed from individual medical savings accounts. Medishield is intended to finance both expensive hospital treatments and out-patient treatments for chronic diseases. In addition, a fund (called Medifund) is used to

support low-income individuals who do not have a medical savings account or who are unable to set aside sufficient savings. Medifund is financed by the state from general taxes.

Implementation of the system of medical savings accounts is not yet complete, because the generation entering into retirement before 1984 was not able to accumulate capital stocks and is therefore financed by family members or by state assistance. For this reason, full implementation will not be achieved until 2030. Apart from medical savings accounts, the low share of health expenditure (3.7 percent of GDP in 2002) may also be attributable to the young population and an incentive scheme of hospital classes. However, several studies indicate that the medical savings accounts have at least made a considerable contribution to this low share (Prescott and Nichols 1998; Schreyögg and Lim 2004).

participation was low: the number of accounts was estimated at 150,000, perhaps because of restrictive legal conditions (Bunce 2001). There is still not enough empirical research for rigorous evaluation of the experimental period.

Although the pilot project was not extended after it ended in 2003, the Bush Administration introduced a new scheme of medical savings accounts, effective on January 1, 2004, for Medicare beneficiaries. According to this scheme an unlimited number of people who are eligible for Medicare are allowed to choose a policy with a minimum deductible of $1,000 for singles and $2,000 for families in combination with medical savings accounts. Employers of all sizes can offer these programs to their employees, but they must be approved by the Medicare program. They are funded by pretax payroll contributions or employer contributions. The idea behind it is that Medicare beneficiaries are able to pay for their "qualified expenses" (such as prescription drugs and doctors' fees), which are not covered or not sufficiently covered by Medicare (Schreyögg 2004).

Various forms of out-of-pocket payments. The introduction of out-of-pocket payments can have merely a financial effect, shifting costs to relieve public financing schemes from cost containment pressure, or they can have an additional behavioral effect, preventing moral hazard (using unnecessary services because they are free or heavily subsidized). For high-income countries, there is evidence from a number of studies in the United States and Europe that out-of-pocket payments, especially copayments, coinsurance, and deductibles, can have the desired effects—if carefully designed (Zweifel and Manning 2001) and if the majority of the population does not have voluntary health insurance to cover these costs. Crucial points for the success of those instruments are the amounts raised and the equity of financing. However, apart from out-of-pocket payments, there are also other ways to direct health resources into the most effective utilization.

Between 1990 and 2002, the five countries with the highest increase in the share of out-of-pocket payments are all European countries (figure 9.2). With the exception of Luxembourg (which had very low out-of-pocket spending in 1990), these countries have predominantly tax-financed health systems. Three of them (Finland, Italy, and Spain) are now among the top five (behind Korea and Switzerland) in out-of-pocket payments as a percentage of total health expenditure. In contrast, countries with a relatively low share of public expenditure (Korea, Switzerland, and the United States) largely reduced their share of out-of-pocket payments. This might be interpreted as a trend toward convergence of countries with high and low shares of out-of-pocket payments as a percentage of total health expenditure.

Organizations collecting resources

Among the social health insurance countries, there is great variety in the types of organizations collecting resources for health care. Sickness funds collect resources

FIGURE 9.2   Changing share of out-of-pocket payments in total health expenditures in high-income countries, 1992 and 2002

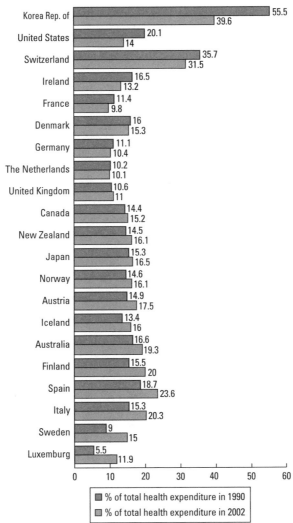

Country	1990	2002
Korea Rep. of	55.5	39.6
United States	20.1	14
Switzerland	35.7	31.5
Ireland	16.5	13.2
France	11.4	9.8
Denmark	16	15.3
Germany	11.1	10.4
The Netherlands	10.2	10.1
United Kingdom	10.6	11
Canada	14.4	15.2
New Zealand	14.5	16.1
Japan	15.3	16.5
Norway	14.6	16.1
Austria	14.9	17.5
Iceland	13.4	16
Australia	16.6	19.3
Finland	15.5	20
Spain	18.7	23.6
Italy	15.3	20.3
Sweden	9	15
Luxemburg	5.5	11.9

■ % of total health expenditure in 1990
□ % of total health expenditure in 2002

Source: OECD 2004a.

directly in Austria, Germany, Japan, Korea, and Switzerland, for example. Other types include associations of funds (Luxembourg), special agencies under government control (Belgium), and the tax authorities directly (the Netherlands) (Busse, Saltman, and Dubois 2004).

There have been changes in collecting organizations in tax-financed systems in the past few years. In Italy and Spain, regional or local governments have received more autonomy for resource collection (though not as much as in Sweden). In many national health service systems, national or regional governments collect resources. For example, Spain and Italy now allow regional governments to collect resources, in addition to the resources they receive from national resource collection on their own. In Italy, 6 of 21 regions added funds from their own taxes to make up for (parts of) the deficit in 2002 (Jommi and Fattore 2003).

Pooling of funds

In most high-income countries, collecting and pooling take place at the central level. In tax-financed systems, two bodies are generally at work: the ministry of finance or the treasury as collecting organization and the ministry of health as the pooling organization (England, Ireland, Italy, and New Zealand). The allocation of responsibility between these two bodies is in most cases more a matter of political agenda setting than of objectively defined allocation. New Zealand is an exception, as it has defined objective allocation criteria. Earmarked taxes, combined with an independent organization responsible for pooling and collecting resources, are another possible approach to overcome the vulnerability of the health system to political priority setting.

Allocating resources from collecting to pooling organizations

Although in tax-financed systems collecting and pooling are mainly centralized, there is a trend toward decentralization of both functions. Regional governments in Italy, Spain, and Sweden have received more autonomy in both collecting and pooling. In Sweden, collection and pooling responsibilities have been strongly decentralized since the 1970s. County councils rely mainly on income taxes, which they collect themselves. In addition, counties receive subsidies from the central government on the basis of an allocation formula (Hjortsberg and others 2001).

In contrast to tax-financed systems, social health insurance systems are increasingly moving away from decentralized pooling organizations. Many countries, such as Belgium, Germany, the Netherlands, and Switzerland, have centralized their pooling organizations in independent organizations at the federal level, such as the Federal Insurance Authority in Germany or the Health Care Insurance Board in the Netherlands. Switzerland is a special case; it pools resources only in each "premia region" (usually on the subcanton level), so that, for example, the high per capita expenditure in Geneva is not shared with the inhabitants of Appenzell, where per capita expenditure is low. Such centralization came in response to the fragmentation and small size of decentralized pools. Small pools (sickness funds) were exposed to high financial risks because of their inability to share risk among a large population, and thus they needed reinsurance or tax subsidies. Now centralized, sickness funds are responsible for only a fraction of health expenditure. They act as purchasing organizations (and in a few countries as collectors). The number of sickness funds has decreased sharply in Belgium, Germany,

Korea, the Netherlands, and Switzerland, in part because of the introduction of competition among funds in their function as purchasing organizations, but also because of the problems and higher administrative costs associated with small pool sizes (Korea is the exception).

The transfer between collecting and pooling organizations is only difficult in social health insurance countries where sickness funds can collect different levels of contributions (Germany and Switzerland). In those countries, pooled resources have to be separated from resources that stay with the sickness fund (for example, for services not taken into account in the pooling or from contribution rates higher than assumed in the pooling calculations).

In addition to transfers from contribution-collection organizations, in some social health insurance countries, pooling organizations receive financial resources from tax authorities. Tax subsidies to the pooling organizations are substantial in Belgium, Luxembourg, and the Netherlands, whereas they are small but rising in Germany. The high Belgian tax component is the result of a policy change in 1981, when social security contributions were lowered by 6.17 percentage points and the value-added tax was increased in an attempt to become internationally more competitive (Busse, Saltman, and Dubois 2004).

Allocating resources from pooling to purchasing organizations

In most countries, the pooling function is centralized, and purchasing bodies usually act at the regional or local level. Common purchasing bodies are regional and local governments, as well as sickness funds.

The allocation of financial resources from pooling to purchasing organizations can either be prospective or retrospective. Under retrospective allocation, pooling organizations allocate according to actual expenditures incurred by purchasing organizations, whereas under prospective allocation a budget is determined for future health expenditure. In Belgium, Luxembourg, and the Netherlands, retrospective allocation according to actual expenditure was the customary approach before reforms in the mid-1990s. Apart from Luxemburg, where this approach is still used for services requiring patient reimbursement, such as physicians' services, these countries have switched to prospective allocation mechanisms. In Korea resources are allocated retrospectively on the basis of a fixed schedule of fees paid to providers, which is negotiated each year (OECD 2003).

In recent decades most countries have moved toward the application of independent criteria of health care needs, frequently referred to as capitation, as the dominant method of allocation. Capitation can be defined as a kind of price paid by the pooling organizations for each individual covered by purchasing organizations with the necessary health services. As individuals' health expenditures vary considerably, depending on personal characteristics such as age, sex, and morbidity, increasing effort is being dedicated to risk adjustment, which seeks an unbiased estimate of the expected expenditure of each individual with certain personal characteristics. Capitation generally increases the degree of equity between different regions of a country, and the pooling responsibility of each region decreases as the predictive value of the applied capitation rises (Rice and Smith 2002).

However, the predictive value of risk adjusters for setting capitations varies widely among the countries reviewed here (tables 9.3 and 9.4). Capitations range from less sophisticated schemes, such as Switzerland's use of only age and sex as risk adjusters, to the very complex, but highly predictive capitations in the Netherlands and Sweden. Sweden, for instance, applies a very advanced matrix approach, using age, sex, marital status, employment status, occupation, and housing tenure, as well as previous high utilization as risk adjusters on an individual level. The Netherlands might be even one step farther ahead since 2002, when it introduced a capitation with age, sex, social security and employment status, region of residence, and even diagnostic and pharmaceutical cost groups as risk adjusters.

Germany shows the typical evolution of capitations. From 1989 to 1995, Germany had a mixed system of pooling expenditure for pensioners while for all other

TABLE 9.3   Risk adjusters in the capitation formulas for resource allocation in countries with social health insurance systems

Country	Year of implementation	Risk adjusters
Austria	None	
Belgium	1995	• Age, sex, social insurance status, employment status, mortality, urbanization, income
	2006	• Age, sex, social insurance status, employment status, mortality, urbanization, income, diagnostic and pharmaceutical cost groups
France	None	
Germany	1994/1995	• Age, sex, disability pension status
	2002	• Age, sex, disability pension status, participation in disease management program
Japan	None	
Korea, Rep. of	None	
Luxembourg	None	
Netherlands	1993	• Age, sex
	1996	• Age, sex, region, disability status
	1999	• Age, sex, social security/employment status, region of residence
	2002	• Age, sex, social security/employment status, region of residence, diagnostic and pharmaceutical cost groups
Switzerland (within canton)	1994	• Age, sex

Source: Adapted from Busse, Saltman, and Dubois 2004 and updated with data from Risk Adjustment Network (RAN).

TABLE 9.4   Risk adjusters in capitation formulas for resource allocation in countries with tax-financed systems

Country	Risk adjusters
Australia	Age, sex, ethnic group, homelessness, mortality, education level, rurality
Canada	Age, sex, socioeconomic status, ethnicity, remoteness
Denmark	Age, number of children in single-parent families, number of rented flats, unemployment, education, immigrants, social status, single elderly people
England	Age, mortality, morbidity, unemployment, elderly people living alone, ethnic origin, socioeconomic status
Finland	Age, disability, morbidity, archipelago, remoteness
Iceland	None
Ireland	Not applicable
Italy	Age, sex, mortality, morbidity, utilization
New Zealand	Age, sex, welfare status, ethnicity, rurality
Norway	Age, sex, mortality, elderly living alone, marital status
Portugal	Based mainly on historical precedent; age, relative burden of illness (diabetes, hypertension, tuberculosis, AIDS)
Spain	Percent of population older than 65, "insularity" (region = islands)
Sweden	Age, sex, marital status, employment status, occupation, housing tenure, high utilizer

Source: Rice and Smith 2002; Mapelli 1999; Järvelin, Rico, and Cetani 2002; Vallgarda, Krasnik, and Vrangbaek 2001.

insured each sickness fund pooled its own resources. The introduction of competition among funds in 1996 was preceded by the introduction of a risk-adjustment mechanism considering age, sex, and disability (Busse 2001). Since then, sickness funds have had to cover all expenditures with the resources allocated from the central pool or else have had to increase their contribution rate. Thus sickness funds have been reduced to their purchasing function, although they still carry a certain financial risk. That risk was further reduced by the extension of the capitation to participation in disease management programs. Other countries, such as the Netherlands and Switzerland, have followed similar approaches.

In summary, nearly every high-income country applies some kind of capitation approach to allocate resources from pooling to purchasing organizations. Even systems such as Korea's, with only one central sickness fund that acts as both the pooling and purchasing organization, needs some mechanism to allocate resources among the regions. Whatever health financing arrangement is chosen, a capitation approach is necessary to redistribute pooled resources equitably. If a system intends to establish competition among sickness funds, capitation also has the regulatory function of equalizing the chances of success for each fund. The higher the predictive value of the capitation, the fairer is the competition and the more equitable is the allocation.

Purchasing and remuneration of providers

Purchasing refers to the transfer of pooled resources to service providers, and *remuneration* refers to the mechanism used to allocate the resources. Purchasing organizations must have the same funds as, but are not necessarily identical to, pooling organizations. Each method for remunerating providers creates different behavioral incentives for service providers. Two main objectives have to be clarified before designing payment systems. First, the market structure has to be taken into account as a framework for activities of purchasing organizations. A single purchaser can cover a whole nation or multiple purchasers can be assigned to fixed areas or compete with each other in the same areas. Second, it is important to be clear about the role assigned to the purchasers: a passive role as a financial intermediary or an active role with full financial power to achieve a defined level of quality and efficiency.

Market structure of purchasing organizations

The number of purchasing organizations, their size, and their market structure vary widely across the countries reviewed here (figure 9.3). Nonetheless, the decentralization wave has reached almost every country over the last three decades, pushing purchasing decisions down from central to regional or local authorities. Only a few countries still retain centralized single-purchaser systems.

During the 1990s, Germany and the Netherlands, which previously had noncompeting multiple-purchaser systems, introduced choice among sickness funds—in this respect joining Belgium and Switzerland. Before the introduction of competition, the members of each sickness fund were defined mainly on the basis of occupation or geographic area. The motivation was not so much a reduction of administrative costs, as is often assumed, but rather an increase of allocative efficiency, a decrease of

FIGURE 9.3 **Market structures for purchasing organizations in high-income countries**

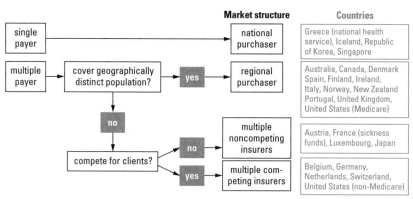

Source: Adapted from Kutzin 2001.

expenditure per insured or an increase in quality of the purchased services. Competition has been accompanied by a large reduction in the number of sickness funds, ranging from cuts of 21 percent in Belgium to 70.6 percent in Germany between 1990 and 2002.

The role of the purchaser

During the 1970s and 1980s, the role of the purchaser was still limited to that of a financial intermediary providing or reimbursing the necessary services on behalf of the population. Because of increasing cost pressure during the late 1980s, however, several countries tried to integrate market mechanisms into their systems to increase the quality and efficiency of provided services. During the 1990s, purchasing organizations in both social health insurance and tax-financed countries gained more autonomy in management and planning, through both contracting and the management of care (not necessarily "managed care" in a narrow sense). Although care management is a rather recent development, many countries with multiple purchaser systems experimented with contracting during the 1990s.

In geographically distinct multiple-payer systems, which are mainly tax-financed systems, an active role of regional purchasing organizations is frequently referred to as an internal market. In 1991 the British national health service embarked on a large-scale experiment of creating an internal or quasi-market within the health system, by separating purchasers from providers and by encouraging competition among providers. Providers became quasi-independent entities managing their own budgets and financing them through contracts with purchasers (Le Grand 1999). There were two types of purchasers: district health authorities and general practitioner (GP) fund-holding schemes. Large GP practices were given a budget from which to purchase a more limited range of secondary care on behalf of their patients. This move reflected the idea that GPs are a better agent for the patient than health authorities, because they have better information on the quality of secondary providers and better knowledge of patients' preferences than health authorities.

Although in efficiency, equity, choice, and responsiveness, the internal market may not have delivered as much as its proponents had hoped, it did not do too badly—especially when its performance is compared with what has happened since it was officially abolished in 1997. GP fund-holding seems to have been particularly effective, with recent research suggesting that it reduced waiting times and referral rates (Dixon, Le Grand, and Smith 2003). Several new problems had also become evident. These included high transaction costs; inequities brought about by splitting purchasing between health authorities and GP fund-holders (Dixon, Le Grand, and Smith 2003); and most worrying, a serious deterioration in clinical outcomes in some instances (Propper, Burgess, and Abraham 2002). Most policy analysts agree that in some unmeasurable ways the national health service had changed fundamentally through the internal market reforms. Changes in culture included extra attention to the concerns of GPs; an overall increase in cost-consciousness; and more clarity about what services should be provided for whom, to what standard, and at what price (Le Grand 1999). Although in 1997 the newly elected Labour government formally abolished the Thatcher internal market, it has developed its own version of an internal market, which maintains the purchaser-provider split. In 2003 it replaced the district health authorities with primary care trusts, in which GPs and other health professionals again hold executive functions. Selected hospitals, called foundation hospitals, are being given more autonomy, and there is a highly controversial scheme to attract private investment for national health service hospitals (Pollock, Shaoul, and Vickers 2002). Thus, the Labour measures have taken the market orientation of the national health service much further than the conservative predecessor government.

Other tax-financed countries have also introduced partial purchaser-provider splits, but mostly on a smaller scale. For example, Sweden introduced internal markets in its national health service in Stockholm County in 1992. Like reforms in the United Kingdom, Sweden's reforms created modest increases in productivity, efficiency, and responsiveness (Quaye 1997). In New Zealand internal markets were introduced in 1993 to achieve greater allocative and technical efficiency and to contain overall health expenditure. Therefore, formerly separate funding streams for general practitioner services and for hospitals and other services were merged, and four regional health authorities (RHA) were established (French, Old, and Healy 2001). In 1996, citing a steep rise in transaction costs after the 1993 reforms, problems with equity of access to care, and substantial deficits in three of the four RHA and many public hospital providers that had to be met by the government (Gauld 1999), a new government decided that the reforms had failed to meet their objectives and decided to merge the four RHA into a single purchasing organization.

Like the move to internal markets in tax-financed countries, selective contracting has developed in some social health insurance countries. In Belgium, France, and Luxembourg, specific benefits are defined by the government, leaving volume and prices to the purchasing organizations. However, the volume of these benefits is quite small. Germany, the Netherlands, and Switzerland even moved one step further. Governments understood that competition among sickness funds cannot work if the single funds have no management instruments to differentiate them in competition. Therefore, sickness funds in all three countries have received more autonomy, not only in selective contracting but also in marketing activities, bonus payments for patients and providers, and other incentive measures.

In the Netherlands, selective contracting has been encouraged since 1992. Under the Anti-Cartel Act, collective contracting in health care has been illegal from 2002 (den Exter and others 2004). Hospitals were exempted from this regulation, but the Anti-Cartel Authority announced that it would sue sickness funds that did not contract ambulatory providers selectively. However, sickness funds still contract providers on a collective basis, mainly because of the high transaction costs in contract negotiations with each single provider. In the Netherlands, as well as in Germany and Switzerland, sickness funds are also allowed to selectively contract with provider networks and to freely negotiate prices for services. The number of selective contracts is low but growing. Since 2004, German sickness funds are required to spend 1 percent of their total expenditure for such contracts with provider networks under the so-called integrated care scheme. This scheme is expected to achieve greater integration of different service sectors that are traditionally separated and thus to prevent duplication of utilization and achieve better outcomes. Selective contracting also breaks up cartels in ambulatory care, wherein physician associations negotiate on behalf of all social health insurance physicians in each region.

In all three countries sickness funds have also received more autonomy to excel in care management activities. In Switzerland, the two biggest funds are offering disease management programs, but the share of participants is rather low, at 5 percent of estimated potential participants (Weber and others 2004). To boost participation rates, the German government followed an innovative approach to increase the attractiveness of programs. Sickness funds are allowed to offer disease management programs, and participants enrolled in approved programs have been treated as a separate category in the risk structure compensation scheme since 2002. Thus, sickness funds with a high share of disease management program participants receive a higher budget from the pooling organization (Federal Insurance Authority). This was expected to stimulate the sickness funds to try to attract and care more about the chronically ill insured (instead of looking at them as "bad risks"). Critics pointed out that the act mainly provides an incentive for the sickness funds to enroll as many chronically ill insured as possible, but not necessarily to improve their care, as the individual sickness funds get compensated for the average expenditure of all disease management program participants across sickness funds (by age and sex) (Busse 2004).

Remuneration of providers

The shift toward purchaser-provider splits in tax-financed health systems and more active purchasing by sickness funds in social health insurance systems has been accompanied by changes in physician and hospital remuneration mechanisms in many countries. The new transparency of service provision that was created by the active contracting process and a heightened cost-consciousness by decision makers, purchasers, and providers alike might have been the main triggers for changes in remuneration mechanisms, rather than purely the desire to control costs.

Historically, provider remuneration has been mainly time- and population-based in tax-financed countries, whereas in social health insurance and mixed systems, (for example, in France, Germany, Japan, and the United States) service-based remuneration methods were and are still commonplace. During the 1980s, global budgets alongside fee-for-service payments for private hospitals or private patients in public hospitals, were still the main mechanism to finance public hospital care in most tax-financed high-income countries. Hospitals received a prospective annual fixed budget with which to cover all their services. Most of the time this budget reflected historical spending rather than service intensity or morbidity of patients cared for. Fee-for-service remains the principal means of paying hospital services in Japan; in some cantons in Switzerland, hospitals are paid according to individual services provided (Docteur and Oxley 2003).

In 1983 the U.S. Medicare program became the first major public payer to introduce a payment per patient episode—the diagnosis-related group (DRG) system. With this type of remuneration mechanism, financing is based on a prospectively specified payment per discharge unit standardized for variation in types of cases or case mix. Different pathologies are grouped into homogeneous cost groups on the basis of either medical conditions or surgical interventions, and average costs of treatment for each group are estimated. When discharged from the hospital, the patient is assigned to a specific group and the hospital receives a lump sum corresponding to the average cost of a patient in this group.

Since then, the majority of tax-financed or social health insurance countries have introduced some form of per case payment systems in their hospital financing systems—most partially and in some combination with global budgets. Tax-financed countries that have developed their own DRG payments or adapted existing systems from other countries and implemented them include Sweden (1985), Finland (1987), Portugal (1989), Canada (1990), Australia (1993), the United Kingdom (1992), Ireland (1993), Italy (1995), Denmark (1999), and Norway (1999). The first social health insurance country to introduce DRG payments was Belgium in 1995, followed by Germany (a partial system in 1995, revised in 2003), France (1997), Austria (1997), Switzerland (1997), the Catalonia region in Spain (1998), and the Netherlands (2003). In Japan (2003) a system called diagnosis procedure combination was introduced. Hospitals receive a defined number of points, each with a fixed value, for each service. Korea has developed its own DRG system, but has not implemented it (Fischer 2003).

Over the years, problems have emerged with per case payment methods, including their administrative and operational complexity, their dependence on the availability of relatively consistent and comprehensive activity and cost data, and the need for incentives to ensure that costs are limited by service type within remuneration boundaries (Langenbrunner and Wiley 2002). On the positive side, prospective pricing systems appear to have encouraged greater cost efficiency in the hospital sector. Evidence from the United States indicates that there have been significant falls in average length of hospital stays compared with other remuneration methods, although this may also have been accompanied by lower intensity of care in certain cases (Chalkley and Malcolmson 2000). In Sweden, a comparison of counties that used prospective remuneration systems with those that did not suggested cost differentials of 10 percent in favor of prospective remuneration (Gerdtham and others 1999; Gerdtham, Rehnberg, and Tambour 1999).

However, the use of these remuneration methods may conflict with overall expenditure control, particularly in the presence of excess supply or productivity reserves. For example, the introduction of DRGs in Stockholm County led to a sharp rise in activity and spending, and as a result, central expenditure control was reimposed through penalties for exceeding volume limits (Docteur and Oxley 2003).

For ambulatory care, the traditional mechanisms of fee-for-service payments in social health insurance systems and salaries in tax-funded systems have been largely replaced by combination systems, which try to outweigh the positive and negative incentives of each individual payment mechanism to encourage providers to align their behavior with the purchaser's objectives. Examples are the mixed capitation payment to physician associations and point-based fee-for-service payment to individual German physicians or the capitation payment to British GPs, which is supplemented by fee-for-service payments for underprovided services, for example, childhood immunizations or cancer screening activities. The same development can be seen in the remuneration of hospital doctors, who now more often receive performance-related payments on top of their salaries.

Endnotes

1. As explained below, medical savings accounts can have the character of compulsory contributions and are therefore subsumed under social security.

2. One must also keep in mind "tax expenditures" resulting from the deductibility of health insurance premiums from corporate and individual taxes as another form of public expenditure. Such deductibles in the United States amount to some 10 percent of total health spending, and if included as a public expenditure significantly increase the U.S. public share.

3. Since the introduction of compulsory health insurance in 1996, Switzerland has had a system of both income- and risk-unrelated per capita health insurance premiums. These premiums differ among insurers but are community-rated for all insured of a particular insurer in a certain region (usually at the subcanton level) (Minder, Schoenholzer, and Amiet 2000).

References

Asher, M. G. 2002. "Pension Reform in an Affluent and Rapidly Ageing Society: The Singapore Case." Paper prepared for the International Symposium on Pension Reforms in Asian Countries, Asian Public Policy Programme, Hitotsubashi University, Tokyo, February 1.

Bärnighausen, T., and R. Sauerborn. 2002. "One Hundred and Eighteen Years of the German Health Insurance System: Are There Any Lessons for Middle- and Low-Income Countries?" *Social Science and Medicine* 54 (10): 1559–87.

Bentes, M., C. Matias Dias, C. Sakellarides, and V. Bankauskaite. 2004. *Health Care Systems in Transition—Portugal.* European Observatory on Health Systems and Policies. Berkshire, U.K.: Open University Press.

Bunce, V. C. 2001. "Medical Savings Accounts—Progress and Problems under HIPAA." Policy Analysis 411, Cato Institute, Washington, D.C.

Busse, R. 2001. "Risk Adjustment Compensation in Germany's Statutory Health Insurance." *European Journal of Public Health* 11 (2): 174–7.

————. 2004. "Disease Management Programs in Germany's Statutory Health Insurance System—A Gordian Solution to the Adverse Selection of Chronically Ill in Competitive Markets?" *Health Affairs* 23 (3): 56–67.

Busse, R., R. B. Saltman, and H. Dubois. 2004. "Organization and Financing of Social Health Insurance Systems—Current Status and Recent Policy Developments." In R. B. Saltman, R. Busse, and J. Figueras, eds., *Social Health Insurance Systems in Western Europe.* European Observatory on Health Systems and Policies. Berkshire, U.K.: Open University Press.

Busse, R., and S. Schlette, eds. 2003. *Health Policy Developments, International Trends, and Analyses,* Issue 1/2003. Gütersloh: Bertelsmann Foundation Publishers.

Carrin, G., and C. James. 2004. "Reaching Universal Coverage via Social Health Insurance: Key Design Features in the Transition Period." Health Financing Policy Issue Paper Series, World Health Organization, Geneva.

CBO (Congressional Budget Office). 2003. *How Many People Lack Health Insurance and for How Long?* Washington, D.C.

Chalkley, M., and J. Malcolmson. 2000. "Government Purchasing of Health Services." In A. Culyer and J. Newhouse, eds., *Handbook of Health Economics.* Amsterdam: Elsevier.

Colombo, F., and N. Tapay. 2003. "Private Health Insurance in Australia—A Case Study." OECD Health Working Paper 8, Organisation for Economic Co-operation and Development, Paris.

den Exter, A., H. Herman, M. Dosljiak, and R. Busse. 2004. *Health Care Systems in Transition—The Netherlands.* European Observatory on Health Systems and Policies. Berkshire, U.K.: Open University Press.

Dixon, J., J. Le Grand, and P. Smith. 2003. *Shaping the National Health Service—Can Market Forces Be Used for Good?* London: King's Fund.

Docteur, E., and H. Oxley. 2003. "Health-Care Systems—Lessons from the Reform Experience." OECD Health Working Papers 9, Organisation for Economic Co-operation and Development, Paris.

Donatini, A., A. Rico, M. G. D'Ambrosio, A. Lo Scalzo, L. Orzella, A. Cicchetti, S. Profili, and T. Cetani. 2001. *Health Care Systems in Transition—Italy.* European Observatory on Health Systems and Policies. Berkshire, U.K.: Open University Press.

Fischer, W. 2003. *Nutzung von DRGs und verwandten Patientenklassifikationssystemen.* [www.fischer-zim.ch/notizen/DRG-Nutzung-2001—0304.htm].

French, S., A. Old, and J. Healy. 2001. *Health Care Systems in Transition—New Zealand.* Copenhagen: European Observatory on Health Care Systems.

Gauld, R. 1999. "Beyond New Zealand's Dual Health Reforms." *Social Policy and Administration* 33 (5): 567–85.

Gerdtham, U. G., M. Löthgren, M. Tambour, and C. Rehnberg. 1999. "Internal Markets and Health-Care Efficiency: A Multiple-Output Stochastic Frontier Analysis." *Health Economics* 8 (2): 151–64.

Gerdtham, U. G., C. Rehnberg, and M. Tambour. 1999. "The Impact of Internal Markets on Health-Care Efficiency: Evidence from Health-Care Reforms in Sweden." *Applied Economics* 31 (8): 935–45.

Gericke, C. A., M. Wismar, and R. Busse. 2004. "Cost-Sharing in the German Health Care System." Discussion paper 2004/4, Faculty of Economics and Management, Technische Universität Berlin. [www.ww.tu-berlin.de/diskussionspapiere/2004/dp04-2004.pdf].

Gibis, B., P. W. Koch-Wulkan, and J. Bultman. 2004. "Shifting Criteria for Benefit Decisions in Social Health Insurance Systems." In R. B. Saltman, R. Busse, and J. Figueras, eds., *Social Health Insurance Systems in Western Europe.* European Observatory on Health Systems and Policies. Berkshire, U.K.: Open University Press.

Halldorsson, M., and V. Bankauskaite. 2003. *Health Care Systems in Transition—Iceland.* European Observatory on Health Systems and Policies. Berkshire, U.K.: Open University Press.

Hilless, M., and J. Healy. 2001. *Health Care Systems in Transition—Australia.* European Observatory on Health Systems and Policies. Berkshire, U.K.: Open University Press.

Hjortsberg, C., O. Ghatnekar, A. Rico, W. Wisbaum, and T. Cetani. 2001. *Health Care Systems in Transition—Sweden.* European Observatory on Health Systems and Policies. Berkshire, U.K.: Open University Press.

Järvelin, J., A. Rico, and T. Cetani. 2002. *Health Care Systems in Transition—Finland.* Copenhagen: European Observatory on Health Systems and Policies. Berkshire, U.K.: Open University Press.

Jommi, C., and G. Fattore. 2003. Regionalisation and Drugs Cost-Sharing in the Italian National Health Service. *EuroObserver* 5 (3): 1–4.

Kaufhold, R., and M. Schneider. 2000. Preisvergleich zahnärztlicher Leistungen im europäischen Kontext. Cologne, Germany: IDZ.

Kupsch, S., A. Kern, C. Klas, B. Kressin, M. Vienonen, and F. Beske. 2000. *Health Service Provision on a Microcosmic Level—An International Comparison.* Results of a WHO/IGSF Survey in 15 European Countries. Kiel, Germany: Institute for Health Systems Research.

Kutzin, J. 2001. "A Descriptive Framework for Country-Level Analysis of Health Care Financing Arrangements." *Health Policy* 56 (3): 171–204.

Langenbrunner, J. C., and M. M. Wiley. 2002. "Hospital Payment Mechanisms: Theory and Practice in Transition Countries." In M. McKee and J. Healy, eds., *Hospitals in a Changing Europe.* European Observatory on Health Systems and Policies. Berkshire, U.K.: Open University Press.

Le Grand, J. 1999. "Competition, Cooperation, or Control? Tales from the British National Health Service." *Health Affairs* 18 (3): 27–40.

Mapelli, V. 1999. *L'allocazione delle risorse nel Servizio Sanitario Nazionale.* Rome: Ministero del Tesoro, del Bilancio e della Programmazione Economica, Commissione Tecnica per la Spesa Pubblica.

McKee, M., M. J. Delnoij, and H. Brand. 2004. "Prevention and Public Health in Social Health Insurance Systems." In R. B. Saltman, R. Busse, and J. Figueras, eds., *Social Health Insurance Systems in Western Europe.* European Observatory on Health Systems and Policies. Berkshire, U.K.: Open University Press.

Minder, A., H. Schoenholzer, and M. Amiet. 2000. *Health Care Systems in Transition—Switzerland.* European Observatory on Health Systems and Policies. Berkshire, U.K.: Open University Press.

OECD (Organisation for Economic Co-operation and Development). 2003. *OECD Reviews of Health Care Systems: Korea.* Paris.

———. 2004a. *OECD Health Data,* 3rd edition. Paris.

———. 2004b. *Private Health Insurance in OECD Countries.* Paris.

Pollock, A. M., J. Shaoul, and N. Vickers. 2002. "Private Finance and Value for Money in NHS Hospitals: A Policy in Search of a Rationale?" *British Medical Journal.*

Prescott, N., and L. M. Nichols. 1998. "International Comparison of Medical Savings Accounts." World Bank Discussion Paper 392: *Choices in Financing Health Care and Old Age Security.* World Bank, Washington, D.C.

Propper, C., S. Burgess, and D. Abraham. 2002. *Competition and Quality: Evidence from the National Health Service Internal Market 1991–1999.* Bristol, U.K.: CMPO, University of Bristol.

Quaye, R. 1997. "Struggle for Control: General Practitioners in the Swedish Health Care System." *European Journal of Public Health* 7 (3): 248–53.

Rice, N., and P. Smith. 2002. "Strategic Resource Allocation and Funding Decisions." In E. Mossialos, A. Dixon, J. Figueras, and J. Kutzin, eds., *Funding Health Care: Options for Europe.* Buckingham, U.K.: Open University Press.

Rico, A., R. Sabes, and W. Wisbaum. 2000. *Health Care Systems in Transition—Spain.* Copenhagen: European Observatory on Health Care Systems.

Sandier, S., V. Paris, D. Polton, S. Thomson, and E. Mossialos. 2004. *Health Care Systems in Transition—France.* Copenhagen: European Observatory on Health Care Systems.

Schreyögg, J. 2004. "Demographic Development and Moral Hazard: Health Insurance with Medical Savings Accounts." *The Geneva Papers on Risk and Insurance* 29 (4): 689–704.

Schreyögg, J., and M. K. Lim. 2004. "Health Care Reforms in Singapore—Twenty Years of Medical Savings Accounts." *Dice-Report—Journal for Institutional Comparisons* 2 (3): 55–60.

Thomson, S., E. Mossialos, and N. Jemiai. 2003. *Cost Sharing for Health Services in the European Union.* Report prepared for the European Commission, Directorate General for Employment and Social Affairs. Copenhagen: European Observatory on Health Care Systems; London: London School of Economics and Political Science.

U.S. Census Bureau. 2003. *Health Insurance Coverage in the United States: 2002.* Washington, D.C.

U.S. GAO (General Accounting Office). 1998. *Comprehensive Study of the Medical Savings Account Demonstration.* GAO/HEHS-98-57. Washington, D.C.

Velasco Garrido, M., and R. Busse. 2005. *Health Technology Assessment—An Introduction to Objectives, Role of Evidence, and Structure in Europe.* Policy Brief. Copenhagen and Brussels: European Observatory on Health Systems and Policies.

Vallgarda, S., A. Krasnik, and K. Vrangbaek. 2001. *Health Care Systems in Transition—Denmark.* Copenhagen: European Observatory on Health Care Systems.

Weber, A., A. S. Götschi, R. Kühne, and D. Meier. 2004. Patientenrekrutierung für Disease Management. *Schweizerische Ärztezeitung* 85 (48): 2581–4.

Zweifel, P., and W. G. Manning. 2001. "Moral Hazard and Consumer Incentives in Health Care." In A. J. Culyer and J. P. Newhouse, eds., *Handbook of Health Economics.* Vol. 1A. North Holland: Elsevier.

Index